SAUNDERS

Medical
Assisting
Exam Review

SAUNDERS

Medical Assisting Exam Review

Second Edition

Deborah E. Barbier Holmes, RN, MLT, CMA-C
Former Medical Assistant Program Chair
Iowa Western Community College
Council Bluffs, Iowa

Joanna Bligh, MEd, RT(R) (ret.), CMA
Senior Medical Writer
Excerpta Medica
Bridgewater, NJ
Guest Lecturer
Medical Assisting Program
Bryman College
Tacoma, Washington
Medical Assisting Program
Dover Business College
Clifton, New Jersey

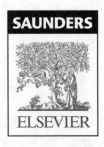

SAUNDERS

ELSEVIER

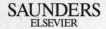

11830 Westline Industrial Drive
St. Louis, Missouri 63146

Saunders Medical Assisting Exam Review, Second Edition

ISBN-13: 978-1-4160-2440-8
ISBN-10: 1-4160-2440-9

Notice

Neither the Publisher nor the Authors assume any responsibility for any loss or injury and/or damage to persons or property arising out of or related to any use of the material contained in this book. It is the responsibility of the treating practitioner, relying on independent expertise and knowledge of the patient, to determine the best treatment and method of application for the patient.

ISBN-13: 978-1-4160-2440-8
ISBN-10: 1-4160-2440-9

Publisher: Michael S. Ledbetter
Senior Developmental Editor: Melissa K. Boyle
Developmental Editor: Jenna Johnson
Publishing Services Manager: Julie Eddy
Project Manager: Andrea Campbell
Design Direction: Teresa McBryan
Cover Design: Maggie Reid

Printed in the Unites States of America

Last digit is the print number: 9 8 7 6 5 4 3 2 1

Working together to grow
libraries in developing countries

www.elsevier.com | www.bookaid.org | www.sabre.org

ELSEVIER   BOOK AID International   Sabre Foundation

Dedication

To
Granny and Jon,
my biggest fans and guardian angels,

and to
my students,
who teach me something new
every day.

Contributors

Joyce Combs, BS, AAS, CMA
Coordinator/Professor
LSAA AH – Medical Assisting
Central Kentucky Technical College
Lexington, Kentucky

Jeanette Goodwin, BS, BSN, CMA
Program Chair/Instructor
Health Division
Southeast Community College
Lincoln, Nebraska

Edith Hamelin, BSN, RN, CMA
Director
Medical Department
Latter Day Saints Business College
Salt Lake City, Utah

Rose Hecht, BS, CMAC
Program Director/Medical Assistant Instructor
Health Science and Medical Technology
Southern California Regional Occupational Center
Torrance, California

Christine Hollander, CMA, BS
Medical Department Director
Health Careers Division
Westwood College of Technology
Denver, Colorado

Preface

Skilled. Compassionate. Healer. Competent.

These a re words that come to mind when describing the medical assistant. As the profession of medical assisting continues to change, the medical assistant must meet these new challenges. Earning a medical assistant credential is the first step.

There are many reasons to achieve this credential. It shows that the student is recognized by the credentialing organization as having met predetermined qualifications. It shows proof of competency, and it shows others a commitment to the profession. This credential will be even more important in the coming years as medical assistants become more and more recognized for the versatile allied health professionals that they are.

Saunders Medical Assisting Exam Review was written to aid the student in studying for a medical assisting credentialing exam and was developed with today's busy student in mind. This textbook presents simplified study materials that focus on all the General, Administrative and Clinical topics from the medical assisting curriculum in preparation for either the Certified Medical Assistant or the Registered Medical Assistant examination.

The book features the following:

- A single, comprehensive guide. This allows for information to be found easily in one text, and eliminates the need for many big, bulky textbooks and stacks of notes.
- An easy-to-follow outline format. Information is organized and presented in this format to allow the student to identify key concepts and facts. All subject areas typically included in a medical assistant Program are covered.
- Three practice pre-tests and a post-test, complete with answers and rationales. These may help assess weak and strong areas. A CD-ROM with different practice exams (as well as the pre-tests from the text) and review questions offers more practice.
- Simple pictures and diagrams to illustrate the text. These may help to clarify concepts.
- Study and test-taking tips to help the student be successful. Included are suggestions on how to prepare to study, how to study, and how to take a multiple-choice exam.

As the practicing medical assistant moves on in his/her career, this text may be used as a source of reference. It is also useful as a reference for educators in creating lecture material, curriculum, or review courses.

The author wishes the best of luck to all who use this text to achieve their credential. Hopefully it helps make the process a little easier.

Acknowledgments

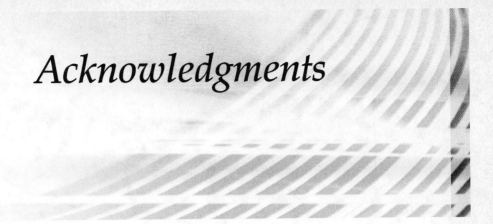

I am deeply grateful to the following people who have given me ideas, encouragement, praise, and support.

My students, past, present, and future—they are THE reason for this project. They have been an endless source of ideas, criticism, support, and inspiration.

Michael Ledbetter and Jenna Johnson at Elsevier—for supporting, understanding, listening to ideas, and helping tremendously. This project started as a discussion at a national convention, and wound up as this book.

Carol Moore, Academic Skills Specialist, Nebraska Methodist College—for providing the test-taking strategies and study skills ideas.

David, Robert and Jennifer—the loves of my life.

Madelyn, Chris and Amy—the newest additions to the Holmes family.

Deborah E. Barbier Holmes

The idea for this book came to me in 1997 when I was the Medical Programs Director at Northeast Career Schools in Manchester, New Hampshire. At that time I was also president of the New Hampshire Society of the American Association of Medical Assistants, and we had just won an important state legislative battle to defeat Bill 281, which limited the medical assistants' scope of practice in New Hampshire. The Academic Director at Northeast Career Schools, Mary Liponis, was instrumental in encouraging me to submit a proposal for this book to the publisher. Mary felt that, after our successful legislative battle, our cohesive group of medical assisting instructors needed another project. I would like to thank the dedicated medical assisting instructors who inspired this project: Nancy Ouellette, CMA; Barbara Massoni, RN, CMA; and Gayle Farley, CMA. Those who contributed need special acknowledgment and thanks: Carolyn Turner, MT(ASCP), CMA, and Enid Harrington, RN, MSW.

Joanna Bligh

Contents

Study Tips: Taking the Medical Assistant Examination

General Examination Descriptions

CMA EXAM

The CMA exam is administered on the last Friday in January, the last Saturday in June, and the fourth Friday in October of each year. Individuals who meet the requirements set by the American Association of Medical Assistants (AAMA) are eligible to sit for this exam. The exam consists of 300 questions in multiple-choice format. Three general areas are covered on the exam, each area consisting of 100 questions. The content of each general area is broken down as follows:

General Medical Knowledge (100 questions)
- Medical terminology
- Anatomy and physiology
- Law
- Ethics
- Patient relations
- Communications

Administrative Knowledge (100 questions)
- Keyboarding concepts
- Correspondence
- Mail
- Appointments
- Phone management
- Filing and records management
- Banking
- Bookkeeping
- Payroll
- Medical coding
- Insurance
- Office automation
- General office management concepts

Clinical Knowledge (100 questions)
- Patient interviewing
- Charting and documentation
- Physical measurements and examinations
- Nutrition
- Physical therapy
- Radiography
- Electrocardiography
- Surgical treatment
- First aid
- Cardiopulmonary resuscitation
- Laboratory orientation
- Urinalysis
- Hematology
- Chemistry
- Serology/Immunology
- Microbiology

You are given four hours to complete the exam. All questions are assigned equal weight. Guessing at answers is not counted against you; the exam is scored according to the number of correct answers versus the total number of questions given. An overall minimum standard score of 445 must be attained to pass the exam. On successfully passing the exam, the medical assistant may wear the CMA credential. For more information on taking the CMA exam, visit the American Association of Medical Assistants Web site at www.aama-ntl.org.

RMA EXAM

The RMA exam is administered throughout the year either by paper and pencil or by computerized test. The paper test is administered at the school with a proctor, and the school sets the time and dates. The computerized test is administered at Pearson Vue locations nationwide any day of the year except Sundays and holidays. Individuals who meet the criteria set forth by the American Medical Technologists (AMT) are eligible to sit for this exam. The exam consists of 200–210 questions in multiple-choice format, covering the same three general areas as the CMA exam. The approximate percentage of material covered from each section and its content is broken down as follows:

General Medical Knowledge (42.5%)
- Anatomy and physiology
- Medical terminology
- Medical law

- Medical ethics
- Human relations
- Patient education

Administrative Knowledge (22.5%)
- Insurance
- Financial bookkeeping
- Medical secretarial-receptionist

Clinical Knowledge (35%)
- Asepsis
- Sterilization
- Instruments
- Vital signs
- Physical examinations
- Clinical pharmacology
- Minor surgery
- Therapeutic modalities
- Laboratory procedures
- Electrocardiography
- First aid

A minimum scaled score of 70 must be attained to pass the exam. On successfully passing the exam, the medical assistant may wear the RMA credential. For more information on taking the RMA exam, visit the American Medical Technologists Web site at www.amt1.com.

Study Tips for The Exam

Taking the medical assistant certification (CMA) or registration (RMA) examination is an important event in the medical assistant's career. This section will guide you in preparing for the examination by offering study techniques and tips and by describing the exam itself and what to expect when exam day arrives.

A great deal of commitment is required on your part to study for the exam. Your performance on the exam will reflect your study habits. If you give an effort of 100%, you should do well; if you halfheartedly study for the exam, you will not do well. The earlier you begin studying for the exam, the better.

It is up to you to determine what study methods work best for you. Once you have done this, discipline yourself and stick to your plan!

1. **Assess your learning capabilities**. This will help you to determine the amount of time you will need to study.
2. **Request a content outline from your certifying agency**. Review the outline and determine the amount of time you will need for your own learning capabilities.
3. **Plot a study schedule**. Divide the outline into subjects. Place the subjects into a study schedule. Allow extra time for subjects that are more difficult for you.
4. **Set up a time schedule**. Retention levels are higher when you study in short sessions.
5. **Prepare to study**.
   - Create the environment:
     Select a place with a desk or table, straight-backed chair, and good lighting. Being too comfortable may encourage sleep.
     Keep the room temperature comfortable—not too warm or too cool.
     Avoid interruptions from family, friends, and telephone.
     Avoid unnecessary noise.
   - Gather study tools:
     Gather all books, notebooks, and flashcards.
     Have extra pens, pencils, and flashcards handy.
6. **Commit to study**. You are preparing to take a national exam for your medical assistant credential!
7. **Study!**
   - Study material you do not know. Do not waste time on the material you do know.
   - Take a break halfway through each session.
   - Study the subject you dislike or are weakest in first and the subject you like or are strongest in last.
   - Do not study after a heavy meal.
   - Take your review book, notes, and/or flashcards with you and answer questions at lunch time, coffee breaks, and in your spare time.
   - Attend an exam review class or join a study group.

The Day Before the Exam

1. Be familiar with the directions and the route to the test site.
2. Review your notes briefly. Do not cram!
3. Go to bed early and get a good night's sleep.
4. Plan to arrive early at the test site. Doors will be locked to latecomers after a certain amount of time.
5. Have pencils and supplies ready to take with you to the exam.

The Day of the Exam

1. Eat a light breakfast.
2. Avoid caffeinated drinks. Caffeine can decrease the attention span and can over-stimulate the metabolism. This reduces concentration!
3. Dress comfortably in layers.
4. Listen to traffic and weather reports beforehand.
5. Bring your flashcards for a last review while waiting to take the exam.
6. Bring test material, photo identification, admission card, and several No. 2 pencils with erasers.

Taking the Exam

As you sit down to take the CMA or RMA exam, remember these important points.

1. Take a deep breath before starting.
2. Read all directions before starting.
3. If permissible, make notes on the exam booklet.
4. Read each question carefully and analyze what is being asked.
5. Pay attention to words that are emphasized by underline, capitalization, bold, or italics.
6. Concentrate on each question. Do not wander off to other questions.

7. Do not leave any blank answers. Guessing gives you a chance to get it right.
8. Be careful when making answers on the answer sheet so that you do not skip a line or mark an incorrect circle.
9. Check your time periodically. Allow one hour per section.
10. Multiple-choice questions have one correct answer. Do not overanalyze. Give the *best* answer to the question as it is written.
11. If you do not know the answer immediately, start eliminating choices to at least two possibilities. Highlight/mark the question on the test booklet so you can return to it after finishing the rest of the test.
12. After completing the exam, check the answer sheet to make sure it is complete. Check your exam booklet for highlighted questions and return to them.
13. Before handing in the test booklet and answer sheet, make sure your identification information is on the answer sheet and that it is correct.

MULTIPLE-CHOICE QUESTIONS

1. Statements that contain words such as "always," "every," "never," and "all" are usually too broad and often incorrect.
2. If two choices have the same or almost the same meaning, they are both incorrect; eliminate both choices when you select your answer.
3. Be aware of directional words such as "but," "except," and "however." They signal opposite meanings.
4. Try to answer the test question before looking at the options.
5. If you do not know the answer, eliminate the choices you know are wrong.
6. Read the question with the answer you selected to hear how they sound together.
7. To answer a multiple-choice question, you need to:
   a. find the main idea
   b. find and remember details that support the main idea
   c. draw conclusions

Scoring the CMA Exam

As you take the practice tests in preparing for the CMA exam, use the following formula to convert your raw test score (number of correct answers) into a standard test score.

(Raw Score × 6.2) + 100

For example: If you have answered 210 questions correctly (out of 300), your raw score is 70% (210 ÷ 300). Take this percentage and compute your standard score as follows:

(70 × 6.2) + 100

a) 70 × 6.2 = 434

b) 434 + 100 = 534

Your standard score is 534 (a passing score).

Note: The above formula is for the purposes of scoring the simulated exams found in this text only and is not promoted by the American Association of Medical Assistants (AAMA).

Scoring the RMA Exam

If you are preparing to take the RMA exam, use the following formula to convert your raw test score (number of correct answers) into a scaled test score.

(Raw Score × 0.75) + 25

For example: If you have answered 134 questions correctly (out of a total 200), your raw score is 67% (134 ÷ 200). Take this percentage and compute your scaled score as follows:

(67 × 0.75) + 25

a) 67 × 0.75 = 50

b) 50 + 25 = 75

Your scaled score is 75 (a passing score).

Note: The above formula is for the purposes of scoring the simulated exams found in this text only and is not promoted by the American Medical Technologists (AMT).

Pre-Test 1

Directions: Each of the following questions is followed by five possible responses. Select the *best* response.

1. An abnormal decrease in the size of a muscle is
   A. Myopathy
   B. Atrophy
   C. Dystrophy
   D. Hypertrophy
   E. Myotrophy

2. The cell from which a muscle develops is called a(n)
   A. Myeloblast
   B. Osteoblast
   C. Myoblast
   D. Myoclast
   E. Erythroblast

3. The abbreviation for *right ear* is
   A. AD
   B. AS
   C. AU
   D. OD
   E. OS

4. An otoscope is used to
   A. Inspect the nasal cavity
   B. Inspect the exterior ear canal
   C. Measure eyeball pressure
   D. Inspect the oral cavity
   E. Measure oxygen levels

5. This procedure is used to puncture the chest and remove fluid.
   A. Spirometry
   B. Bronchoscopy
   C. Intubation
   D. Thoracentesis
   E. Tracheostomy

6. Which of the following laboratory tests would be abnormal for a patient with anemia?
   A. Differential
   B. Hematocrit and hemoglobin
   C. Blood glucose
   D. Total cholesterol
   E. White blood cell count

7. Hyperparathyroidism may be treated by which medical specialist?
   A. Cardiologist
   B. Emergency medical technician
   C. Endocrinologist
   D. Hematologist
   E. Obstetrician

8. An abnormal increase in total number of white blood cells is called
   A. Anemia
   B. Leukopenia
   C. Leukosis
   D. Leukocytosis
   E. Polycythemia

9. The term for extremely rapid breathing is
   A. Hyperpnea
   B. Hypopnea
   C. Dyspnea
   D. Apnea
   E. Hypertension

10. Which of the following suffixes refers to pain?
    A. -phagia
    B. -desis
    C. -pnea
    D. -algia
    E. -lysis

11. A suffix used to denote a surgical repair is
    A. -pexy
    B. -desis
    C. -plasty
    D. -lysis
    E. -centesis

12. A mammogram is a radiograph of the
    A. Chest
    B. Bladder
    C. Breast
    D. Lymph nodes
    E. Axilla

13. The term *alopecia* is synonymous with
    A. Excessive hair growth
    B. Itching
    C. Myopia
    D. Baldness
    E. A whitish pigmentation of the skin

14. Another term for chewing is
    A. Mastication
    B. Obstipation
    C. Deglutition
    D. Peristalsis
    E. Regurgitation

15. A nevus in the antecubital area is a
    A. Mass on the shoulder
    B. Polyp on the lower back
    C. Wart on the ankle
    D. Scar on the knee
    E. Mole on the inside of the elbow

16. An inflammation of a joint is called
    A. Arthrodesis
    B. Arthrodynia
    C. Arthroclasis
    D. Arthritis
    E. Arthrocentesis

17. Fat is the main component of
    A. The epidermis
    B. Adipose tissue
    C. Muscle tissue
    D. Tendons
    E. Lymphatic tissue

18. The study of the cause of disease is referred to as
    A. Biology
    B. Epidemiology
    C. Pathology
    D. Etiology
    E. Physiology

19. The main function of the olfactory nerve is
    A. Touching
    B. Tasting
    C. Smelling
    D. Seeing
    E. Hearing

20. An oophorectomy is a surgical procedure performed on the
    A. Uterus
    B. Ovaries
    C. Knee
    D. Vagina
    E. Ear

21. The medical specialty that is involved with diseases and treatment of the male and female urinary systems is
    A. Nephrology
    B. Oncology
    C. Urology
    D. Proctology
    E. Gynecology

22. This diagnostic procedure allows for visualization of the urinary bladder.
    A. Urethral dilation
    B. Intravenous pyelogram (IVP)
    C. Cystography
    D. Cystoscopy
    E. Transurethral resection of the prostate (TURP)

23. The correct medical term for hives is
    A. Urticaria
    B. Verruca
    C. A nevus
    D. Shingles
    E. Alopecia

24. The membrane that surrounds the heart is the
    A. Endocardium
    B. Endometrium
    C. Pericardium
    D. Perineum
    E. Myocardium

25. A mucous membrane
    A. Lines closed cavities of the body
    B. Covers the lungs
    C. Lines the abdominal cavity
    D. Lines body cavities that open to the outside
    E. Surrounds the heart

26. The ventral region of the body is described as
    A. Superior
    B. Lateral
    C. Medial
    D. Anterior
    E. Posterior

27. The body cavity that contains the intestines is the
    A. Thoracic
    B. Spinal
    C. Abdominal
    D. Pleural
    E. Peritoneal

28. Movement of a body part toward the midline of the body is
    A. Supination
    B. Pronation
    C. Adduction
    D. Abduction
    E. Rotation

29. The plane that divides the body into front and back halves is
    A. Frontal
    B. Horizontal
    C. Median
    D. Oblique
    E. Transverse

30. Reye's syndrome
    A. Can follow a viral illness in children
    B. Is caused by high fever
    C. Is a symptom of acquired immunodeficiency syndrome (AIDS)
    D. Causes muscular dystrophy
    E. Is the common cold

31. The vertebrae located in the lower back are the
    A. Cervical
    B. Thoracic
    C. Lumbar
    D. Sacral
    E. Coccyx

32. This acute infectious skin disease is caused by staphylococci.
    A. Impetigo
    B. Psoriasis
    C. Athlete's foot
    D. Melanoma
    E. Eczema

33. The bone located in the posterior of the skull is the
    A. Frontal
    B. Ethmoid
    C. Temporal
    D. Occipital
    E. Mandible

34. The type of bone fracture in which the bone is bent and partially broken is a
    A. Simple fracture
    B. Compound fracture
    C. Greenstick fracture
    D. Comminuted fracture
    E. Complete fracture

35. The peripheral nervous system is composed of how many pairs of spinal nerves?
    A. 2
    B. 5
    C. 12
    D. 20
    E. 31

36. The pons and medulla make up the
    A. Brainstem
    B. Cerebellum
    C. Cerebrum
    D. Thalamus
    E. Right hemisphere

37. The failure of bone marrow to produce red blood cells results in which type of anemia?
    A. Aplastic
    B. Hemolytic
    C. Pernicious
    D. Microcytic
    E. Leukemia

38. Protrusion of a part of the stomach through the esophageal opening in the diaphragm is a(n)
    A. Esophageal aneurysm
    B. Esophageal varices
    C. Hiatal hernia
    D. Pyloric stenosis
    E. Gastroesophageal reflux disease (GERD)

39. Another name for the tympanic membrane is the
    A. Ossicle
    B. Cochlea
    C. Auricle
    D. Eardrum
    E. Organ of Corti

40. The largest artery in the body is the
    A. Brachial artery
    B. Temporal artery
    C. Radial artery
    D. Aorta
    E. Femoral artery

41. The sinoatrial node
    A. Stimulates the diaphragm
    B. Is the same as the atrioventricular node
    C. Is the pacemaker of the heart
    D. Divides the heart into right and left sides
    E. Regulates blood flow to the brain

42. An x-ray taken to confirm a fracture of the distal forearm would include the
    A. Tibia and fibula
    B. Radius and ulna
    C. Femur and trochanter
    D. Calcaneus and malleolus
    E. Humerus and scapula

43. Which of the following demonstrates an involuntary muscle action?
    A. Heartbeat
    B. Breathing
    C. Peristalsis
    D. Pupil dilation
    E. All of the above

44. Which of the following organs is located in the right upper quadrant?
    A. Liver
    B. Right ovary
    C. Appendix
    D. Uterus
    E. Stomach

45. Which of the following nerves stimulates the diaphragm?
    A. Trochlear
    B. Accessory
    C. Sciatic
    D. Phrenic
    E. Vagus

46. An abnormal lateral curvature of the spine is known as
    A. Spondylosis
    B. Kyphosis
    C. Scoliosis
    D. Ankylosis
    E. Lordosis

47. The alpha cells in the pancreas are responsible for the production of
    A. Insulin
    B. Glucagon
    C. Hydrochloric acid (HCl)
    D. Pepsin
    E. Gastrin

48. The surgical removal of the gallbladder is a
    A. Cholectomy
    B. Colostomy
    C. Cholecystectomy
    D. Laparoscopy
    E. Gastrectomy

49. Which of the following cranial nerves is involved in blindness?
    A. Abducens
    B. Oculomotor
    C. Trigeminal
    D. Olfactory
    E. Optic

50. The number of permanent teeth is
    A. 20
    B. 24
    C. 28
    D. 32
    E. 36

51. Legally, a physician
    A. May not refuse treatment in an emergency situation
    B. May refuse to provide follow-up care after initial treatment
    C. Must provide a diagnosis to a patient's employer if requested
    D. Must provide a medical history to the patient's insurance company if the insurance company requests it
    E. May refuse to accept a patient if he or she chooses

52. An itinerary
    A. Is a yearly schedule
    B. Is a travel guide
    C. Contains tickets
    D. Is a detailed outline of a trip
    E. Makes travel arrangements

53. Professionalism may best be displayed by
    A. Keeping emotions to one's self
    B. Staying calm when dealing with angry patients
    C. Showing no consideration for other members of the team
    D. Referring all problems to the physician
    E. Arriving late or leaving early

54. The ability to imagine taking the place of the patient and accepting the patient's behavior is
    A. Objectivity
    B. Empathy
    C. Sympathy
    D. Industry
    E. Subjectivity

55. The patient's medical record belongs to
    A. The patient's spouse
    B. The physician
    C. The patient
    D. The patient's attorney
    E. The state medical board

56. A breast mass is found in a woman whose mother and sister have died from breast cancer. She cancels her next three follow-up appointments. Which defense mechanism is she using?
    A. Denial
    B. Anxiety
    C. Acceptance
    D. Isolation
    E. Suppression

57. Personality differences are due to
    A. Age
    B. Experience
    C. Heredity
    D. Environment
    E. All of the above

58. Which of the following is *not* a characteristic desirable in a medical assistant?
    A. Appreciation
    B. Impatience
    C. Flexibility
    D. Friendliness
    E. Concern

59. Which of the following is *not* an example of stereotyping?
    A. Similar people have similar needs
    B. Elderly patients have hearing deficits
    C. Medicaid patients are lazy
    D. Educated patients have no fear of illness
    E. Young children react differently to stressful situations

60. To release medical information
    A. The physician must sign a waiver
    B. The insurance company must make the request in writing
    C. The patient must sign a release form
    D. A certified record technician must be employed by the office
    E. The patient must deliver the records in person to the requester

61. Which of the following should be reported to the health department?
    A. Otitis media
    B. Strep throat
    C. Influenza
    D. Vaginal yeast infection
    E. Human immunodeficiency virus (HIV)

62. Which of the following is an example of objective data?
    A. Family history
    B. Vital signs
    C. Past surgical history
    D. Last menstrual period (LMP)
    E. Insurance information

63. Which of the following telephone calls should be given immediately to the physician?
    A. Another physician
    B. An angry patient
    C. A patient's family member
    D. A salesperson
    E. An insurance company

64. In Maslow's hierarchy of needs, the need to be loved and free from loneliness is a
    A. Physiologic need
    B. Safety need
    C. Social need
    D. Self-esteem need
    E. Self-actualization need

65. If a patient refuses to consent to treatment, the medical assistant should
    A. Schedule the patient for another appointment
    B. Force treatment on the patient
    C. Force the patient to consent
    D. Delay treatment and inform or consult with the physician
    E. Terminate the patient

66. An enforceable contract contains
    A. An offer
    B. An acceptance
    C. A consideration
    D. A capacity
    E. All of the above

67. The opposite of anterior is
   A. Distal
   B. Medial
   C. Proximal
   D. Posterior
   E. Lateral

68. Informed consent includes which of the following elements?
   A. Benefits and risks of the treatment
   B. Purpose of treatment
   C. Nature of the patient's condition
   D. Assessment of the patient's understanding of the treatment
   E. All of the above

69. All of the following are reasons for revoking a physician's license *except*
   A. Mental incapacity
   B. Physical incapacity
   C. Conviction of a crime
   D. Unprofessional conduct
   E. Providing atypical care

70. The control center of a cell is
   A. DNA
   B. Organelles
   C. Nucleus
   D. Ribosomes
   E. Cell membrane

71. Subcutaneous tissue
   A. Is found under the skin
   B. Contains fat
   C. Is an injection site
   D. Connects the dermis to the muscle surface
   E. All of the above

72. Which of the following is *not* a bone of the lower extremity?
   A. Femur
   B. Humerus
   C. Tibia
   D. Fibula
   E. Metatarsals

73. The muscle in the upper extremity that is used as an injection site is the
   A. Deltoid
   B. Biceps brachii
   C. Triceps brachii
   D. Trapezius
   E. Gluteus medius

74. The pacemaker of the heart is the
   A. Septum
   B. Sinoatrial node
   C. Atrioventricular node
   D. Left atrium
   E. Mitral valve

75. Gas exchange in the lungs takes place in the
   A. Pharynx
   B. Bronchi
   C. Trachea
   D. Bronchiole
   E. Alveoli

76. The liver
   A. Makes bile
   B. Detoxifies harmful substances
   C. Produces heparin
   D. Stores glycogen
   E. All of the above

77. The fertilized ovum implants into the
   A. Cervix
   B. Endometrium
   C. Myometrium
   D. Epimetrium
   E. Oviducts

78. In the male, testosterone is produced in the
   A. Ovaries
   B. Testes
   C. Epididymis
   D. Seminal vesicles
   E. Prostate gland

79. The largest portion of the brain is the
   A. Cerebrum
   B. Cerebellum
   C. Medulla oblongata
   D. Brainstem
   E. Hypothalamus

80. There are _____ pairs of spinal nerves.
   A. 100
   B. 10
   C. 12
   D. 25
   E. 31

81. Gustatory receptors are located in the
   A. Mouth
   B. Nose
   C. Eye
   D. Ear
   E. Skin

82. Insulin
    A. Is produced by the liver
    B. Controls metabolism
    C. Increases blood sugar levels
    D. Decreases blood sugar levels
    E. Controls blood calcium levels

83. A decrease in the total number of white blood cells is called
    A. Leukocyte
    B. Leukoderma
    C. Leukocytosis
    D. Anemia
    E. Leukopenia

84. The abbreviation meaning *immediately* is
    A. prn
    B. stat
    C. qod
    D. ad lib
    E. dc

85. The physician is legally obligated to report
    A. Deaths
    B. Births
    C. Communicable diseases
    D. Abuse
    E. All of the above

86. The prefix *brady-* denotes
    A. Slow
    B. Fast
    C. Hard
    D. Soft
    E. Difficult

87. The opposite of superficial is
    A. Ventral
    B. Proximal
    C. Deep
    D. Distal
    E. Dorsal

88. An authorization in advance to withdraw artificial life support is
    A. Assault
    B. Battery
    C. An advanced directive
    D. Uniform Anatomical Gift Act
    E. Good Samaritan Act

89. Unconsciously avoiding the reality of an unpleasant event is
    A. Regression
    B. Denial
    C. Repression
    D. Suppression
    E. Rationalization

90. "Tell me more about it" is an example of
    A. An open-ended statement
    B. A closed statement
    C. Clarification
    D. Feedback
    E. Reflection

91. The study of the cause of disease is
    A. Epidemiology
    B. Pathology
    C. Etiology
    D. Symptomology
    E. Risk management

92. Nonverbal communication may be conveyed by
    A. Touch
    B. Eye contact
    C. Body position
    D. Silence
    E. All of the above

93. Bulimia is
    A. A mass of food
    B. An eating disorder
    C. Loss of appetite
    D. A blood condition
    E. An arrhythmia

94. A cerebral vascular accident can also be called a(n)
    A. Arrhythmia
    B. Heart attack
    C. Aneurysm
    D. Stroke
    E. Thrombus

95. Rubeola is
    A. Herpes simplex virus I
    B. Scarlet fever
    C. Whooping cough
    D. Measles
    E. Chicken pox

96. A sexually transmitted disease caused by a protozoal infestation is
    A. Herpes
    B. Gonorrhea
    C. Trichomoniasis
    D. Crabs
    E. Syphilis

97. An electrolyte that has an important influence on the activity of the heart muscle is
    A. Chloride
    B. Magnesium
    C. Peptase
    D. Phosphorus
    E. Potassium

98. Which of the following respiratory disorders is characterized by a loss of lung capacity?
    A. Asthma
    B. Emphysema
    C. Bronchitis
    D. Tuberculosis
    E. Psoriasis

99. The type of membrane that lines cavities of the body that open to the outside is
    A. Cutaneous
    B. Synovial
    C. Mucous
    D. Pleural
    E. Peritoneum

100. Another name for an open fracture is a
    A. Comminuted fracture
    B. Closed fracture
    C. Simple fracture
    D. Greenstick fracture
    E. Compound fracture

Pre-Test 2

Directions: Each of the following questions is followed by five possible responses. Select the *best* response.

1. Which of the following types of scheduling allows for the most efficient use of staff, materials, and facilities?
   A. Open appointments
   B. Double-booking
   C. Wave
   D. Modified wave
   E. Grouping

2. What piece of mail should be placed on top when sorting the physician's mail?
   A. First-class mail
   B. Journals
   C. Envelope marked *Personal*
   D. Bills and statements
   E. Equipment catalogs

3. Open punctuation is characterized by
   A. Enclosure notation
   B. Absence of punctuation after the salutation and a comma after the complimentary close
   C. Modified block style
   D. Use of a colon after the salutation
   E. Block style

4. The federal insurance program that provides for the medically indigent is
   A. CHAMPUS
   B. Medicare
   C. Blue Shield
   D. Medicaid
   E. HMO

5. The process of transferring an amount from the day sheet to the ledger is
   A. Journalizing
   B. Charting
   C. Posting
   D. Crediting
   E. Debiting

6. A numeric filing system requires the use of
   A. Lateral files
   B. An alphabetical cross-reference
   C. Color-coding
   D. A tickler file
   E. Subject headings

7. The file folder label for Jennie Holmes-Mathis should be
   A. Jennie, Holmes-Mathis
   B. Mathis, Jennie Holmes
   C. Holmes, Jennie-Mathis
   D. Holmes-Mathis, Jennie
   E. Mathis, Jennie (nee Holmes)

8. Third-party participation in an office indicates the relationships among the
   A. Physician, patient, and medical assistant
   B. Physician, medical assistant, and insurance company
   C. Physician, patient, and insurance company
   D. Physician, hospital, and insurance company
   E. Physician, patient, and hospital

9. A claim may be rejected by an insurance company because of the omission of
   A. Complete diagnosis
   B. Policy number
   C. Patient birth date
   D. Itemization of charges
   E. All of the above

10. How much postage is required for a first-class letter that weighs 3 oz if the first ounce costs $0.34 and each additional ounce is $0.25?
    A. $1.00
    B. $0.50
    C. $0.34
    D. $0.84
    E. $0.75

11. When the word *Confidential* is to be typed on the envelope, it should be placed
    A. In the lower right corner
    B. Below the zip code
    C. In the lower left corner
    D. Below the return address
    E. Both C and D

12. The most formal of complimentary closings is
    A. Very truly yours
    B. Warm wishes
    C. Sincerely
    D. Sincerely yours
    E. As always

13. When making an appointment, which of the following is *not* needed?
    A. Patient's name
    B. Telephone number
    C. Reason for visit
    D. Insurance information
    E. Availability

14. This type of call allows more than one person in more than one place to talk simultaneously.
    A. Person-to-person
    B. Conference call
    C. Three-party billing
    D. Appointment call
    E. Collect call

15. This procedure protects against the loss of data.
    A. Buffering
    B. Debugging
    C. Backing up
    D. Initializing
    E. Formatting

16. A tickler file is
    A. A guide for processing insurance claims
    B. A list of procedures for equipment maintenance
    C. A type of color-coding
    D. A physician referral service
    E. Future events arranged in chronologic order

17. All of the following would require a Current Procedural Terminology (CPT) code *except*
    A. Diarrhea
    B. Mastectomy
    C. Otoplasty
    D. Hysterectomy
    E. Sigmoidoscopy

18. Which of the following characteristics of a receptionist might make an impression on a patient?
    A. Appearance
    B. Professionalism
    C. Manners
    D. Attitude
    E. All of the above

19. A direction to consider additional codes is
    A. NEC
    B. NOS
    C. See also
    D. See condition
    E. See category

20. A V-code
    A. Refers to specific health conditions
    B. Refers to specific body systems
    C. Refers to factors that influence health status
    D. Refers to neoplasms
    E. Refers to injuries

21. Mail that is opened accidentally should be
    A. Hand delivered immediately
    B. Put at the bottom of the stack
    C. Left as is
    D. Resealed with tape and noted as *opened in error*
    E. Placed in another envelope

22. Which of the following are Evaluation and Management (E&M) descriptors?
    A. Physical examination
    B. School physical
    C. Well-baby check-up
    D. Preoperative physical
    E. All of the above

23. Which is an example of a third-party payor?
    A. Health Maintenance Organization (HMO)
    B. Medicare
    C. Preferred Provider Organization (PPO)
    D. Patient's spouse
    E. Patient's parent

24. In the problem-oriented medical record (POMR) system, the initial database includes
    A. A list of past medical problems
    B. A complete physical examination
    C. A numbered list of present problems
    D. The patient's progress
    E. A list of social problems

25. A trial balance is a comparison of
    A. Cash on hand and cash received
    B. Daily charges and payments
    C. Balance sheet and income sheet
    D. Ledger card totals and account-receivable balance
    E. Owners' equity and liabilities

26. When adding information to the medical record, new notes are added
    A. In alphabetical order
    B. In subject order
    C. Newest to the front
    D. Newest to the back
    E. To a newly created file

27. Which of the following calls require immediate transfer to the physician?
    A. A young child with a high fever
    B. A patient with a possible medical allergy
    C. Another physician
    D. An adult with a low-grade fever
    E. A patient with questions about a mammogram

28. Appointments should be scheduled
    A. For 15 minutes each with 15-minute open slots in between
    B. Every 15 minutes
    C. Either all in the morning or all in the afternoon
    D. In consecutive order without large gaps
    E. So that patients with similar problems are seen on the same day

29. Which is *not* part of basic information obtained at the patient's first visit?
    A. Insurance information
    B. Name, address, and telephone number
    C. Name of person who referred the patient
    D. Business address and business telephone number
    E. Diagnosis

30. Standard-size paper and envelope for business correspondence is
    A. 8½ × 11; no. 10 envelope
    B. 7¼ × 10-½; no. 7¾ envelope
    C. 5½ × 8½; 3½ × 6 envelope
    D. 6¼ × 9¼; no. 6¾ envelope
    E. 11 × 14; no. 10 envelope

31. Patient's ledger cards should be kept
    A. With the patient's chart
    B. In a general ledger
    C. In a separate ledger file
    D. In a job ledger
    E. With insurance forms

32. The bank statement is reconciled with
    A. The checkbook
    B. The day sheet
    C. Accounts receivable
    D. The payment record
    E. Both A and D

33. The record of the proceedings of a meeting is the
    A. Agenda
    B. *Roberts Rules of Order*
    C. Itinerary
    D. Minutes
    E. Format

34. Which of the following protects data from loss?
    A. Booting up the system
    B. Initializing disks
    C. Backing up
    D. Virus check
    E. Debugging

35. The scheduling system based on scheduling similar appointments or procedures together is called
    A. Wave
    B. Modified wave
    C. Grouping
    D. Double-booking
    E. Open scheduling

36. Appropriate information to include in a patient information brochure would be
    A. Information about the scope of the practice
    B. Physician's fees
    C. Billing information
    D. Employee's names and telephone numbers
    E. Coding information

37. A new employee must complete which of the following?
    A. 501 Form
    B. W-4 Form
    C. W-3 Form
    D. W-2 Form
    E. FICA Form

38. Which of the following abbreviations is *not* correct?
    A. pH
    B. mEq
    C. PKU
    D. HGB
    E. Kg

39. Patient information that is released without patient's authorization might result in legal charge of
    A. Fraud
    B. Battery
    C. Invasion of privacy
    D. Abandonment
    E. Libel

40. A correctly addressed envelope includes
    A. Omission of all punctuation
    B. Periods after abbreviation
    C. Periods after initials
    D. Comma between city and state
    E. Comma between street name and numbers

41. Which of the following circumstances would waive the need for a written release of medical records?
    A. Requested from other practices
    B. A subpoena
    C. Attorney request
    D. Hospital request
    E. Insurance company request

42. In double-entry bookkeeping, the original entry is put onto the
    A. Patient ledger card
    B. Daily log
    C. General ledger
    D. Account ledger
    E. Appointment book

43. The correct way to indicate an enclosure notation is
    A. encl:
    B. Enclosure
    C. enclosure
    D. enc
    E. encl

44. A superbill provides which of the following?
    A. Insurance claim
    B. Fee schedule
    C. Deposit slip
    D. Dictation
    E. Abnormal test results

45. Which of the following is the purpose of records management?
    A. Storage
    B. Arranging
    C. Accessibility
    D. Classifying
    E. All of the above

46. Which coding system is *not* associated with medical procedures?
    A. CPT
    B. *International Classification of Diseases*, ninth edition, Clinical Modification (ICD-9-CM)
    C. Health Care Financing Administration Common Procedure Coding System (HCPCS)
    D. Relative value scale (RVS)
    E. Resource-based RVS (RBRVS)

47. Which is *not* an indexing rule?
    A. Unit 1 is the surname
    B. A hyphen is disregarded
    C. Initials come before complete names
    D. Apostrophes are disregarded
    E. Names are divided into units

48. ICD-9-CM codes that refer to factors that may influence the patient's health status are
    A. Human immunodeficiency virus (HIV) codes
    B. Volume I codes
    C. Volume II codes
    D. E-codes
    E. V-codes

49. The smallest piece of information that the computer can process is a(n)
    A. Output
    B. Bit
    C. Byte
    D. Font
    E. Icon

50. The index of files on a disk is the
    A. Window
    B. Menu
    C. Byte
    D. Directory
    E. Icon

51. The appointment system of the office should take into account the needs of the
    A. Staff
    B. Physician
    C. Patients
    D. A and B only
    E. B and C only

52. *Dear Mrs. May:* is an example of
    A. Open punctuation
    B. Mixed punctuation
    C. Block punctuation
    D. Semiblock punctuation
    E. Modified block

53. A master list of equipment inventory includes all of the following *except* the
    A. Date of purchase
    B. Cost
    C. Operating manuals
    D. Estimated life of the piece
    E. Description

54. Which of the following hospital records may be released by the authorization of the attending surgeon only?
    A. Nurses' notes
    B. Operative notes
    C. Laboratory reports
    D. Radiology reports
    E. Billing information

55. An illness that existed before an insurance policy is written is known as a(n)
    A. Special risk
    B. Exclusion
    C. Preexisting condition
    D. Waiting period
    E. Prior authorization required

56. A patient has not been seen in the office for 2 years. The patient's record would be found in the
    A. Basement
    B. Active files
    C. Open files
    D. Inactive files
    E. Closed files

57. An important consideration when deciding how to position the computer monitor at the reception desk is
    A. Patient confidentiality
    B. Staff access
    C. Lighting
    D. Position of the printer
    E. Availability of patient records

58. Which group of patients should be escorted to the examination room and given instructions on what they are to do?
    A. Children
    B. New patients
    C. Established patients
    D. Older adults
    E. All of the above

59. Which information is *not* essential for the surgery scheduler when requesting a surgery date?
    A. Type of procedure
    B. Name of the assisting physician
    C. Name of patient
    D. Age of patient
    E. Telephone number of the patient

60. The notation *c: Julia Jones, MD* means
    A. A copy is made for Dr. Jones
    B. A copy of the letter is sent to Dr. Jones
    C. The receiver had been advised that a copy has been sent to Dr. Jones
    D. Dr. Jones will answer the letter
    E. The copy was sent to Dr. Jones by certified mail

61. A *history and physical* usually contains all of the following *except*
    A. Results of laboratory tests
    B. Reason for the visit
    C. Vital signs
    D. Review of body systems
    E. General appearance of patient

62. Under a managed care plan, the physician agrees to
    A. Set fees within certain ranges provided by the plan
    B. Accept predetermined fees
    C. Charge fees based on community average
    D. Base fees on the national average
    E. Limit the number of patients seen

63. Which type of insurance organization uses the fee-for-services concept?
    A. Health Maintenance Organization (HMO)
    B. Managed care
    C. Independent practice association
    D. Preferred Provider Organization (PPO)
    E. Medicaid

64. Which factor is *not* included when determining the level of service for E&M codes?
    A. Cost of services
    B. Level of decision making required of the physician
    C. Health history of patient
    D. Type of examination
    E. Type of laboratory tests

65. When money is placed in an account, which of the following documents is prepared?
    A. Check
    B. Statement
    C. Debit slip
    D. Credit slip
    E. Deposit slip

66. The most common color-coding system color codes the
    A. Patient's Social Security number
    B. Patient's date of birth
    C. Patient's given name
    D. Patient's surname
    E. Patient's account number

67. Who is the legal owner of the information in a patient's medical record?
    A. The physician
    B. The patient
    C. The insurance company
    D. The patient and physician
    E. The physician and the insurance company

68. When preparing the appointment matrix, the first action is to indicate
    A. Hospital calls
    B. Times available
    C. Times not available
    D. Facilities available
    E. Staff available

69. Scheduling patients with the same medical complaints on the same day is
    A. Wave scheduling
    B. Modified wave scheduling
    C. Open hours
    D. Group scheduling
    E. Double-booking

70. A major advantage of using a computer for word processing is
    A. Extensive editing capability
    B. Speed of processing
    C. Spell-check
    D. Column layout
    E. Storage capacity

71. Which is *not* true of certified mail?
    A. Insurance coverage is available
    B. Receipt of delivery can be obtained for a fee
    C. Only first-class mail can be certified
    D. Record of delivery is kept by the post office
    E. Restricted delivery can be obtained for a fee

72. Which of the following must be sent by first-class mail?
    A. Magazines
    B. Books
    C. Printed materials
    D. Personal letters and postcards
    E. Equipment catalogues

73. A Medicare claim for a deceased beneficiary may be paid directly to the physician if
    A. The physician accepts assignment
    B. The spouse assigns benefits to the physician
    C. Social Security verifies Medicare coverage
    D. Charges are paid by the intermediary
    E. The estate is billed

74. All checks received as payment for charges should be endorsed
    A. Immediately
    B. At the end of the day
    C. When they are deposited
    D. After they are posted
    E. Monthly

75. In an alphabetic file, which is filed first?
    A. A. R. Stephenson
    B. John Stephenson
    C. George Stephens
    D. Ann Stephenson-Bailey
    E. Andrew Stephen

76. Which is correct for an inside address?
    A. Dr. David Roberts
    B. Dr. David Roberts, M.D.
    C. Mr. David Roberts, M.D.
    D. Roberts, David, M.D.
    E. David Roberts, M.D.

77. Which is *not* true about a postage meter?
    A. It prints its own postage
    B. Some can seal the envelope
    C. It locks when the postage is used up
    D. The mailer leases the machine and purchases the postage
    E. A license must be obtained from the post office

78. The two-letter abbreviation for Nebraska is
    A. NB
    B. NE
    C. NA
    D. NR
    E. NK

79. Which letter style requires the complimentary closing and typed signature be placed in line with the left margin of the body of the letter?
    A. Block style
    B. Semiblock style
    C. Full block style
    D. Indented style
    E. Semi-indented style

80. Which of the following is *not* included in a memorandum?
    A. Date
    B. Subject
    C. Complimentary close
    D. Writer's name
    E. Reference initials

81. The second page of a two-page letter contains which of the following in the heading?
    A. Name and date
    B. Name and page number
    C. Name, page number, and date
    D. Name, page number, date, and subject
    E. Name, writer's name, subject, and date

82. The complimentary close of a letter is typed how many lines below the last line of the body?
    A. Two
    B. Three
    C. Four
    D. Five
    E. Ten

83. A fee profile is derived from
    A. Insurance payments
    B. Patient's payments
    C. Government payments
    D. Physician charges
    E. Insurance charges

84. Which of the following is demographic information included in a medical record?
    A. Present illness
    B. Date of birth
    C. Laboratory reports
    D. X-ray findings
    E. Complete physical examination

85. Which of the following requires an ICD-9-CM code?
    A. Proctoscopy
    B. Pap smear
    C. Appendectomy
    D. Irritable bowel syndrome
    E. Mastectomy

86. When it is 4:00 PM in New York City, what time is it in Seattle, WA?
    A. 12:00 PM
    B. 1:00 PM
    C. 2:00 PM
    D. 3:00 PM
    E. 4:00 PM

87. Ideally, a telephone should be answered before the
    A. First ring
    B. Third ring
    C. Fourth ring
    D. Fifth ring
    E. Other line picks up the call

88. An E code in the ICD-9-CM coding system
    A. Refers to external causes
    B. Refers to hypertension
    C. Refers to neoplasms
    D. Refers to suicide attempt
    E. Refers to disease

89. The universal claim form developed by Health Care Financing Administration (HCFA) is
    A. Form 1904
    B. ICD-9
    C. Form 1040
    D. CMS-1500
    E. HCFA-1999

90. Patients who are always late or who habitually cancel appointments should be scheduled
    A. First in the morning
    B. Right before lunch
    C. Midafternoon
    D. At the end of the day
    E. On Fridays

91. An error was made in charting the patient's record. The method used to correct the error is to
    A. Erase the error and write in the correction
    B. Reenter the notation on the next line
    C. Draw a single line through the error, write the word *error*, make the correction, and date and initial the entry
    D. Cross out the error, and make the correction in the margin
    E. Cross out the entry, and correct it

92. SOAP is an acronym for
    A. Child protection services
    B. A medical assistant society
    C. Source-oriented medical records
    D. Problem-oriented progress notes
    E. Traditional medical records

93. A patient refuses to follow medical advice and the physician decides to terminate the relationship. The letter to the patient should state all of the following *except*
    A. A referral to another physician
    B. An offer to make records available
    C. That the physician withdraws from the case
    D. A future date after which the physician is not available
    E. That the patient still needs medical care

94. When the medical office works on a fixed appointment schedule and a patient arrives without an appointment requesting to see the physician, the patient
    A. Should be sent away
    B. Should be referred to another physician
    C. Should be called as soon as a cancellation has been made
    D. Should be told to come back tomorrow
    E. Should be squeezed in for a brief visit so the physician can decide what the next treatment step should be

95. If a patient calls to cancel his or her appointment
    A. Express regret
    B. Immediately offer a new appointment time
    C. Have the patient speak to the office manager
    D. Discourage cancellations sternly
    E. All of the above

96. A good telephone technique is a
    A. High-pitched voice
    B. Low-pitched and expressive voice
    C. Monotone voice
    D. Breathless and excited voice
    E. Soft-spoken voice

97. If a patient's account has been turned over to a collection agency and the patient calls about the bill, the patient should be told
    A. To remit payment to the physician's office
    B. To deal with the collection agency
    C. To talk with the office manager
    D. To disregard further statements
    E. To find another physician

98. The entry, editing, manipulation, and storage of text using the computer is
    A. Telecommunications
    B. Documentation
    C. Interfacing
    D. Word processing
    E. Formatting

99. When a shipment of supplies is received, the supplies should be checked against the
    A. Advertised prices
    B. Enclosed packing slip
    C. Invoice
    D. Requisition slip
    E. Inventory

100. A credit balance on an account occurs when
    A. The patient's check was returned for insufficient funds
    B. The insurance company disallows the claim
    C. The patient pays in advance
    D. A discount is given
    E. The patient is sent to collection

Pre-Test 3

Directions: Each of the following questions is followed by five possible responses. Select the *best* response.

1. *Standard precautions* are designed to be used for
   A. Patients known to be infected
   B. Patients suspected of being infected
   C. All patients
   D. Patients recovering from an infectious disease
   E. Infected health care workers

2. Disposable single-use gloves should be worn
   A. When taking a blood pressure
   B. When handling specimens
   C. When performing venipuncture
   D. All of the above
   E. B and C

3. Normal oral temperature, in degrees, is
   A. 96.8°F
   B. 97.6°F
   C. 98.6°F
   D. 36°C
   E. 38°C

4. Normal respiratory rate for an adult is
   A. 10 to 16 breaths per minute
   B. 14 to 20 breaths per minute
   C. 20 to 26 breaths per minute
   D. 30 to 38 breaths per minute
   E. 30 to 60 breaths per minute

5. Vital signs include
   A. Temperature
   B. Blood pressure
   C. TPR
   D. A and B
   E. B and C

6. The pulse rate is
   A. Usually higher in adults than in children
   B. Usually higher in children than in adults
   C. The same for both
   D. Lower at birth than at 1 year
   E. Higher in adults over 60 than in a child under 7 years of age

7. Pulse rate is decreased by
   A. Sleep
   B. Brain injury, causing increased pressure
   C. Hypothyroidism
   D. A and B
   E. All of the above

8. A high fever occurs when the body temperature, in degrees, is
   A. 98° to 99°F
   B. 99° to 101°F
   C. 101° to 103°F
   D. 103° to 105°F
   E. 38.3° to 39.5°C

9. The pulse pressure is
   A. The difference between the systolic and the diastolic blood pressure
   B. An occasional missed beat
   C. Absence of a carotid pulse
   D. Alternating weak and strong beats
   E. The difference between apical and radial pulses

10. A patient who weighs 45 kg also weighs how many pounds?
    A. 45
    B. 99
    C. 105
    D. 145
    E. 150

11. A patient who is 72 inches tall is
    A. 6 feet
    B. 6 feet, 2 inches
    C. 6 feet, 4 inches
    D. 5 feet, 2 inches
    E. 5 feet, 6 inches

12. During a physical examination, percussion is most commonly used to examine the
    A. Chest and back
    B. Mouth and throat
    C. Eyes and ears
    D. Breasts
    E. Nose and neck

13. A patient's reaction to stress, use of defense mechanisms, and resources for support would be recorded under
    A. Chief complaint
    B. Past history
    C. History of present illness
    D. Social history
    E. Family history

14. Subjective findings include
    A. How the patient feels
    B. Information about the patient's family
    C. Previous pregnancies
    D. All of the above
    E. A and B

15. Visual acuity is
    A. Pressure in the eyeball
    B. Nearsightedness
    C. Farsightedness
    D. Color vision
    E. Clearness of vision

16. The purpose of a proctoscopy is to examine the
    A. Prostate gland
    B. Uterus
    C. Rectum
    D. Sigmoid colon
    E. Esophagus

17. A patient in the Sims' position is lying on the
    A. Right side, with left leg flexed
    B. Left side and chest, with right leg flexed
    C. Back, with both legs bent
    D. Right side, with right leg flexed
    E. Left side, with left leg flexed

18. A patient lying flat on the abdomen is in the
    A. Dorsal position
    B. Lithotomy position
    C. Supine position
    D. Prone position
    E. Fowler's position

19. The physician uses which of the following to examine the patient's eyes?
    A. Ophthalmoscope
    B. Percussion hammer
    C. Tonometer
    D. Otoscope
    E. Speculum

20. The patient should be placed in which of the following positions for examination of the head and neck?
    A. Standing
    B. Sitting
    C. Prone
    D. Supine
    E. Sims'

21. For an obstetrics examination, urine is routinely checked for the presence of
    A. Glucose and protein
    B. Glucose and ketones
    C. Human chorionic gonadotropin (HCG)
    D. Protein and ketones
    E. Blood and glucose

22. A patient should be taught that the best time to perform breast self-examination is approximately
    A. 1 week after her period
    B. The sixth day of every month
    C. 1 week before her period
    D. 2 weeks after her period
    E. 2 weeks before her period

23. An infection that has a rapid onset, severe symptoms, and subsides in a short period is called
    A. Acute
    B. Chronic
    C. Local
    D. Systemic
    E. Contagious

24. Sterile-wrapped items can be safely stored, and considered sterile, for up to
    A. 7 to 14 days
    B. 14 to 21 days
    C. 21 to 28 days
    D. 28 to 30 days
    E. Indefinitely

25. When removing a pack from the autoclave, you notice that the sterilization indicator has not changed color. You should
    A. Do nothing
    B. Place the pack back in the autoclave and resterilize
    C. Place a new indicator on the pack and resterilize
    D. Place the pack back in the autoclave but in a different location
    E. Unwrap the pack, rewrap the pack, replace the indicator, and resterilize

26. Scrubbing an item with soap and water before sterilization is
    A. Cleaning
    B. Sanitization
    C. Disinfection
    D. Sterilization
    E. Antisepsis

27. The type of immunity that develops from having the disease is
    A. Natural active
    B. Natural passive
    C. Acquired active
    D. Acquired passive
    E. Congenital

28. When opening a sterile pack, the top flap should be opened
    A. Toward the body
    B. Away from the body
    C. Toward the right side
    D. Toward the left side
    E. In any direction

29. The finest suture material of the following list is
    A. 0
    B. 00
    C. 000
    D. 4-0
    E. 8-0

30. A type of instrument that is used to grasp or hold tissues or objects is a
    A. Probe
    B. Scalpel
    C. Scissors
    D. Forceps
    E. Retractor

31. Betadine (povidone-iodine) should not be used on the skin of a patient who is allergic to
    A. Alcohol
    B. Metal
    C. Iodine
    D. Soap
    E. Latex

32. Wound drainage that contains pus is charted as
    A. Serous
    B. Normal
    C. Serosanguineous
    D. Sanguinous
    E. Purulent

33. The angle for the insertion of the needle for an intradermal injection is
    A. 10 to 15 degrees
    B. 20 to 30 degrees
    C. 45 degrees
    D. 90 degrees
    E. Not important

34. A medication that is placed under the tongue is being administered by which technique?
    A. By mouth
    B. Buccal
    C. Sublingual
    D. Instillation
    E. Topical

35. To administer an intramuscular injection, which needle would you use?
    A. 1 inch, 25 gauge
    B. 1½ inch, 21 gauge
    C. 1 inch, 18 gauge
    D. ½ inch, 22 gauge
    E. 2 inch, 20 gauge

36. A type of drug that increases urinary output is a(n)
    A. Emetic
    B. Diuretic
    C. Miotic
    D. Cathartic
    E. Antibiotic

37. The physician orders 250 mg amoxicillin intramuscularly. The vial reads *500 mg per 1 mL*. How much would be given to the patient?
    A. 0.5 mL
    B. 1 mL
    C. 2 mL
    D. 3 mL
    E. 5 mL

38. When a specimen is placed in a centrifuge, a tube of similar size containing a liquid of similar weight should be placed
    A. On the counter
    B. Directly opposite from the specimen
    C. Directly beside the specimen
    D. In all empty spaces in the centrifuge
    E. To the right side of the specimen

39. Microscopic examination of a urine sample should be performed
    A. Within ½ hour of collection
    B. Within 1 hour of collection
    C. Within 1½ hours of collection
    D. Within 2 hours of collection
    E. Within 3 hours of collection

40. The absence of urine formation is termed
    A. Anuria
    B. Polyuria
    C. Dysuria
    D. Oliguria
    E. Ketonuria

41. Normal specific gravity is generally between
    A. 1.000 and 1.005
    B. 1.010 and 1.050
    C. 1.025 and 1.500
    D. 1.005 and 1.050
    E. 1.010 and 1.025

42. A complete blood count (CBC) includes
    A. Platelet count
    B. Hemoglobin and hematocrit
    C. White blood cell count
    D. All of the above
    E. A and C

43. Capillary blood is usually obtained
    A. From a skin puncture
    B. From a venipuncture
    C. From an arterial puncture
    D. All of the above
    E. B and C

44. A cholecystogram is used to view the
    A. Urinary bladder
    B. Liver
    C. Gallbladder
    D. Kidneys
    E. Ureters

45. Application of heat
    A. Dilates blood vessels
    B. Constricts blood vessels
    C. Elevates blood pressure
    D. Decreases respiration
    E. Produces weight loss

46. The wave on an electrocardiogram that represents contraction of the atria is
    A. P
    B. QRS
    C. T
    D. V
    E. R

47. The pacemaker of the heart is the
    A. Myocardium
    B. Sinoatrial node
    C. Atrioventricular node
    D. Purkinje fibers
    E. Bundle of His

48. A standard electrocardiogram has how many leads?
    A. 4
    B. 8
    C. 10
    D. 12
    E. 14

49. The standard speed for recording an electrocardiogram is
    A. 5 mm/sec
    B. 10 mm/sec
    C. 20 mm/sec
    D. 25 mm/sec
    E. 50 mm/sec

50. To cauterize a small lesion on the oral mucosa, the physician may use an applicator with
    A. Silver nitrate
    B. Alcohol
    C. Formalin
    D. Betadine
    E. Zephiran chloride

51. A common laboratory test that may be ordered for a patient on Coumadin therapy is
    A. Prothrombin time
    B. Erythrocyte sedimentation rate (ESR)
    C. White blood cell (WBC) count
    D. Hematocrit
    E. Complete blood count (CBC)

52. Which one of the following types of suture material is absorbable?
    A. Steel
    B. Cotton
    C. Catgut
    D. Nylon
    E. Silk

53. The minimum number of cells to be counted in a differential blood smear is
    A. 50
    B. 100
    C. 150
    D. 200
    E. Unlimited; count them all

54. A hemoglobin of 10 g/dL is approximately equivalent to a hematocrit of
    A. 10%
    B. 20%
    C. 30%
    D. 36%
    E. 40%

55. Which of the following laboratory results should be called to the attention of the physician?
  A. White blood cell count: 7200/mm³
  B. Red blood cell count: 4.4 million/mm³
  C. Hemoglobin: 12 g/dL
  D. Erythrocyte sedimentation rate: 30 mm/hr
  E. Total cholesterol: 180 mg

56. The stain used to identify bacteria on a prepared slide is the
  A. Gram stain
  B. Wright's stain
  C. Giemsa stain
  D. India ink
  E. All of the above

57. After sitting for a long time, a urine sample becomes
  A. Clear
  B. Alkaline
  C. Acid
  D. Neutral
  E. Darker

58. A blood sample for serum is collected in which of the following tubes?
  A. Blue-stoppered
  B. Lavender-stoppered
  C. Green-stoppered
  D. Red-stoppered (tiger)
  E. Black-stoppered

59. Which of the following are categories to classify instruments used in surgery?
  A. Probing and dilating
  B. Cutting and dissecting
  C. Grasping and clamping
  D. Retracting
  E. All of the above

60. The first thing that should be done in an emergent situation involving an unconscious person is to
  A. Assess the victim's airway
  B. Control any bleeding
  C. Apply a tourniquet
  D. Dial 911
  E. Give the patient breaths

61. A physical examination of a urine sample includes
  A. Odor
  B. Color
  C. Transparency
  D. Specific gravity
  E. All of the above

62. Most drugs are metabolized in the
  A. Lungs
  B. Blood
  C. Stomach
  D. Liver
  E. Intestines

63. The Ishihara test
  A. Tests for visual acuity
  B. Tests for glaucoma
  C. Tests for color-blindness
  D. Tests for presbyopia
  E. Tests for nerve deafness

64. Which is *not* a common symptom of a myocardial infarction?
  A. Nausea
  B. Angina
  C. Dyspnea
  D. Diaphoresis
  E. Polyuria

65. Hemostats are a type of
  A. Forceps
  B. Probe
  C. Applicator
  D. Scissors
  E. Retractors

66. The normal ratio for respiration to pulse is
  A. 1 to 6
  B. 1 to 2
  C. 1 to 4
  D. 2 to 4
  E. 4 to 1

67. Symptoms of insulin shock include
  A. Restless and confusion
  B. Cold, clammy skin
  C. Profuse sweating
  D. Rapid, weak pulse
  E. All of the above

68. Which is the most important route for eliminating drugs from the body?
  A. Kidneys
  B. Skin
  C. Mammary glands
  D. Lungs
  E. Digestive system

69. Prozac is an example of an
  A. Antihistamine
  B. Antidiuretic
  C. Antidepressant
  D. Antifungal
  E. Antibiotic

70. The two most important factors in performing effective hand washing are
   A. Temperature of water and soap
   B. Friction and running water
   C. Position of hands and hot water
   D. Length of time and soap
   E. Friction and soap

71. At which age is the first mumps, measles, and rubella (MMR) vaccination recommended?
   A. Birth
   B. 2 months
   C. 4 months
   D. 12 months
   E. 5 years

72. If a patient describes an aura before the onset of a severe headache, this is often a sign of
   A. Cerebrovascular accident
   B. Migraine
   C. Hay fever
   D. Brain tumor
   E. Seizure

73. A function of hemoglobin is
   A. To repair cells
   B. To destroy cells
   C. To prevent blood loss
   D. To carry oxygen and carbon dioxide
   E. To fight off infection

74. A quality assurance program in the laboratory
   A. Ensures the accuracy of results
   B. Requires less paperwork
   C. Eliminates outside laboratory tests
   D. Increases convenience
   E. Provides quick results

75. The reaction of the purified protein derivative (PPD) test is read
   A. 12 to 24 hours after it has been placed
   B. 48 to 72 hours after it has been placed
   C. Immediately after it has been placed
   D. 24 to 36 hours after it has been placed
   E. 4 to 8 hours after it has been placed

76. The abbreviation for *both ears* is
   A. AS
   B. AD
   C. AU
   D. BE
   E. AS/AD

77. The blood type known as the *universal donor* is
   A. A
   B. B
   C. AB
   D. O
   E. All of the above

78. A lower gastrointestinal (GI) series is performed to outline the
   A. Esophagus
   B. Stomach
   C. Ileum
   D. Duodenum
   E. Colon

79. A technique that provides soft-tissue images in three dimensions is
   A. Ultrasound
   B. Computed tomographic (CT) scan
   C. Myelography
   D. Tomography
   E. Intravenous pyelogram (IVP)

80. Massive and prolonged exposure to radiation can result in
   A. Cancer
   B. Increased number of white blood cells
   C. Increased number of red blood cells
   D. Arthritis
   E. Death

81. Which is the first group of leads to be recorded on an electrocardiogram?
   A. Augmented leads
   B. Leads I, II, and III
   C. aVR, aVL, and aVF
   D. Leads V_1 through V_3
   E. Leads V_1 through V_6

82. Streptococci are arranged in
   A. Clusters
   B. Chains
   C. Circles
   D. Pairs
   E. Fours

83. Pulse rate may be increased in all of the following *except*
   A. Fear
   B. Anger
   C. Anxiety
   D. Increasing age
   E. Exercise

84. The electrode that is used for grounding in an electrocardiogram is placed on the
    A. LA
    B. RA
    C. LL
    D. RL
    E. C

85. Which federal agency oversees the safety of health facilities?
    A. OSHA
    B. CLIA '88
    C. CDC
    D. DEA
    E. COLA

86. A drug reference contains all of the following information *except*
    A. Description
    B. Indications
    C. Contraindications
    D. Dose
    E. Cost

87. Ibuprofen has analgesic and antipyretic properties and is used to treat
    A. Pain
    B. Arthritis
    C. Headache
    D. Dysmenorrhea
    E. All of the above

88. Which of the following patient instructions is critical for a successful Holter monitor recording interpretation?
    A. Avoid stress
    B. Refrain from exercise
    C. Keep a written record of all daily activities
    D. Wear the monitor for 5 days
    E. Do not take any medications

89. The involuntary muscular action that moves food along the gastrointestinal tract is called
    A. Digestion
    B. Indigestion
    C. Mastication
    D. Peristalsis
    E. Deglutition

90. The first dose of diphtheria tetanus acellular pertussis (DTaP) vaccine should be administered at
    A. 2 months
    B. 4 months
    C. 12 months
    D. 5 years
    E. 12 years

91. Tissue samples removed during a biopsy would be sent to which department of the laboratory?
    A. Serology
    B. Cytology
    C. Histology
    D. Chemistry
    E. Microbiology

92. Which of the following would be *least* likely to contaminate the sterile field?
    A. Talking over the field
    B. Hair not pulled back
    C. A nonsterile person entering the room
    D. A sterile instrument touching the edge of the field
    E. Moisture on the sterile field

93. An antihistamine that may be used to treat an allergic reaction is
    A. Bactrim
    B. Motrin
    C. Benadryl
    D. Inderal
    E. Indocin

94. Each of the following abbreviations is correctly defined *except*
    A. bid (twice a day)
    B. tid (three times a day)
    C. OD (right eye)
    D. qod (every day)
    E. ac (before meals)

95. Surgical asepsis should be maintained when performing which of the following?
    A. Dipstick urinalysis
    B. Pelvic examination
    C. Snellen test
    D. Needle biopsy
    E. Blood pressure

96. How often should quality control tests be performed in the laboratory?
    A. Daily
    B. Weekly
    C. Monthly
    D. When necessary
    E. Before each test

97. An infectious inflammatory skin disease caused by staphylococci and characterized by vesicles that later crust is called
    A. Vitiligo
    B. Impetigo
    C. Tinea
    D. Cellulitis
    E. Acne

98. A decrease in bone density may indicate
- **A.** Osteolysis
- **B.** Osteoclasis
- **C.** Osteoporosis
- **D.** Crepitus
- **E.** Osteomyelitis

99. A disorder of accommodation usually associated with aging is known as
- **A.** Myopia
- **B.** Hyperopia
- **C.** Astigmatism
- **D.** Presbyopia
- **E.** Macular degeneration

100. An infection of the middle ear may be charted as
- **A.** Otitis media
- **B.** Tinnitus
- **C.** Conjunctivitis
- **D.** Mastoiditis
- **E.** Tympanitis

1 | *Medical Terminology*

- Language of medicine
- Mostly Latin and Greek origins
- Made up of word parts:
  1. Root word
     - Core of the word
     - Tells the fundamental meaning of the word
     - More than one root word may exist in a medical term
  2. Suffix
     - Word part attached to the end of a root word
     - Changes or modifies its meaning
     - Can be:
       - Symptomatic: describes evidence of illness
       - Diagnostic: names a medical condition
       - Operative: describes a surgical treatment
       - General: general applications
  3. Prefix
     - Word part attached to the beginning of a root word
     - Changes or modifies its meaning
  4. Combining vowel or form
     - Used between two root words or between a root word and a suffix to make pronunciation easier
     - Not used between a prefix and the root word
     - Usually an *o*
     - Combining form is a root word with the combining vowel attached

  To analyze a medical term:
  - Divide the word into word parts.
  - Divide the word by slashes, and label each word part.

    Example: leukocytosis
    leuk/o/cyt/osis
    rw/cv/rw/s

  To define a medical term:
  - Give each word part a meaning.
  - Begin by defining the suffix, then the prefix, then the root word.

  To build a medical term, use the same procedure as previously described.

A. BODY STRUCTURE COMBINING FORMS

1. blast/o	immature form; developing cell
2. carcin/o	cancer
cancer/o	
3. cyt/o	cell
4. epitheli/o	epithelium
5. eti/o	cause
6. gno/o	knowledge
7. hist/o	tissue
8. iatr/o	physician; medicine
9. kary/o	nucleus
10. lei/o	smooth
11. lip/o	fat
12. my/o	muscle
13. neur/o	nerve
14. onc/o	tumor
15. organ/o	organ
16. path/o	disease
17. rhabd/o	rod shaped
18. sarc/o	flesh; connective tissue
19. somat/o	body
20. system/o	system
21. viscer/o	internal organs; viscera

B. INTEGUMENTARY SYSTEM COMBINING FORMS

1. aden/o	gland
2. aut/o	self
3. bi/o	life
4. coni/o	dust
5. crypt/o	hidden
6. cutane/o	skin
derm/o	
dermat/o	
7. fibr/o	fibrous tissue; fiber
8. heter/o	other
9. hidr/o	sweat
10. kerat/o	hard; horny tissue
11. myc/o	fungus
12. necr/o	death

13. onych/o   nail
    ungu/o
14. pachy/o   thick
15. rhytid/o   wrinkle
16. seb/o   sebum (oil)
17. staphyl/o   grapelike clusters
18. strept/o   chainlike
19. trich/o   hair
20. xer/o   dry

C. MUSCULOSKELETAL SYSTEM COMBINING FORMS

1. ankyl/o   stiff
2. aponeur/o   aponeurosis
3. arthr/o   joint
4. burs/o   bursa
5. carp/o   carpals
6. chondr/o   cartilage
7. clavic/o   clavicle
   clavicul/o
8. cost/o   rib
9. crani/o   skull
10. disk/o   intervertebral disk
11. femor/o   femur
12. fibul/o   fibula
13. humer/o   humerus
14. ili/o   ilium
15. ischi/o   ischium
16. kinesi/o   movement
17. kyph/o   hump
18. lamin/o   thin, flat layer
19. lord/o   bent forward; abnormal convexity
                     of the spine
20. mandibul/o   mandible
21. maxill/o   maxilla
22. menisc/o   meniscus
23. myel/o   bone marrow; spinal cord
    myelon/o
24. my/o   muscle
    myos/o
25. oste/o   bone
26. patell/o   patella
27. phalang/o   phalanges
28. pub/o   pubis
29. radi/o   radius
30. scapul/o   scapula
31. scoli/o   bent; curved
32. stern/o   sternum
33. synovi/o   synovial fluid; synovial membrane
34. tars/o   tarsals
35. ten/o   tendon
    tend/o
    tendin/o
36. tibi/o   tibia
37. uln/o   ulna
38. vertebr/o   vertebrae; vertebral column
    rachi/o
    spondyl/o

D. NERVOUS SYSTEM COMBINING FORMS

1. cerebell/o   cerebellum
2. cerebr/o   cerebrum
3. dur/o   dura mater
4. encephal/o   brain
5. esthesi/o   feeling; sensation; sensitivity
6. gangli/o   ganglion
   ganglion/o
7. meningi/o   meninges
   mening/o
8. mon/o   one; single
9. myel/o   spinal cord
10. neur/o   nerve
11. phas/o   speech
12. poli/o   gray; gray matter
13. psych/o   mind
    ment/o
    phren/o
14. quadr/i   four

E. CARDIOVASCULAR AND LYMPHATIC SYSTEMS COMBINING FORMS

1. angi/o   vessel
2. aort/o   aorta
3. arteri/o   artery
4. ather/o   fatty deposit
5. bacteri/o   bacteria
6. cardi/o   heart
7. ech/o   sound
8. electr/o   electrical activity; electricity
9. hem/o   blood
   hemat/o
10. isch/o   blockage; deficiency
11. lymph/o   lymph
12. phleb/o   vein
    ven/o
13. plasm/o   plasma
14. sphygm/o   pulse
15. splen/o   spleen
16. therm/o   heat
17. thromb/o   clot
18. thym/o   thymus gland
19. valv/o   valve
    valvul/o
20. ventricul/o   ventricle

F. RESPIRATORY SYSTEM COMBINING FORMS

1. adenoid/o   adenoid
2. alveol/o   alveolus
3. atel/o   incomplete; imperfect
4. bronchi/o   bronchus
   bronch/o
5. bronchiol/o   bronchiole
6. diaphragmat/o   diaphragm
7. epiglott/o   epiglottis
8. laryng/o   larynx
9. lob/o   lobe
10. muc/o   mucus

11.	nas/o	nose
	rhin/o	
12.	orth/o	straight
13.	ox/o	oxygen
	ox/i	
14.	pharyng/o	pharynx
15.	pleur/o	pleura
16.	pneum/o	lung; air
	pneumat/o	
	pneumon/o	
17.	pulmon/o	lung
18.	py/o	pus
19.	sinus/o	sinus
20.	sept/o	septum; wall off
21.	spir/o	breathe; breathing
22.	thorac/o	thorax; chest
23.	tonsill/o	tonsil
24.	trache/o	trachea

G. DIGESTIVE SYSTEM COMBINING FORMS

1.	an/o	anus
2.	appendic/o	appendix
3.	cec/o	cecum
4.	duoden/o	duodenum
5.	chol/e	bile; gall
6.	cholecyst/o	gallbladder
7.	cholangi/o	bile duct
8.	choledoch/o	common bile duct
9.	col/o	colon
10.	dent/i	tooth
11.	diverticul/o	diverticulum; blind pouch extending from an organ
12.	duoden/o	duodenum
13.	enter/o	small intestines
14.	esophag/o	esophagus
15.	gastr/o	stomach
16.	gingiv/o	gum
17.	gloss/o	tongue
	lingu/o	
18.	hepat/o	liver
19.	herni/o	hernia
20.	ile/o	ileum
21.	jejun/o	jejunum
22.	lapar/o	abdomen
	abdomin/o	
	celi/o	
23.	palat/o	palate
24.	pancreat/o	pancreas
25.	peritone/o	peritoneum
26.	proct/o	rectum
	rect/o	
27.	polyp/o	polyp; small growth on a stalk
28.	pylor/o	pylorus; pyloric sphincter
29.	sial/o	saliva
30.	sigmoid/o	sigmoid colon
31.	stomat/o	mouth
	or/o	
32.	uvul/o	uvula

H. URINARY SYSTEM COMBINING FORMS

1.	albumin/o	albumin
2.	azot/o	urea; nitrogen
3.	cyst/o	bladder; sac
	vesic/o	
4.	glomerul/o	glomerulus
5.	glyc/o	sugar
	glycos/o	
6.	hydr/o	water
7.	lith/o	stone; calculus
8.	meat/o	meatus; opening
9.	nephr/o	kidney
	ren/o	
10.	noct/i	night
11.	olig/o	scanty; few
12.	pyel/o	renal pelvis
13.	son/o	sound
14.	ureter/o	ureter
15.	urethr/o	urethra
16.	urin/o	urine; urinary tract
	ur/o	

I. ENDOCRINE SYSTEM COMBINING FORMS

1.	acr/o	extremities
2.	adeno/o	gland
3.	adren/o	adrenal glands
	adrenal/o	
4.	calc/i	calcium
5.	cortic/o	cortex
6.	dips/o	thirst
7.	endocrin/o	endocrine
8.	hormon/o	hormone
9.	kal/i	potassium
10.	natr/o	sodium
11.	parathyroid/o	parathyroid glands
12.	thyroid/o	thyroid gland
	thyr/o	
13.	toxic/o	poison

J. MALE REPRODUCTIVE SYSTEM COMBINING FORMS

1.	andr/o	male; man
2.	balan/o	glans penis
3.	epididym/o	epididymis
4.	prostat/o	prostate gland
5.	vas/o	vessel; duct
6.	vesicul/o	seminal vesicles
7.	orchid/o	testicle; testes
	orchi/o	
	orch/o	
8.	sperm/o	sperm
	spermat/o	
9.	test/o	testicle; testes

K. FEMALE REPRODUCTIVE SYSTEM COMBINING FORMS

1.	arche/o	beginning; first
2.	cervic/o	cervix
3.	colp/o	vagina
	vagin/o	

4. gynec/o   female; woman
   gyn/o
5. hymen/o   hymen
6. hyster/o   uterus
   metr/o
   metri/o
   uter/o
7. lact/o   milk
8. mamm/o   breast
   mast/o
9. men/o   menstruation
10. oophor/o   ovary
11. ov/o   egg; ovum
    ov/i
12. perine/o   perineum
13. salping/o   fallopian tubes
14. vulv/o   vulva
    episi/o

L. COMBINING FORMS INDICATING COLORS

1. albin/o   white
   leuk/o
2. chlor/o   green
3. cyan/o   blue
4. erythr/o   red
5. melan/o   black
6. xanth/o   yellow

M. SUFFIXES USED TO INDICATE PATHOLOGICAL CONDITIONS

1. -algia   pain
   -dynia
2. -cele   hernia
3. -ectasis   dilation; swelling
4. -edema   swelling
5. -emesis   vomiting
6. -emia   blood condition
7. -ia   state of; condition
8. -iasis   abnormal condition
9. -itis   inflammation
10. -lith   stone; calculus
11. -lysis   destruction; separation; breakdown
12. -malacia   softening
13. -megaly   enlargement
14. -oma   tumor; mass
15. -osis   abnormal increase; abnormal condition
16. -pathy   disease process
17. -penia   decrease; deficiency
18. -phobia   irrational fear
19. -plegia   paralysis
20. -ptosis   drooping; sagging prolapse
21. -ptysis   spitting
22. -rrhage   bursting forth
    -rrhagia

23. -rrhea   flow; discharge
24. -rrhexis   rupture
25. -sclerosis   hardening
26. -spasm   involuntary contraction
27. -stenosis   narrowing
28. -y   process; state; condition

N. SUFFIXES USED TO INDICATE DIAGNOSTIC AND SURGICAL PROCEDURES

1. -centesis   surgical puncture to remove fluid
2. -desis   surgical binding; surgical fusion
3. -ectomy   excision; surgical removal
4. -gram   record; writing
5. -graph   instrument used to record
6. -graphy   process of recording; producing images
7. -meter   instrument used to measure
8. -metry   to measure; measurement
9. -opsy   to view
10. -pexy   surgical fixation
11. -plasty   surgical repair; surgical reconstruction
12. -rrhaphy   suture; sew
13. -scope   instrument used to visually examine
14. -scopy   process of visually examining
15. -stasis   stoppage; stopping; controlling
16. -stomy   new opening
17. -tome   instrument used to cut
18. -tomy   process of cutting; incision into
19. -tripsy   surgical crushing

O. GENERAL SUFFIXES

1. -ase   enzyme
2. -blast   immature form
3. -cyte   cell
4. -er   specialist; one who
   -or   specializes
   -ician
   -logist
   -ist
5. -ion   process
6. -ium   membrane
7. -logy   study of
8. -ose   sugar
9. -phagia   to eat; swallow
10. -phasia   speech
11. -plasia   formation; development
12. -pnea   breathing
13. -poiesis   production; formation
14. -trophy   development; growth
15. -uria   urine

P. SUFFIXES USED TO CREATE ADJECTIVE FORMS

1. -ac   pertaining to
   -al
   -ar
   -ary
   -eal

-ic
-ine
-ior
-ose
-ous
-tic

2. -genous   produced by; producing
   -genic
3. -oid   like; resembling
4. -ole   small
   -ule

Q. PREFIXES USED TO INDICATE DIRECTION AND POSITION

1. ab-   away from
2. ad-   toward
3. ante-   before
4. circum-   around
5. dia-   complete; through
6. ecto-   outside
7. endo-   within
8. e-   out; outward; outside
   ex-
   exo-
   extra-
9. epi-   upon; on; above
10. eso-   inward; within
11. hyper-   above; excessive
12. hypo-   below; under; deficient
13. in-   in; into
14. infra-   below; beneath
15. inter-   between
16. intra-   within
17. meta-   beyond; change
18. para-   beside; near
19. per-   through
20. peri-   around
21. post-   after
22. pre-   before; in front of
23. pro-   before
24. retro-   back; behind
25. sub-   under; below
26. supra-   above
27. trans-   across

R. PREFIXES REFERRING TO NUMBER OR MEASUREMENT

1. bi-   two
   di-
2. hemi-   half
   semi-
3. mono-   one
   uni-
4. multi-   many
   poly-
5. nulli-   none
6. primi-   first

7. quadri-   four
8. tri-   three

S. MISCELLANEOUS PREFIXES

1. a-   no; not; lack of; without
   an-
2. ana-   apart
3. anti-   against
4. auto-   self
5. brady-   slow
6. contra-   against
7. dys-   bad; abnormal; difficult; painful
8. in-   not
   ir-
   im-
9. macro-   large
10. mal-   bad
11. micro-   small
12. neo-   new
13. pan-   all
14. syn-   together; joined; with
    sym-
15. tachy-   fast; rapid

T. PLURALS

To form a plural, change the:

a as in burs**a**	→	**ae** as in burs**ae**
ax as in thor**ax**	→	**aces** as in thor**aces**
en as in foram**en**	→	**ina** as in foram**ina**
is as in cris**is**	→	**es** as in cris**es**
is as in ir**is**	→	**ides** as in ir**ides**
is as in femor**is**	→	**a** as in femor**a**
ix as in append**ix**	→	**ices** as in append**ices**
nx as in phala**nx**	→	**ges** an in phalan**ges**
on as in spermatozo**on**	→	**a** as in spermatozo**a**
um as in ov**um**	→	**a** as in ov**a**
us as in nucle**us**	→	**i** as in nucle**i**
y as in arter**y**	→	**ies** as in arter**ies**

Abbreviations

Follow the institution's policies for use of abbreviations. Some institutions do not use abbreviations because of the increased chance of errors.

A. CHARTING TERMS

abd	abdomen
ADL	activities of daily living
approx	approximately
ASAP	as soon as possible
ax	axillary
BE	barium enema
BM	bowel movement
BP, B/P	blood pressure
BSE	breast self-examination
bx	biopsy
cath	catheterization; catheter
CC	chief complaint

chemo	chemotherapy
c/o	complains of
CSF	cerebrospinal fluid
D&C	dilatation (dilation) and curettage
disc, d/c, dc	discontinue
DOB	date of birth
Dr.	doctor
drsg, dsg	dressing
dx	diagnosis
EDC, EDD	estimated date of confinement (due date); estimated date of delivery
EEG	electroencephalogram
EKG, ECG	electrocardiogram
ETOH	ethyl alcohol
FB	foreign body
FH	family history
FU	follow up
fx	fracture
GI	gastrointestinal
GP	general practitioner
grav, gravida	pregnancy
GYN	gynecology
H&P	history and physical
HEENT	head, eye, ear, nose, throat
hr	hour
hs	hour of sleep; bedtime
ht	height
hx	history
I&D	incision and drainage
ID	intradermal
IM	intramuscular
IV	intravenous
KUB	kidney, ureter, bladder
Ⓛ	left
LLQ	left lower quadrant
LMP	last menstrual period
LUQ	left upper quadrant
med(s)	medication(s)
mets	metastasis
MRI	magnetic resonance imaging
N&V	nausea and vomiting
NKA	no known allergies
NPO	nothing by mouth
NVD	nausea, vomiting, diarrhea
OB	obstetrics
OC	oral contraceptives
OR	operating room
os	opening
P	pulse
para	live birth
PE, px	physical examination
Peds	pediatrics
PERLA	pupils equally reactive to light and accommodation

PERRLA	pupils equal, round, react to light and accommodation
PH	past history
pt	patient
R	respiration
®	right
RLQ	right lower quadrant
r/o	rule out
ROM	range of motion
RUQ	right upper quadrant
Rx	prescription
SOAP	subjective, objective, assessment, plan
SQ, subQ, SC	subcutaneous
stat	immediately
sx	symptoms
T	temperature
T&A	tonsilloadenoidectomy (tonsils and adenoids)
TLC	tender loving care
tx	treatment, therapy
UCHD	usual childhood diseases
vo	verbal order
VS	vital signs
WDWN	well-developed, well-nourished
WNL	within normal limits
wt	weight

B. DIAGNOSTIC TERMS

AIDS	acquired immune deficiency syndrome
ADD	attention deficit disorder
ADHD	attention deficit hyperactivity disorder
ASHD	arteriosclerotic heart disease
CA, Ca	cancer
CHF	congestive heart failure
COPD	chronic obstructive pulmonary disease
CVA	cerebral vascular accident
FTT	failure to thrive
GERD	gastroesophageal reflux disease
HAV	hepatitis A virus
HBV	hepatitis B virus
HCV	hepatitis C virus
HIV	human immunodeficiency virus
IDDM	insulin-dependent diabetes mellitus
MI	myocardial infarction
NIDDM	non–insulin-dependent diabetes mellitus
PMS	premenstrual syndrome
SIDS	sudden infant death syndrome
SOB	shortness of breath
STD	sexually transmitted disease
TB	tuberculosis

URI	upper respiratory infection
UTI	urinary tract infection

C. PRESCRIPTION TERMS

aa	of each
ac	before meals
AD	right ear
ad lib	as desired
AM	morning
amt	amount
AS	left ear
ASA	aspirin
ASAP	as soon as possible
AU	both ears
bid	twice daily, two times a day
c̄	with
et	and
noct	night
OD	right eye
OS	left eye
OU	both eyes
p̄	after
pc	after meals
po	by mouth
PM	afternoon
prn	as needed
q̄	every
qd	every day
qh	every hour
qid	four times daily, four times a day
qod	every other day
qoh	every other hour
s̄	without
s̄s̄	half
tab	tablet
tid	three times daily, three times a day

D. LABORATORY TERMS

ABO	main blood grouping system
AP	anterior/posterior (x-ray)
BUN	blood urea nitrogen
CBC	complete blood count
C&S	culture and sensitivity
diff, dif	differential white blood cell count
ESR	erythrocyte sedimentation rate; sed rate
FBS	fasting blood sugar
GTT	glucose tolerance test
H&H	hemoglobin and hematocrit
hct	hematocrit
hgb	hemoglobin
HCG	human chorionic gonadotropin
HDL	high-density lipoprotein
GTT	glucose tolerance test
lat	lateral (x-ray)

LDL	low-density lipoprotein
O&P	ova and parasites
obl	oblique (x-ray)
Pap	Pap smear
pH	degree of acidity or alkalinity
PKU	phenylketonuria
QNS	quantity not sufficient
RBC	red blood cell
UA	urinalysis
WBC	white blood cell

E. MEASURES

C	centigrade
cc	cubic centimeter
cm	centimeter
dr	dram
F	Fahrenheit
g, gm	gram
gr	grain
gtt(s)	drop(s)
kg	kilogram
L	liter
lb, #	pound
mcg, μ	microgram
mg	milligram
mL	milliliter
mn	minum
oz	ounce
pt	pint
qt	quart
tbsp, T	tablespoon
tsp, t	teaspoon
U	unit

F. COMPOUNDS AND CHEMICALS

Ba	barium
Ca	calcium
Cl	chloride
CO_2	carbon dioxide
Fe	iron
H	hydrogen
H_2O	water
Hg	mercury
K	potassium
KOH	potassium hydrochloride
Na	sodium
NaCl	sodium chloride
O_2	oxygen

G. SYMBOLS

♂	male
♀	female
>	greater than
<	less than
↑	increase, above
↓	decrease, below
×	times (multiply by)

%	percent	⊕	positive
=	equal	⊖	negative
+	plus	♀	standing
−	minus		sitting
:	ratio		lying down
::	proportion	Δ	change

2 | Anatomy and Physiology

I. Introduction to the Body

A. GENERAL
1. Anatomy: the study of body structures
2. Physiology: the study of body functions

B. LEVELS OF ORGANIZATION (ARRANGED FROM SMALLEST TO LARGEST)
1. Chemical: includes atoms and molecules
2. Cell: basic unit of all life
3. Tissue: group of cells with similar structure and function
4. Organ: group of tissues that work together to perform a function
5. System: group of organs working together to accomplish a set of functions
6. Organism: made up of systems that work together to maintain life

C. ORGAN SYSTEMS (EACH WITH A SPECIFIC FUNCTION, YET ALL SYSTEMS WORKING TOGETHER)
1. Integumentary system
   a. Made up of skin and accessory organs
   b. Provides protection, temperature regulation, chemical synthesis, water balance, and sensory reception
2. Skeletal system
   a. Made up of bones, joints, tendons, and ligaments
   b. Provides protection, provides a framework for the body, assists with movement, stores minerals, hemopoiesis
3. Muscular system
   a. Made up of muscles
   b. Provides movement, body heat, and storage of energy
4. Nervous system
   a. Made up of brain, spinal cord, and nerves
   b. Coordinates all body activities and detects changes in the outside environment
5. Endocrine system
   a. Made up of glands that secrete chemical messengers (hormones)
   b. Coordinates and balances body activities and regulates reproductive systems
6. Cardiovascular system
   a. Made up of heart and blood vessels
   b. Transports substances to the tissues and removes waste products from tissues
7. Lymphatic system
   a. Made up of lymph, lymph vessels, lymph nodes, and lymphoid organs
   b. Removes excess fluid and helps protect the body against disease
8. Digestive system
   a. Made up of mouth, esophagus, stomach, intestines, rectum, liver, gallbladder, and pancreas
   b. Takes in food and processes it into molecules that can be used by the body; eliminates solid waste products
9. Urinary system
   a. Made up of kidneys, ureters, bladder, and urethra
   b. Removes liquid nitrogenous waste products and helps regulate water balance
10. Respiratory system
    a. Made up of nose, pharynx, larynx, trachea, bronchi, and lungs
    b. Brings oxygen (O_2) into the lungs and removes carbon dioxide (CO_2) from the body
11. Reproductive system
    a. Made up of gonads (ovaries and testes), duct systems, accessory glands, and support structures
    b. Produces new individuals

D. LIFE PROCESSES
1. Characteristics that distinguish a living organism from a nonliving organism

2. Organization: each part has a function and cooperates with all other parts
3. Metabolism: all chemical reactions in the body
4. Responsiveness: ability to detect changes in the internal and external environment and respond to them
5. Movement: all activities accomplished by the muscular system
6. Reproduction: formation of new cells; formation of a new individual
7. Growth: increase in size by an increase in the number of cells
8. Respiration: exchange of O_2 and CO_2
9. Digestion: ability to break down complex foodstuffs into simpler molecules that the body can use
10. Excretion: process of removing waste products from the body
11. Maintaining boundaries: keeping the inside environment separate from the outside

E. SURVIVAL NEEDS
1. Requirements of an organism to sustain life
2. Physical factors that come from the environment
3. Water
   a. Probably more necessary than food
   b. Provides a medium for all chemical reactions
   c. Provides a fluid base for body secretions and excretions
   d. Makes up approximately 60% of body weight
4. Oxygen: necessary for metabolic reactions
5. Nutrients
   a. Taken in from diet
   b. Provide raw materials necessary for growth, replacement, and repair
   c. Provide energy for body processes
6. Temperature
   a. Necessary for chemical reactions to occur
   b. Optimum is 98.6° F
7. Pressure
   a. Application of a force
   b. Necessary for breathing and blood pressure

F. HOMEOSTASIS
1. Body's ability to maintain a constant internal environment, regardless of the external environment
2. When the body is healthy, the internal environment remains stable within limited normal ranges
3. Lack of homeostasis can lead to disease and eventually death

G. ANATOMICAL TERMS
1. Universal language
2. Used to describe directions and regions of the body
3. Anatomical position
   a. Beginning position for point of reference
   b. Body is standing erect, face forward, arms at sides with palms facing forward, and toes pointing forward

4. Directions in the body (see Figure 2-1)
   a. Superior: part above another part; toward the head
   b. Inferior: part below another part; toward the feet
   c. Anterior (ventral): toward the front
   d. Posterior (dorsal): toward the back
   e. Medial: toward or near the midline of the body
   f. Lateral: toward or near the side of the body; away from the midline
   g. Proximal: closer to the point of attachment
   h. Distal: farther away from the point of attachment
   i. Superficial: on or near the surface
   j. Deep: away from the surface
5. Planes and sections of the body (see Figure 2-1)
   a. Used to visualize spatial relationships of body parts
   b. Sagittal plane: divides the body into left and right parts
   c. Midsagittal plane: divides the body into equal right and left halves
   d. Transverse plane: divides the body into upper and lower parts; cross-section
   e. Frontal (coronal) plane: divides the body into front and back parts
6. Body cavities (see Figure 2-2): hollow body spaces that contain internal organs
   a. Dorsal cavity: made up of two cavities along the back of the body:
      1) Cranial cavity: contains the brain
      2) Spinal cavity: contains the spinal cord
   b. Ventral cavity: made up of two cavities along the front of the body:
      1) Thoracic cavity: contains heart, lungs, esophagus, and trachea
      2) Abdominopelvic cavity: contains organs below the diaphragm
   c. Diaphragm: separates the thoracic and abdominopelvic cavities
7. Abdominal regions (see Figure 2-3, p. 40): two methods used to describe locations of body organs or pain
   a. Quadrants: divides abdomen into four regions
      1) Right upper quadrant (RUQ)
      2) Left upper quadrant (LUQ)
      3) Right lower quadrant (RLQ)
      4) Left lower quadrant (LLQ)
   b. Nine regions: more specific
      1) Epigastric
      2) Umbilical
      3) Hypogastric
      4,5) Right and left hypochondriac
      6,7) Right and left lumbar
      8,9) Right and left iliac
8. Body areas
   a. Abdominal: portion of trunk below diaphragm; between thorax and pelvis
   b. Antebrachial: forearm; region between elbow and wrist
   c. Antecubital: space in front of elbow

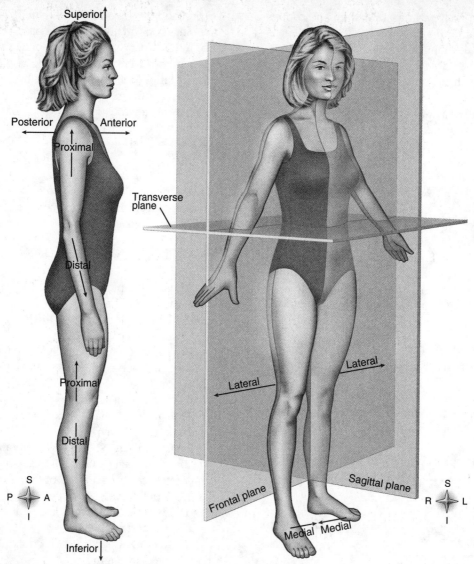

FIGURE 2-1.   Directions and planes of the body. (Barbara Cousins, from Thibodeau GA, Patton KT: *The human body in health and disease,* ed 4, St. Louis, 2005, Mosby.)

d. Axillary: armpit area
e. Brachial: arm; region between elbow and shoulder
f. Buccal: cheek area
g. Carpal: wrist area
h. Celiac: abdomen
i. Cephalic: head
j. Cervical: neck area; cervix
k. Costal: ribs
l. Cranial: skull
m. Cutaneous: skin
n. Femoral: thigh area; region between the hip and knee
o. Frontal: forehead
p. Gluteal: buttock area
q. Inguinal: groin
r. Lumbar: lower back area between ribs and pelvis
s. Mammary: breast
t. Occipital: lower portion of back of head

u. Ophthalmic: eyes
v. Oral: mouth
w. Otic: ears
x. Palmar: palm of the hand
y. Pectoral: chest area
z. Pedal: foot
aa. Pelvic: inferior region of abdominal cavity
bb. Perineal: region between the anus and pubic symphysis; includes region of external reproductive organs
cc. Plantar: sole of the foot
dd. Popliteal: area behind the knee
ee. Sacral: posterior region between hipbones
ff. Sternal: anterior midline of thorax
gg. Tarsal: ankle area
hh. Thoracic: chest
ii. Umbilical: navel
jj. Vertebral: backbone

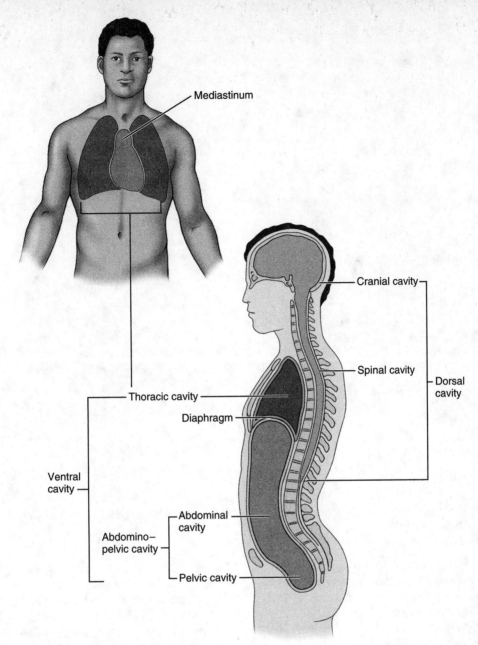

FIGURE 2-2. Major body cavities. (Herlihy B, Maebius N: *The human body in health and illness,* ed 2, Philadelphia, 2003, Saunders.)

II.   Cell

A. GENERAL
1. Basic structural and functional unit of the body
2. Vary in size, shape, and function
3. Very well organized in structure

B. STRUCTURE (see Figure 2-4)
1. Cell membrane
   a. Thin, flexible, outermost barrier of the cell
   b. Made up of a double layer of phospholipids
   c. Allows water and chemicals to pass in and out
   d. Permeable and selective

2. Cytoplasm
   a. Cytosol
   b. Thick, semisolid substance that contains mostly water
   c. Site of cellular activity
   d. Holds organelles in place
3. Nuclear membrane: encloses the nucleus
4. Nucleus
   a. Control center of the cell
   b. Contains genetic material (deoxyribonucleic acid [DNA])
5. Nucleolus
   a. Small, dense structure located in the nucleus
   b. Important in the synthesis of ribosomes

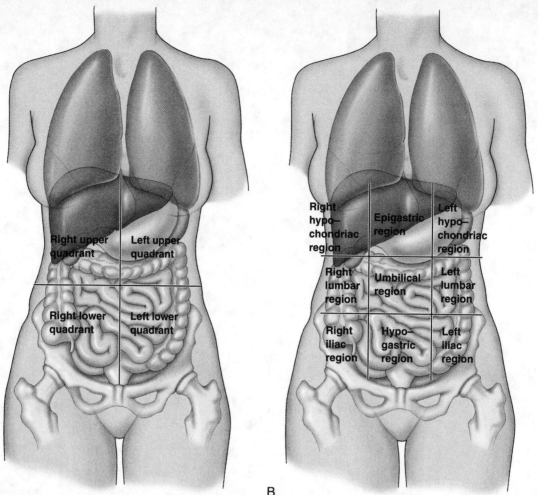

FIGURE 2-3. Areas of the abdomen. **A,** Four quadrants. **B,** Nine regions. (Herlihy B, Maebius N: *The human body in health and illness,* ed 2, Philadelphia, 2003, Saunders.)

6. Centrioles
   a. Hollow, rod-shaped structures found in the cyto-plasm near the nucleus
   b. Play an important role in cell division
7. Endoplasmic reticulum
   a. Complex network of tubular channels
   b. *"Transportation system"* of the cell
   c. Allows molecules to move from one part of the cell to the other
   d. Two types
      1) Rough: ribosomes attached; transports proteins
      2) Smooth: without ribosomes; manufactures lipids and hormones
8. Golgi apparatus
   a. Stack of flattened sacs
   b. Located near the nucleus
   c. Processes and packages proteins
9. Lysosomes
   a. Sacs of various sizes and shapes
   b. Contain strong chemicals that digest various substances that enter the cytoplasm
10. Mitochondria
   a. Sausage-shaped sacs

   b. Inner layer arranged in folds
   c. *"Powerhouse"* of the cell
   d. Source of energy for cells and tissues
11. Microtubules
   a. Extremely small, hollow tubes
   b. Crisscross cytoplasm to form a "skeleton"
   c. Give cells strength and shape
12. Peroxisomes
   a. Membranous sacs that resemble lysosomes
   b. Contain enzymes that detoxify harmful sub-stances
13. Ribosomes
   a. Composed of ribonucleic acid (RNA) and protein
   b. Form amino acids into new protein molecules
   c. Some are free floating in the cytoplasm; some are attached to endoplasmic reticulum
14. Vacuoles
   a. Membrane-bound sacs that appear in the cyto-plasm when the cell membrane folds inward on itself
   b. Contain fluid or solid substances
   c. Lysosomes can empty their enzymes into the sac
   d. Aid in metabolic activity of the cell

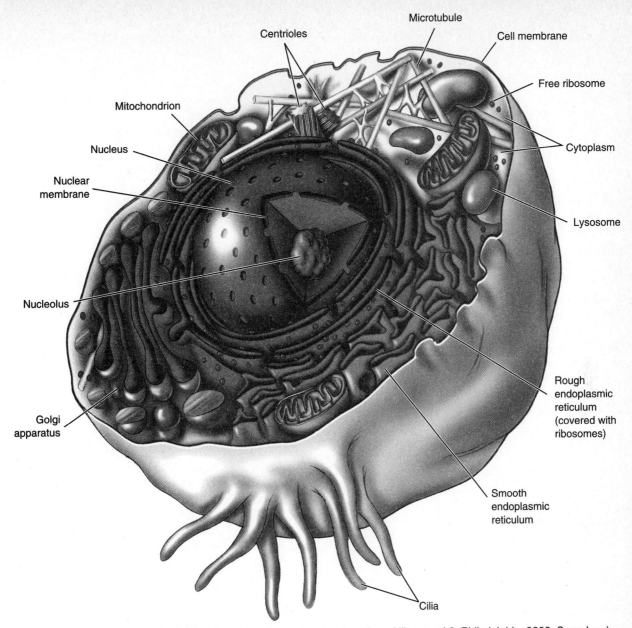

FIGURE 2-4. A typical cell. (Herlihy B, Maebius N: *The human body in health and illness,* ed 2, Philadelphia, 2003, Saunders.)

15. Microvilli
    a. Tiny fingerlike extensions that project from the surface of certain cells
    b. Increase absorptive surface of cell
16. Cilia
    a. Hairlike projections on the surface of the cell
    b. Move substances along the cell surface
17. Flagella
    a. Hairlike projection from surface of the cell
    b. Provides movement

C. TYPES OF MOVEMENT ACROSS THE CELL MEMBRANE
1. Ability of the cell to carry out its function depends on movement or exchange of fluids, particles, and molecules

2. Movement controlled and facilitated by cell membrane
   a. Diffusion
      1) Movement of solids from an area of higher concentration to an area of lower concentration
      2) Does not require cellular energy
   b. Filtration
      1) Movement of a fluid by hydrostatic pressure
      2) Does not require cellular energy
   c. Osmosis
      1) Movement of water from an area of higher concentration to an area of lower concentration
      2) Does not require cellular energy

d. Phagocytosis
  1) *"Cell eating"*; cell engulfs particles
  2) Requires cellular energy
e. Pinocytosis
  1) *"Cell drinking"*; cell engulfs fluid
  2) Requires cellular energy
f. Active transport
  1) Movement of substances from an area of lower concentration to an area of higher concentration
  2) Requires cellular energy

D. CELL DIVISION
1. Mitosis
2. Results in two identical daughter cells
3. Consists of two separate operations:
   a. Division of the nucleus (karyokinesis)
   b. Division of cytoplasm (cytokinesis)
4. Entire process has several phases:
   a. Interphase: chromosomes double
   b. Prophase: centrioles move to opposite ends of the cell, trailing a thin, threadlike substance that forms a structure resembling a spindle
   c. Metaphase: chromosomes line up across the spindles and begin to move toward the opposite ends of the cell
   d. Telophase: nuclear area becomes pinched in the middle until two regions have formed; similar change happens in the cell membrane; the cell eventually splits in two
5. Meiosis: division of gametes producing half the number of chromosomes (23) as in mitosis when fertilization occurs; nuclei of sperm and egg come together to produce a zygote with full number of chromosomes (46)

III. Tissues and Membranes

A. GENERAL
1. Group of cells similar in structure and function
2. Organized into four general types

B. TYPES OF TISSUES
1. Connective tissue
   a. Variety of forms throughout the body
   b. Serves as a framework for other tissues
   c. Combines to form more complex tissues (organs)
   d. Provides support and protection
   e. Serves as storage sites
   f. Fills in spaces between body structures
   g. Types include:
      1) Loose (areolar)
         a) Attaches skin to underlying tissues
         b) Surrounds blood and lymph vessels
         c) Fills spaces around muscles and other organs
      2) Dense
         a) Provides great strength
         b) Makes up tendons and ligaments
      3) Elastic: capable of stretching
      4) Adipose
         a) Stores fat
         b) Serves to insulate body and as an energy reserve
      5) Reticular: associated with the formation of blood
      6) Cartilage
         a) Rigid connective tissue
         b) Forms sliding surface for joints
         c) Contains no blood vessels
         d) Three types:
            ■ Hyaline cartilage
            ■ Elastic cartilage
            ■ Fibrocartilage
      7) Bone (osseous)
         a) Compact and rigid
         b) Calcium deposits in fibers give it hardness and strength
2. Epithelial tissue
   a. Epithelium
   b. Provides covering and lining for surfaces
   c. Classified according to number of cells, arrangement of cells, location of tissue, and shape of cells at the surface of the tissue
3. Muscle tissue
   a. Makes up muscles
   b. Has ability to contract (shorten)
   c. Basis of and provides for movement
   d. Three kinds:
      1) Skeletal muscle tissue
         a) Attaches to bone and produces movement
         b) Voluntary (under conscious control)
      2) Smooth muscle
         a) Found in internal organs
         b) Involuntary (not under conscious control)
      3) Cardiac muscle tissue
         a) Found in the heart
         b) Complex network of cells
         c) Involuntary
4. Nervous tissue
   a. Composed of cells that can respond to surroundings
   b. Cells called neurons: supported and nourished by neuroglial cells
   c. Regulates all activities and functions of the body

C. MEMBRANES (see Figure 2-5)
1. Thin sheet of tissue
2. Can cover a surface, serve as a partition, line organs and cavities, or anchor an organ
   a. Serous membrane
      1) Serosa
      2) Lines walls of body cavities that do not open to the outside
      3) Has two layers:
         a) Parietal layer: layer attached to the wall of the cavity or sac

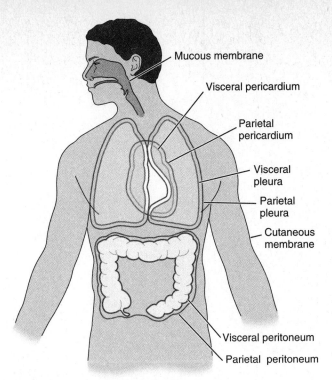

FIGURE 2-5. Epithelial membranes: cutaneous membrane (skin), mucous membranes, and serous membranes (pleura, pericardium, and peritoneum). (Herlihy B, Maebius N: *The human body in health and illness,* ed 2, Philadelphia, 2003, Saunders.)

Mucous membrane
Visceral pericardium
Parietal pericardium
Visceral pleura
Parietal pleura
Cutaneous membrane
Visceral peritoneum
Parietal peritoneum

    b) Visceral layer: layer attached to the internal organ
   4) Three main serous membranes
    a) Pleura: lines thoracic cavity and covers the lungs
    b) Pericardium: sac that encloses the heart
    c) Peritoneum: largest serous membrane; lines the wall of the abdominal cavity and covers the abdominal organs
  b. Mucous membrane
   1) Mucosa
   2) Lines the walls of body cavities that open to the outside
   3) Produces a thick, sticky substance (mucus)
  c. Cutaneous membrane: the skin
  d. Synovial membrane
   1) Lines joint cavities
   2) Secretes a lubricating fluid that reduces friction

IV. Integumentary System

A. GENERAL
  1. Considered to be the largest system and organ of the body
  2. Made up of skin and its appendages (hair, glands, nails)
  3. Forms outer boundary of the body

B. FUNCTIONS
  1. Protection from radiation, water loss, drying, and invasion of microorganisms
  2. Control of body temperature

  3. Detection of sensation
  4. Secretion of waste products
  5. Production of vitamin D

C. STRUCTURE (see Figure 2-6)
  1. Two main layers:
   a. Epidermis
    1) Outer layer
    2) Made up of four to five sublayers (strata)
    3) Innermost layer continuously supplies cells that move up to the next strata
    4) Cells continue to pick up keratin as they pass through the strata
    5) Outermost layer contains lifeless, keratin-filled cells that continually slough off
    6) Contains melanocytes that produce pigment (melanin), which gives skin color
    7) Contains no blood supply
   b. Dermis
    1) Corium; *"true skin"*
    2) Innermost layer
    3) Contains nerve and blood supply
    4) Also contains appendages of the skin
    5) Provides strength to the skin
    6) Stores water and electrolytes
  2. Appendages: special structures that perform a variety of functions
   a. Sudoriferous glands
    1) Sweat glands
    2) Coiled, tubelike structures in the dermis
    3) Produce and transport sweat to the skin surface
    4) Sweat then evaporates and cools the body
   b. Ceruminous glands
    1) Modified sweat glands found in the ear
    2) Secrete cerumen (earwax)
   c. Sebaceous glands
    1) Oil glands
    2) Connected to hair follicle
    3) Secrete sebum that oils the hair and lubricates the skin
   d. Hair
    1) Covers most of the body
    2) Made up of dead, keratinized tissue
    3) Connected to small muscles (erector pili)
   e. Nails
    1) Hard, keratinized structures found on the fingertips and tips of toes
    2) Protective function
  3. Subcutaneous tissue
   a. Layer of tissue below the dermis
   b. Connects dermis to the surface of muscles
   c. Made up of adipose tissue, elastic fibers, and fibers
   d. Injection site

D. DISEASES AND DISORDERS
  1. Abrasion: scrape
  2. Abscess: localized collection of pus within a circumscribed area; associated with tissue destruction

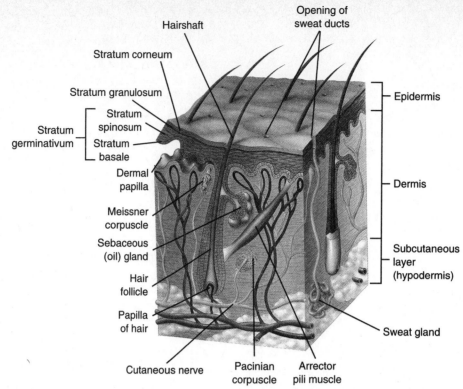

FIGURE 2-6. Normal skin. (Rolin Graphics, from Thibodeau GA, Patton KT: *Structure and function of the body,* ed 12, St.Louis, 2004, Mosby.)

3. Acne vulgaris: inflammation of a sebaceous gland; characterized by papules, pustules, and comedos
4. Actinic keratosis: premalignant lesion of the skin caused by excess exposure to sunlight
5. Albinism: whiteness of skin caused by lack of melanin
6. Alopecia: baldness
7. Avulsion: torn-away tissue
8. Bulla: large vesicle
9. Burn: tissue injury resulting from thermal, chemical, electrical, or radioactive agents
   a. First degree: superficial involvement of epidermis; characterized by erythema, tenderness, and pain
   b. Second degree: involves epidermis and dermis; characterized by vesicles
   c. Third degree: involves epidermis, dermis, and injury to underlying tissues; characterized by charring, tissue damage, and loss of fluid
   d. Rule of Nines: method of determining percentage of body surface area affected:
      1) Head and neck = 9%
      2) Torso = 36%
      3) Arms = 18%
      4) Legs = 36%
      5) Genitals = 1%
10. Callus: thickened area of epidermis caused by pressure or friction

11. Carcinoma: skin cancer: caused by exposure to ultraviolet (UV) rays and radiation; types include:
    a. Basal cell: malignant tumor of the basal cell layer of epidermis
    b. Squamous cell: malignant tumor of the squamous epithelial cells of the epidermis
    c. Malignant melanoma: cancerous growth of melanocytes
12. Cellulitis: infection of connective tissue with severe inflammation within the skin layers
13. Comedo (pl. *comedos*): papule having a small, dark central region (blackhead) or pale region (whitehead)
14. Cyanosis: blue coloration of the skin due to lack of O_2
15. Cyst: raised or flat fluid-filled or solid-filled sac
16. Decubitus ulcer: bedsore; open lesion caused by poor or no circulation to the area resulting from pressure against the tissue
17. Dermatitis: inflammation of the skin; characterized by pruritus, various lesions, and erythema
    a. Seborrheic dermatitis: chronic dermatitis; caused by an increase in sebaceous secretions; characterized by greasy scales, pruritus, dandruff
    b. Atopic dermatitis: inflammation with rash
    c. Eczema: dry, leathery vesicles in adults; characteristic pattern on face, neck, elbows, and knees

d. Contact dermatitis: inflammation caused by irritant

18. Dermatophytosis: superficial fungal infection; caused by *Tinea* species: lesions are round, scaly, and/or ring-shaped
    a. *Tinea corporis:* ringworm; involves exposed skin
    b. *Tinea unguium:* involves toenail
    c. *Tinea pedis:* athlete's foot
    d. *Tinea cruris:* jock itch
19. Ecchymosis: purplish area caused by bleeding within the skin; a bruise
20. Eczema: an acute or chronic skin inflammation characterized by redness, scales, crusts, and itching
21. Erythema: redness caused by local inflammation or irritation
22. Excoriation: scratch
23. Fissure: crack, groove, or crevice
24. Furuncle: boil
25. Hematoma: bruise; caused by collection of blood under the tissue from a blood vessel injury
26. Herpes simplex: cold sore or fever blister; small painful vesicles that erupt around the mouth, lips, nose, or mucous membranes; caused by herpes simplex virus type I
27. Herpes zoster: shingles; acute inflammatory eruption of painful vesicles along the course of a peripheral nerve; caused by herpes zoster virus
28. Hirsutism: excessive hairiness
29. Impetigo: infectious bacterial infection caused by staphylococci or streptococci; vesicles dry to form crusts especially around the mouth and nose
30. Jaundice: yellowing of the skin; can be caused by liver, blood, or gallbladder disorders
31. Keloid: abnormal scar formation
32. Lesion: any injury, wound, or area of disease
33. Macule: flat lesion (freckle)
34. Nevus: mole
35. Nodule: raised lesion made of a solid tissue mass
36. Papule: firm, raised lesion (pimple)
37. Pediculosis: infestation by lice (genus: *Pediculus*)
    a. *Pediculosis capitas:* head lice
    b. *Pediculosis corporis:* body lice
    c. *Pediculosis palpebrarum:* infestation of eyebrows and lashes
    d. *Pediculosis pubis:* "crabs" (genital lice)
38. Polyp: cyst on a stalk
39. Pruritus: itching
40. Psoriasis: chronic disease characterized by red lesions and silvery scales; may be autoimmune
41. Pustule: pus-filled vesicle
42. Rosacea: chronic condition of unknown cause that produces redness, tiny pimples and broken blood vessels
43. Scleroderma: thick, dense, fibrous skin
44. Sebaceous cyst: cyst of a sebaceous gland containing yellow, fatty material

45. Skin tags: small, flesh-colored or light brown growths that hang from the body by fine stalks
46. Ulcer: open sore
47. Urticaria: hives; usually caused by allergic reaction
48. Verruca (verrucae): warts; caused by papilloma virus
49. Vesicle: fluid-filled lesion (blister)
50. Vitiligo: white patches on skin caused by lack of melanin production
51. Wheal: circular, raised lesion having central pallor and circumscribed redness

V. Skeletal System

A. GENERAL (see Figure 2-7)
1. Composed of bones, cartilage, and ligaments
2. Adult skeleton composed of 206 bones

B. FUNCTIONS
1. Provides a framework for the body: shape and support for other structures

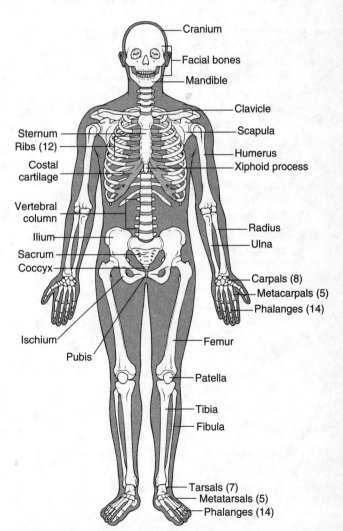

FIGURE 2-7. Normal skeletal system (anterior view). (Frazier MS, Drzymkowski JW: *Essentials of human diseases and conditions,* ed 3, Philadelphia, 2004, Saunders.)

2. Provides for movement: places for muscles to attach
3. Provides protection: surrounds body cavities
4. Provides hematopoiesis: blood cell formation in marrow
5. Provides storage: inorganic minerals (calcium [Ca], phosphorus [P], magnesium [Mg], potassium [K], sodium [Na]) stored in matrix and released into circulation as needed

C. ANATOMY OF LONG BONE

1. Diaphysis: shaft of the long bone; made up of compact and cancellous bone
2. Epiphysis: ends of the long bone
3. Epiphyseal cartilage (plate): *"growth plate"*; layer of cartilage between the diaphysis and epiphysis where the growth in length occurs
4. Articular cartilage: thin sheet of cartilage that covers the end of the epiphysis; provides a cushion and lubrication for joint
5. Periosteum: tough, vascular covering of the bone; made up of fibrous connective tissue; does not cover the epiphysis
6. Endosteum: lining of the medullary cavity
7. Medullary cavity: cavity in the center of long bones; contains marrow
   a. Red marrow: produces red blood cells
   b. Yellow marrow: made up of fat
8. Process: bony projection on the surface of a bone
9. Foramen: an opening in a bone
10. Sinus: bony cavity in a bone

D. BONE CLASSIFICATIONS

1. Long: length exceeds width
2. Short: smaller than long bone with expanded ends
3. Flat: thin, sheetlike
4. Sesamoid: rounded bones embedded in tendons; round bones
5. Irregular: various shapes

E. ORGANIZATION OF THE SKELETON

1. Axial skeleton: consists of bones of the skull, spine, and chest (see Figure 2-8)
   a. Cranium: bones enclose the brain
      1) Frontal: forms forehead
      2) Parietal: forms sides and top
      3) Temporal: forms lower sides and floor; contains ossicles (bones of middle ear): malleus, incus, and stapes; external auditory meatus (opening into middle ear)
      4) Mastoid process: projection located on temporal bone
      5) Styloid process: sharp projection inferior to external auditory meatus
      6) Zygomatic process: projects anteriorly to form prominence of cheek
      7) Occipital: single bone forming the posterior of cranium; contains foramen magnum where spinal cord exits skull

      8) Sphenoid: butterfly-shaped bone that bridges the temporal regions to form the floor of the cranium; contains sella turcica where the pituitary gland sits
      9) Ethmoid: single bone that forms most of bony area between the nasal cavity and orbits
   b. Facial: forms the basic framework for the face
      1) Nasal: two bones forming the bridge of the nose
      2) Vomer: thin bone that forms the inferior nasal septum
      3) Lacrimal: located in the medial walls of the orbits; contains the lacrimal glands
      4) Zygomatic: forms the arch of the cheekbone
      5) Palatine: forms the posterior of the hard palate
      6) Mandible: lower jawbone (only movable bone in the face)
      7) Hyoid: U-shaped bone that supports the tongue; only bone that does not articulate with another
   c. Spinal column: composed of 26 vertebrae separated by pads of cartilage (intervertebral disks); houses the spinal cord; four distinct curves; common structural pattern (see Figure 2-9)
      1) Cervical vertebrae: first seven, C-1 through C-7; forms the neck
         a) C-1: atlas; supports the skull
         b) C-2: axis; allows for rotation of skull
      2) Thoracic vertebrae: next 12, T-1 through T-12; articulate with the ribs
      3) Lumbar vertebrae: next five, L-1 through L-5; forms the small of the back
      4) Sacrum: triangular-shaped bone; forms the posterior wall of the pelvic cavity
      5) Coccyx: tailbone
   d. Thorax: thoracic cage; protects heart, lungs, and great vessels (see Figure 2-10, p. 49)
      1) Sternum: breastbone; three parts:
         a) Manubrium: superior, triangular part
         b) Body: middle, slender part
         c) Xiphoid process: projection at end of body; landmark for cardiopulmonary resuscitation (CPR)
      2) Ribs
         a) Curved, flat bones that form the lateral sides of thorax
         b) 12 pairs
            ■ True ribs; first seven pairs; articulate with the sternum by means of costal cartilage
            ■ False ribs: next three pairs; articulate with the seventh rib by means of costal cartilage
            ■ Floating ribs: last two pairs; do not articulate with the sternum
2. Appendicular skeleton: made up of bones of upper and lower extremities and girdles that are anchored to the axial skeleton (see Figure 2-11, p. 50)
   a. Shoulder girdle

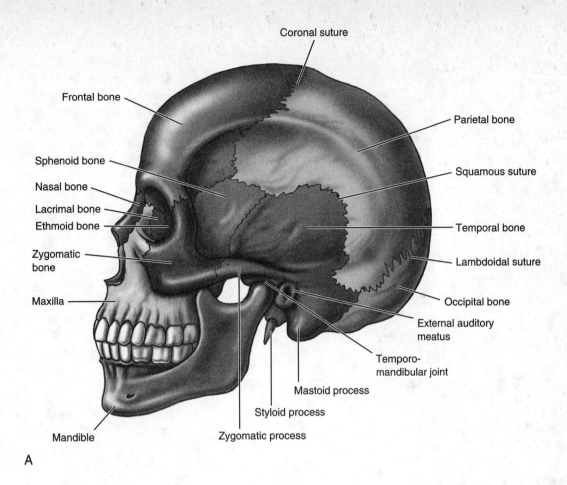

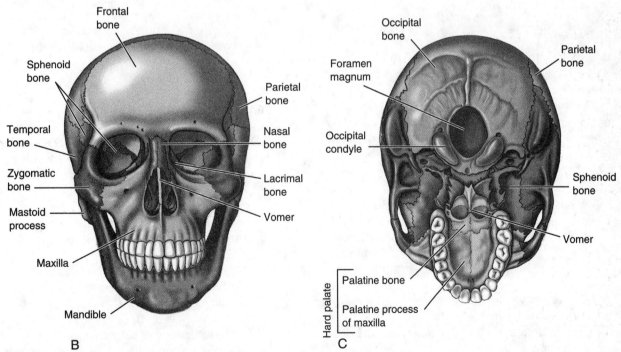

FIGURE 2-8. Bones of the skull. **A,** Side view. **B,** Front view. **C,** Base of the skull. (Herlihy B, Maebius N: *The human body in health and illness,* ed 2, Philadelphia, 2003, Saunders.)

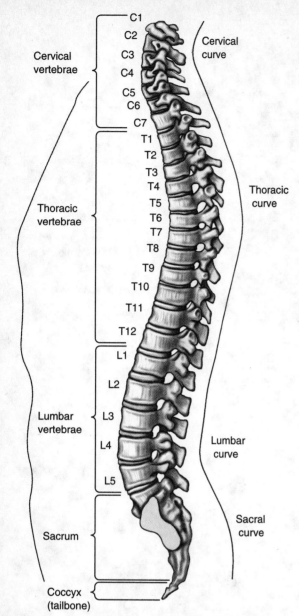

Cervical
vertebrae

C1
C2
C3
C4
C5
C6
C7

Cervical
curve

Thoracic
vertebrae

T1
T2
T3
T4
T5
T6
T7
T8
T9
T10
T11
T12

Thoracic
curve

Lumbar
vertebrae

L1
L2
L3
L4
L5

Lumbar
curve

Sacrum

Sacral
curve

Coccyx
(tailbone)

FIGURE 2-9. The vertebral column. (Herlihy B, Maebius N: *The human body in health and illness,* ed 2, Philadelphia, 2003, Saunders.)

1) Clavicle: collarbone (two); forms a bridge between shoulder blades and breastbone
2) Scapula (two): shoulder blade
3) Humerus: bone of the upper arm
4) Radius: lateral bone of the forearm (thumb side)
5) Ulna: medial bone of the forearm (little finger side)
6) Carpals: two rows of four bones tightly bound by ligaments; make up the wrist
7) Metacarpals: five bones that make up the hand
8) Phalanges
   a) Three bones in each finger (proximal, medial, and distal)
   b) Two bones in each thumb (proximal and distal)

b. Pelvic girdle: attaches lower extremities to axial skeleton (see Figure 2-12, p. 51)
   1) Pelvis: os coxae basin-shaped bones on floor of trunk; three parts:
      a) Ilium: superior, wing-shaped bones of hips
      b) Ischium: inferior portion; *"sit-down"* bone
      c) Pubis: anterior portion; right and left sides join at symphysis pubis (pad of cartilage)
   2) Femur: thighbone; largest, longest, and strongest bone in the body
   3) Patella: kneecap; triangular-shaped, enclosed in tendon
   4) Tibia: shinbone
      a) Lateral malleolus: bulge on outside of ankle
      b) Medial malleolus: bulge on inside of ankle
   5) Fibula: smaller leg bone lateral to the tibia
   6) Tarsals: seven bones that make up the ankle; largest is the calcaneous (heel bone)
   7) Metatarsals: five bones that make up the instep of the foot
   8) Phalanges: 14 bones that make up the toe
      a) Three in each toe (proximal, medial, and distal)
      b) Two in each great toe (proximal and distal)
c. Articulations: joints; where two bones come together; classified by the amount of movement allowed (see Figure 2-13, p. 52)
   1) Synarthroses: immovable joints (example: sutures in skull)
   2) Amphiarthroses: slightly movable joints; bones are connected by cartilage (example: symphysis pubis)
   3) Diarthroses: freely movable joints; ends covered with cartilage; separated by a space containing synovial fluid for lubrication (example: elbow)

F. DISEASES AND DISORDERS
1. Abnormal spinal curvatures
   a. Scoliosis: abnormal lateral curvature of the spine
   b. Kyphosis: humpback; abnormal outward curvature of the spine
   c. Lordosis: swayback; abnormal inward curvature of the spine
2. Arthritis: inflammation of the joints
   a. Osteoarthritis
      1) Chronic inflammation of joint
      2) Results in degeneration of cartilage, which causes hypertrophy of bone
   b. Rheumatoid arthritis
      1) Chronic, systemic inflammatory disease of joint
      2) Causes erosion of cartilage
   c. Ankylosing spondylitis: rheumatoid arthritis of the spine
   d. Gout: arthritis caused by deposit of uric acid in joint
3. Bursitis: inflammation of the bursa (thin sac that helps tendons and muscles move over bones)

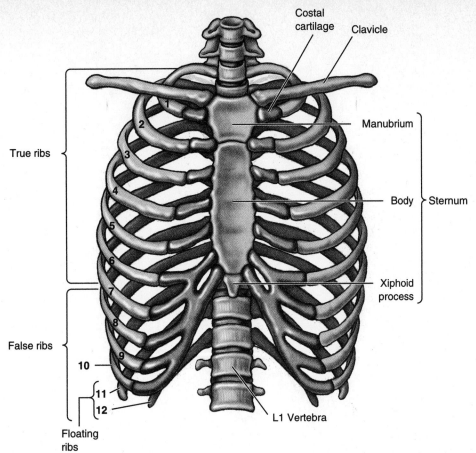

FIGURE 2-10. The thoracic cage. (Herlihy B, Maebius N: *The human body in health and illness,* ed 2, Philadelphia, 2003, Saunders.)

4. Fractures: crack or break in a bone
   a. Simple (closed): fracture with no external wound
   b. Compound (open): fracture with external break in the skin
   c. Greenstick: incomplete break
   d. Comminuted: shattering of the bone (bone fragments)
   e. Impacted: one broken end is forced into the other
5. Neoplasms
   a. Osteosarcoma: malignant tumor of connective tissue arising from the bone
   b. Osteochondroma: tumor of bone and cartilage
   c. Chondrosarcoma: tumor of cartilage
6. Osteomalacia: condition of softening of bones; caused by low level of vitamin D
7. Osteomyelitis: inflammation of bone, usually following compound fracture or symptoms
8. Osteoporosis: condition of porous, brittle bones, especially in menopausal women; caused by low levels of calcium and potassium
9. Paget's disease: osteitis deformans; chronic metabolic disease causing bones to thicken and soften
10. Spina bifida: congenital abnormality characterized by failure of vertebrae to close around the spinal cord
12. Sprain: acute partial tear of a muscle, tendon, or ligament

13. Strain: result of overuse, overstretching, or excessive forcible stretching of a muscle
14. Talipes: club foot

VI. Muscular System

A. GENERAL
1. Approximately 650 muscles in the body
2. Makes up approximately 40% of body weight

B. FUNCTIONS
1. Movement: contractions (shortening) allows movement of bone
2. Protection: sheets of muscle protect internal organs
3. Posture: provides position and alignment of body parts
4. Heat production: movement produces heat
5. Shape: muscles plus bones give the body shape

C. TYPES OF MUSCLE TISSUE (see Figure 2-14, p.53)
1. Skeletal: under conscious control (voluntary); appears striated (striped); provides movement of body
2. Smooth: involuntary muscles (operate automatically); appears nonstriated; helps with metabolic functions
3. Cardiac: found only in the heart; involuntary; causes contraction of heart muscle to maintain blood flow

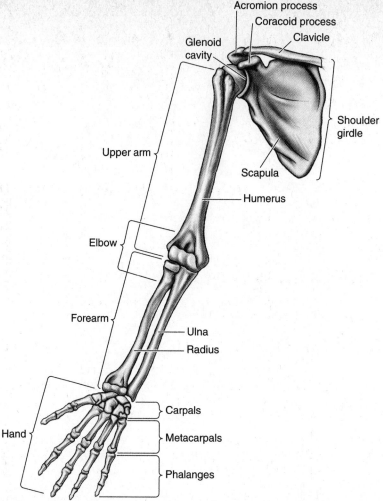

FIGURE 2-11. Bones of the upper limb. (Herlihy B, Maebius N: *The human body in health and illness*, ed 2, Philadelphia, 2003, Saunders.)

D. CHARACTERISTICS OF MUSCLE

1. Excitability: ability to receive and respond to a stimulus
2. Contractility: ability to shorten (contract)
3. Extensibility: ability to stretch
4. Elasticity: ability to return to original shape and length

E. SKELETAL MUSCLE STRUCTURE

1. Composed of bundles of fibers held together by fibrous connective tissue
   a. Fiber: skeletal muscle cell
   b. Endomysium: connective tissue membrane that covers a muscle fiber
   c. Fasciculus: bundle of muscle fibers
   d. Perimysium: connective tissue membrane that surrounds the fasciculus
   e. Epimysium: tough tissue membrane that covers the entire muscle
   f. Fascia: connective tissue outside of the epimysium; surrounds and separates the muscles
   g. Tendon: strong, cordlike structure that attaches muscles to bones
   h. Aponeurosis: sheetlike tendon that attaches muscle to muscle

F. NAMING OF MUSCLES

1. May be named according to the following:
   a. Size: maximus, medius, longus
   b. Shape: deltoid, latus
   c. Fiber direction: rectus, oblique
   d. Points of attachment:
      1) Origin: point of attachment that does not move on contraction
      2) Insertion: point of attachment that moves on contraction
   e. Number of attachments: biceps, quadriceps
   f. Action of muscle: adductor, flexor, and levator

G. MUSCLE ACTIONS

1. Prime mover: provides movement
2. Antagonist: opposes prime mover; can cause opposite movement or provide more control and precision to prime mover
3. Synergist: helps prime mover work more efficiently and effectively
4. Fixator: stabilizes the origin of the prime mover

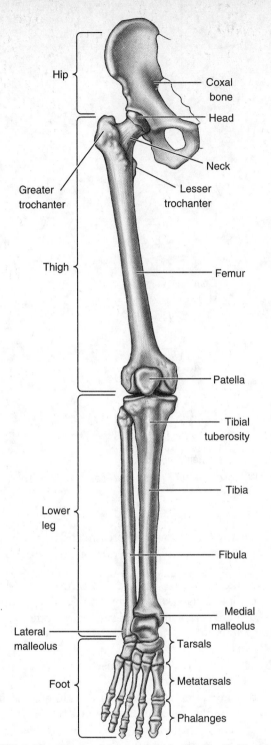

FIGURE 2-12. Bones of the lower limb. (Herlihy B, Maebius N: *The human body in health and illness,* ed 2, Philadelphia, 2003, Saunders.)

H. MOVEMENT

1. Caused by contraction (shortening) of muscle
2. Complex series of events based on chemical reactions at cellular level
3. Begins with stimulation by nerve cell and ends when the muscle is relaxed
4. Requires adenosine triphosphate (ATP) for energy source

I. TYPES OF MOVEMENTS (see Figure 2-15, p.54)

1. Flexion: to bend; brings two bones closer together and decreases the angle between them
2. Extension: to straighten; opposite of flexion; increases the angle between bones
3. Hyperextension: extension beyond the anatomical position; joint angle in excess of 180 degrees
4. Abduction: to take away; movement of a bone or limb away from the midline of the body
5. Adduction: to bring together; opposite of abduction; movement of a bone or limb toward the midline of the body
6. Circumduction: circular motion of a body part or segment; the proximal end is stationary, whereas the distal end outlines a large circle
7. Rotation: movement of a bone around its own axis
8. Inversion: turning a body part inward
9. Eversion: opposite of inversion; turning a body part outward
10. Supination: movement of a body part to face upward
11. Pronation: opposite of supination; movement of a body part to face downward

J. MAJOR SKELETAL MUSCLES

(see Figures 2-16 and 2-17, pp. 55-56)
1. Muscles of facial expression
   a. Frontalis: over the frontal bone; raises eyebrows and wrinkles forehead
   b. Orbicularis oris: circular muscle that surrounds mouth; closes mouth, forms words, puckers lips
   c. Orbicularis oculi: circular muscle that surrounds the eye; helps in winking, blinking, and squinting
   d. Buccinator: principle muscle of the cheek; helps in whistling, sucking, and blowing out air
   e. Zygomaticus: extends from the zygomatic arch to corner of mouth; raises the corners of the mouth when smiling
2. Muscles of mastication (chewing)
   a. Temporalis: largest; inserts in mandible; responsible for chewing
   b. Masseter: inserts in mandible; used for chewing
3. Neck muscles
   a. Sternocleidomastoid: runs across front of neck from the sternum to clavicle to mastoid process; flexes neck
   b. Trapezius: extends from occipital bone to end of thoracic vertebrae; extends head
4. Vertebral column muscles
   a. Erector spinae: group of muscles on each side of vertebral column from sacrum to skull; keeps vertebral column erect
   b. Quadratus lumborum (deep back muscles): short muscles between vertebrae; responsible for movement of vertebral column
5. Thoracic wall muscles
   a. Intercostal muscles (internal and external): located between ribs; helps with breathing

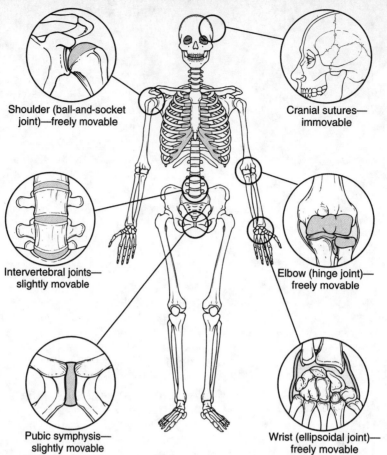

FIGURE 2-13. Examples of types of joints. (Frazier MS, Drzymkowski JW: *Essentials of human diseases and conditions*, ed 3, Philadelphia, 2004, Saunders.)

b. Diaphragm: dome-shaped muscle located between thorax and abdomen; muscle of respiration

6. Abdominal wall muscles
   a. External oblique: fibers run medially and inferiorally
   b. Internal oblique: fibers run opposite of external obliques
   c. Transversus abdominus: fibers run horizontally
   d. Rectus abdominus: fibers run vertically

7. Muscles that move the shoulder and arm
   a. Trapezius: large, triangular muscle of the back; used to shrug shoulders
   b. Serratus anterior: located on side of chest; used in pushing
   c. Pectoralis major: superficial muscle on anterior chest; adductor; moves arm medially across chest
   d. Latissimus dorsi: large superficial muscle of lower back
   e. Deltoid: large triangular muscle that covers the shoulder; used to abduct arm; injection site
   f. Rotator cuff muscles: infraspinatus, supraspinatus, subscapularis, teres minor; assists with movement of the humerus; form cuff over proximal humerus

8. Muscles that move the forearm and hand
   a. Triceps brachii: posterior of arm; extends the forearm
   b. Biceps brachii: flexes the forearm
   c. Brachialis: flexes the forearm
   d. Brachioradialis: lateral side of forearm; flexes the forearm

9. Muscles that move the thigh
   a. Gluteus maximus: forms the buttocks; extends and straightens the thigh at the hip
   b. Gluteus medius: deep to the gluteus maximus; common injection site; abducts the thigh
   c. Gluteus minimus: deepest of gluteal group; abducts the thigh
   d. Iliopsoas: anterior muscle; flexes the thigh
   e. Adductor longus: medial muscle; adducts the thigh
   f. Adductor brevis: medial muscle; adducts the thigh
   g. Adductor magnus: medial muscle; adducts the thigh
   h. Gracilis: medial muscle; adducts the thigh

10. Muscles that move the leg
    a. Quadriceps femoris: group of muscles located on anterior and lateral sides of thigh; extend the leg and straighten the leg at the knee

Cellular appearance:

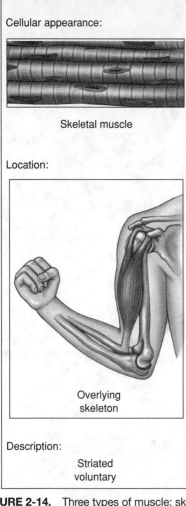

Skeletal muscle

Smooth muscle

Tight junctions

Cardiac muscle

Location:

Overlying
skeleton

Organs or
viscera (stomach)

Heart

Description:

Striated
voluntary

Nonstriated
involuntary

Striated
involuntary

FIGURE 2-14. Three types of muscle: skeletal, smooth, and cardiac. (Herlihy B, Maebius N: *The human body in health and illness,* ed 2, Philadelphia, 2003, Saunders.)

1) Vastus lateralis: injection site for infants and children; extends leg and supports knee joint
2) Vastus intermedius: extends leg
3) Vastus medialis: extends leg
4) Rectus femoris: extends leg
b. Sartorius: longest muscle in the body; runs obliquely over the quad group; flexes and medially rotates the legs (to sit cross-legged)
c. Hamstrings: posterior to the thigh; flexes the leg at the knee; strong tendons; includes:
1) Biceps femoris
2) Semitendinosus
3) Semimembranosus
11. Muscles that move the ankle and foot
a. Tibialis anterior: primary muscle of anterior group; dorsiflexion of foot
b. Peroneus longus: lateral to the leg; everts the foot
c. Gastrocnemius: posterior to leg (calf); plantar flexion ("*toe-dancer's*" muscles)
d. Soleus: posterior to the leg (calf)
e. Achilles tendon: common tendon for gastrocnemius and soleus; connects muscles to calcaneus; largest tendon in body

K. DISEASES AND DISORDERS
1. Muscular dystrophy: congenital disorder; characterized by progressive wasting of muscle tissue
2. Myasthenia gravis: chronic, progressive neuromuscular disease; may be autoimmune; characterized by muscle weakness, dysphagia, and blepharoptosis
3. Tendinitis (sometimes spelled *tendonitis*): inflammation of tendon

VII. Nervous System

A. GENERAL
1. Major controlling, regulating, and communicating system of the body
2. Works with the endocrine system to regulate and maintain homeostasis

B. FUNCTIONS
1. Control: regulates internal body functions and processes
2. Communication: directs processes among body systems
3. Mental processes: generates thoughts, feelings, perception, sensations, and emotions

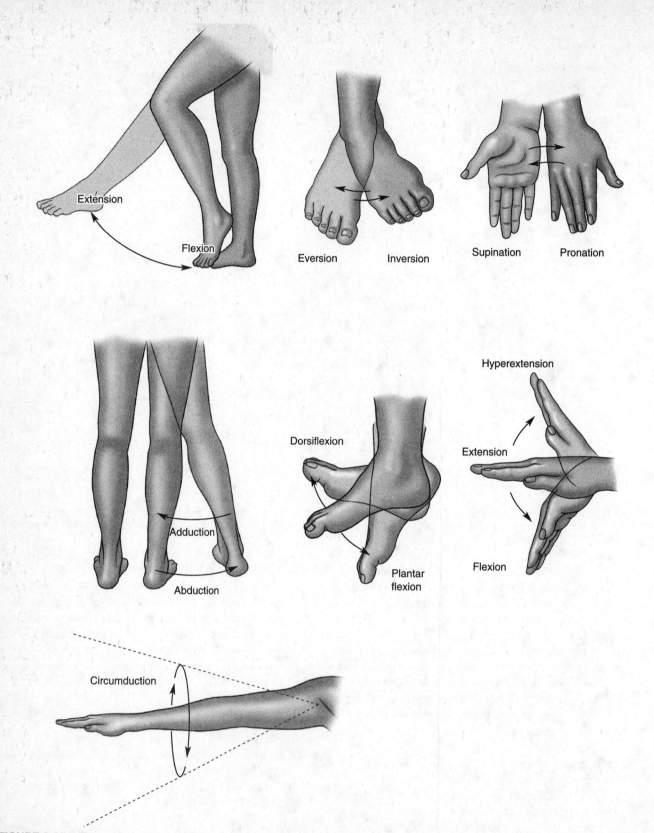

FIGURE 2-15.   Types of movements at joints. (Herlihy B, Maebius N: *The human body in health and illness,* ed 2, Philadelphia, 2003, Saunders.)

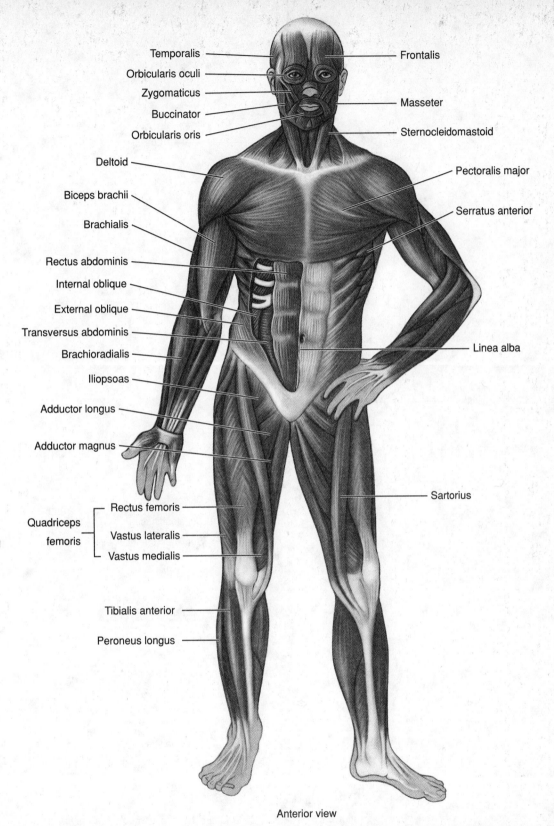

Temporalis
Orbicularis oculi
Zygomaticus
Buccinator
Orbicularis oris

Frontalis
Masseter
Sternocleidomastoid

Deltoid
Biceps brachii
Brachialis
Rectus abdominis
Internal oblique
External oblique
Transversus abdominis
Brachioradialis
Iliopsoas
Adductor longus
Adductor magnus

Pectoralis major
Serratus anterior

Linea alba

Quadriceps femoris
Rectus femoris
Vastus lateralis
Vastus medialis

Sartorius

Tibialis anterior
Peroneus longus

Anterior view

FIGURE 2-16. Major muscles of the body, anterior view. (Herlihy B, Maebius N: *The human body in health and illness,* ed 2, Philadelphia, 2003, Saunders.)

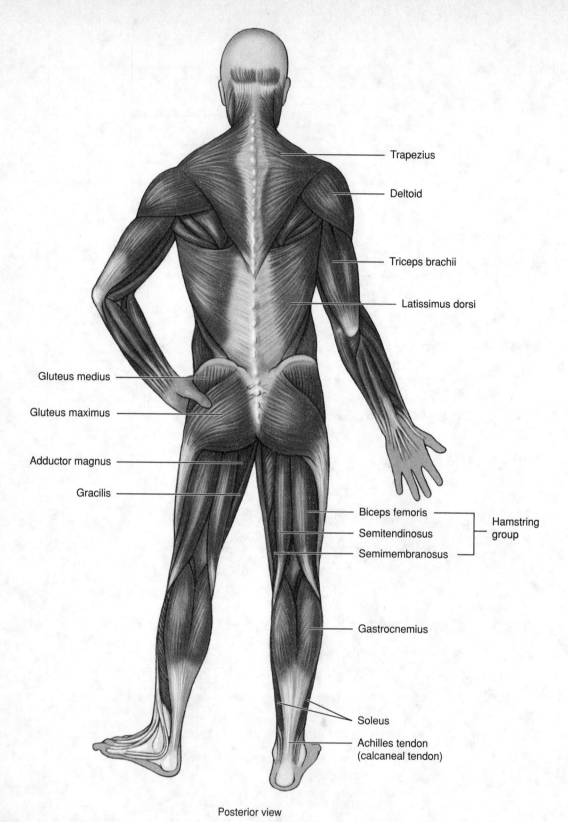

Posterior view

FIGURE 2-17. Major muscles of the body (posterior view). (Herlihy B, Maebius N: *The human body in health and illness,* ed 2, Philadelphia, 2003, Saunders.)

C. ORGANIZATION (see Figure 2-18)

1. Central nervous system (CNS): made up of brain and spinal cord
2. Peripheral nervous system (PNS): made up of nerves and ganglia; includes
   a. 12 pairs of cranial nerves originating in the brain
   b. 31 pairs of spinal nerves originating from spinal cord
   c. Afferent (sensory) division: transmits information to brain
   d. Efferent (motor) division: transmits information from brain to organs and body parts
   e. Somatic nervous system: transmits impulses to voluntary muscles
   f. Autonomic nervous system: transmits impulses to involuntary muscles and glands
   g. Sympathetic nervous system: prepares the body for stressful conditions
   h. Parasympathetic nervous system: coordinates the normal resting activities

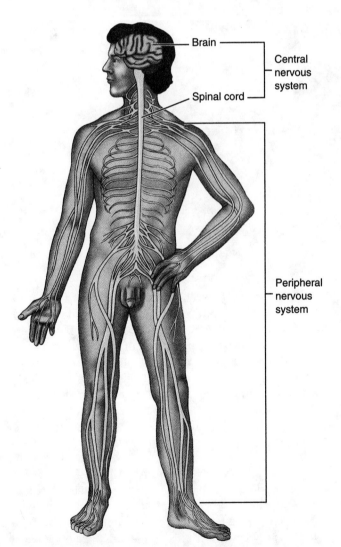

FIGURE 2-18. Divisions of the nervous system: central and peripheral. (Herlihy B, Maebius N: *The human body in health and illness*, ed 2, Philadelphia, 2003, Saunders.)

D. ORGANS OF THE NERVOUS SYSTEM (see Figure 2-19)

1. Neuron: nerve cell; structural and functional unit of nerve tissue; highly specialized; if destroyed, cannot be replaced (does not go through mitosis)
   a. Cell body: contains nucleus and organelles
   b. Dendrites: one or more branching extensions; receives signals from other neurons and brings them to the cell body
   c. Axon: single extension from the cell body; carries impulses away from the cell body
   d. Myelin sheath: white, segmented, fatty substance that surrounds axons; produced by Schwann cells that cover the axons; serves as an insulator and to speed the conduction of nerve impulses; gives white appearance to fibers (white matter)
   e. Neurilemma: outer membrane of axon
   f. Nodes of Ranvier: gaps in myelin sheath
   g. Neurotransmitter: chemical substance that allows neurons to communicate with each other
2. Neuroglia: *"nerve glue"*; nonconductive cells of nerve tissue; provides support system (nourishment and protection) for neurons; more numerous than neurons; different types with specialized functions; capable of mitosis
3. Nerves: collection of nerve fibers held together by layers of connective tissue
   a. Afferent (sensory): carry impulses from PNS to CNS
   b. Efferent (motor): carry impulses from CNS to PNS
4. Brain (see Figure 2-20)
   a. Cerebrum: largest superior portion; consists of thin layer of gray matter (cerebral cortex) and white matter (bulk of cerebrum)
      1) Cortex: makes us *"human"*; concerned with memory, language, reasoning, intelligence, personality, and other factors associated with human life
      2) Divided into two halves (hemispheres) by longitudinal fissure
         a) Right hemisphere: controls the left side of the body; responsible for auditory perception, tactile perception, and interpretation of spatial relationships
         b) Left hemisphere: controls the right side of the body; responsible for language and hand movements; hemispheres divided into five lobes
      3) Each hemisphere is divided into five lobes named for bones that cover them (except for the insula)
         a) Frontal lobe: controls voluntary muscle movements and speech
         b) Parietal lobe: receives and integrates sensory output
         c) Temporal lobe: interprets sound; involved with personality, emotion, memory, and behavior

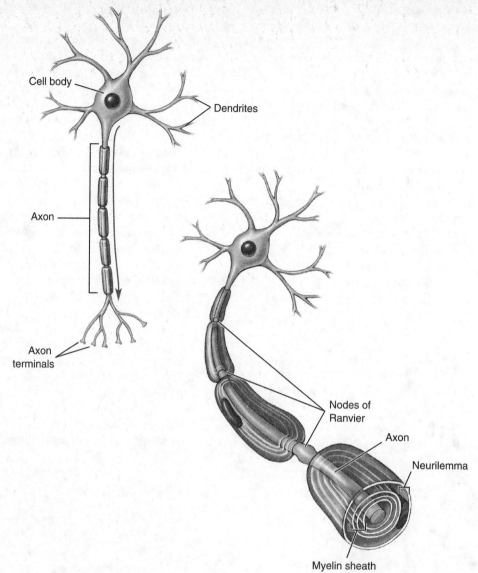

Cell body

Dendrites

Axon

Axon
terminals

Nodes of
Ranvier

Axon

Neurilemma

Myelin sheath

FIGURE 2-19. Structure of a neuron. (Herlihy B, Maebius N: *The human body in health and illness,* ed 2, Philadelphia, 2003, Saunders.)

d) Occipital lobe: interprets sight
e) Insula: visceral effects
4) Ventricles: cavities within each hemisphere that make and store cerebrospinal fluid (CSF)
b. Diencephalon: centrally located; surrounded by cerebral hemispheres
1) Thalamus: relay station for all sensory input; associated with pain, temperature, and touch sensations; located between cerebrum and midbrain
2) Hypothalamus: located below thalamus; important role in regulating heart rate, blood pressure, body temperature, water balance, hunger, sleep, and wakefulness
c. Brainstem
1) Medulla oblongata: lowest portion of brain, connects to spinal cord; contains vital centers for control of heartbeat, respiration, and blood pressure

2) Pons: bulge at the base of the brain; links the cerebellum to the rest of the nervous system; nerve fibers cross here; one side of the brain controls the other side of the body
3) Midbrain: upper portion of the brainstem; correlates information about muscle tone and posture; relay center for certain eye and ear reflexes
d. Cerebellum: second largest portion of the brain, located below the cerebrum; responsible for coordination of voluntary movement, posture, and balance
e. Spinal cord: extends from the brainstem through the foramen magnum into the vertebral column to the second lumbar vertebra; approximately 17 inches long; conducts nerve impulses to and from brain; center for spinal reflexes; 31 pairs of spinal nerves connected to cord
f. Meninges: protective membrane covering brain and spinal cord; three layers

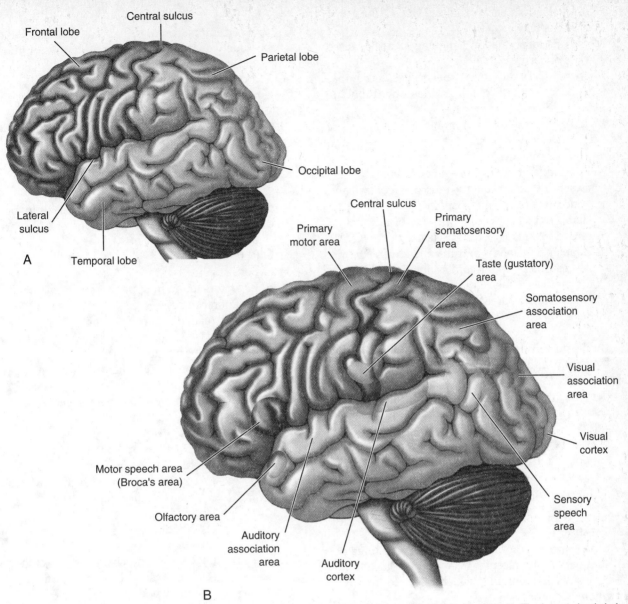

FIGURE 2-20. **A,** The lobes of the cerebrum. **B,** The functional areas of the cerebrum. (Herlihy B, Maebius N: *The human body in health and illness,* ed 2, Philadelphia, 2003, Saunders.)

1) Dura mater: strong, fibrous outer layer
2) Arachnoid: middle, delicate weblike layer that allows for movement of CSF
3) Pia mater: thin inner layer; contains blood vessels to supply the brain

g. Meningeal spaces
   1) Epidural space: located between dura mater and bone (skull or vertebra); acts as a cushion
   2) Subdural space: located between dura mater and arachnoid; contains serous fluid for lubrication
   3) Subarachnoid space: located between arachnoid and pia mater; contains CSF

h. Cerebrospinal fluid (CSF): clear, colorless, watery fluid found in subarachnoid space and in the ventricles of the brain; is constantly circulating; provides protective cushion for the brain; can detect physiologic changes in the body

E. DISEASES AND DISORDERS OF THE BRAIN

1. Alzheimer's disease: senile dementia; chronic organic brain syndrome; characterized by degeneration of nervous tissue resulting in lowered intellectual functioning and untimely death
2. Amyotrophic lateral sclerosis (ALS); also known as Lou Gehrig's disease; affects motor neurons; characterized by muscle atrophy and weakness
3. Cerebral palsy: caused by congenital brain defects or injury at birth; characterized by loss of sensation and/or control of muscle movements
4. Encephalitis: inflammation of the brain
5. Epilepsy: abnormal electrical activity of the brain; characterized by random, intense electrical discharges that result in seizure activity
6. Guillain-Barré syndrome: acute rapidly progressive disease of the spinal nerves

7. Hydrocephalus: excessive amount of CSF causing macroencephaly
8. Meningitis: inflammation of meninges; can be caused by virus or bacteria
9. Migraine: periodic severe headaches; accompanied by nausea and vomiting, auras, and throbbing pain
10. Multiple sclerosis (MS): chronic inflammation of CNS; attacks myelin sheath causing sensory and motor abnormalities
11. Neuritis: inflammation of peripheral nerves
12. Paralysis: loss of voluntary muscular control and sensation to a body part or organ
    a. Hemiplegia: paralysis of one side of body, often caused by stroke (cerebrovascular accident [CVA])
    b. Paraplegia: paralysis of trunk and lower extremities, caused by spinal cord injury; the area below the injury is paralyzed
    c. Quadriplegia: paralysis of all four extremities
    d. Bell's palsy: paralysis of muscles on one side of face
13. Parkinson's disease: chronic disease; characterized by tremors and muscle rigidity
14. Stroke: CVA; *"brain attack"*; caused by occlusion or hemorrhage of blood vessels supplying the brain; results in impairment and paralysis of the affected side
15. Transient ischemic attack (TIA): *"mini"* stroke; temporary, recurrent episodes of impaired neurological activity; caused by lack of blood flow to the brain

VIII. Special Senses

A. GENERAL
1. Variety of receptors located in various structures
2. Stimulation of a receptor by an appropriate stimulus results in an impulse, which is sent to the CNS, where it is processed
3. Allows the human to be aware of the world around him or her
4. Depends on sensory receptors classified as:
   a. General (widely distributed)
   b. Special (localized in a specific area)

B. GENERAL SENSES: SOMATIC SENSES; FOUND THROUGHOUT THE BODY (see Figure 2-21)
1. Touch and pressure
   a. Mechanoreceptor (responds to a bending, or a change in the shape of, a cell)
   b. Widely distributed in skin
   c. Includes free nerve endings, Meissner's corpuscles (touch), Pacinian corpuscles (pressure)
2. Position and orientation: proprioceptors
3. Temperature
   a. Thermoreceptor (detects change in temperature)
   b. Found immediately under the skin
   c. Ten times more cold receptors than heat receptors

4. Pain
   a. Nociceptors (responds to tissue damage)
   b. Widely distributed in skin and tissues of internal organs
   c. Protective function

C. SPECIAL SENSES: LOCATED WITHIN SPECIAL ORGANS
1. Gustatory sense
   a. Sense of taste
   b. Organs of taste (taste buds) localized on the surface of tongue
   c. Chemoreceptors (sensitive to chemicals in food)
   d. Includes receptors for sensations of salty, sweet, sour, and bitter
2. Olfactory sense
   a. Sense of smell
   b. Receptors found in upper nose
   c. Chemoreceptors
   d. Closely related to sense of taste
3. Visual sense (see Figure 2-22):
   a. Receptors located in the eye
   b. Photoreceptors (detects light)
      1) Eye
         a) Found in protective bony socket (orbit)
         b) Three layers (tunics)
            ■ Sclera
               (1) Outer layer; white of the eye
               (2) Made of tough fibrous tissue
               (3) Anterior portion covered by cornea, which focuses light rays
            ■ Choroid
               (1) Middle layer
               (2) Highly vascular
               (3) Ciliary body; changes shape of the lens
               (4) Suspensory ligament: connects the ciliary body to lens
               (5) Iris: colored portion of the eye
                  (a) Doughnut-shaped muscle with hole in the middle (pupil)
                  (b) Continually contracts and relaxes to regulate the amount of light entering the eye
            ■ Retina
               (1) Innermost layer
               (2) Posterior portion of the eye
               (3) Contains
                  (a) Rods: receptors sensitive to shades of gray
                  (b) Cones: receptors sensitive to color
               (4) Fovea centralis: area of closely packed cones that function as the area of sharpest vision
               (5) Optic disk: area on the retina where the optic nerve exits the eye; the *"blind spot"*

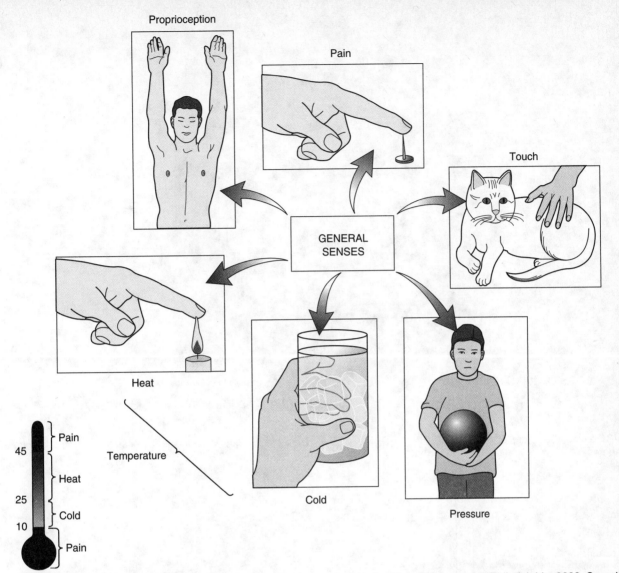

FIGURE 2-21. The general senses. (Herlihy B, Maebius N: *The human body in health and illness,* ed 2, Philadelphia, 2003, Saunders.)

2) Cavities
  a) Anterior cavity: anterior space between the lens and the cornea; filled with aqueous humor (maintains shape and internal pressure)
  b) Posterior cavity: between lens and the retina; filled with gel-like substance (vitreous humor); keeps retina against the wall of the eye, supports parts of the eye and helps maintain shape
3) Accessory structures
  a) Eyebrows and eyelashes: protects against foreign objects
  b) Eyelids: opens and closes eye to keep foreign objects out and to keep eye moist
  c) Lacrimal apparatus: lacrimal glands make tears to lubricate, moisten, and cleanse the eye; nasolacrimal duct drains tears into the nasal cavity
  d) Conjunctiva: mucous membrane that lines the inner eyelids and anterior eyeball

4) Muscles of the eye
  a) Extrinsic muscles: skeletal muscles attached to the orbital bones and outer eye
  b) Intrinsic muscles: smooth muscles located in the eye
5) Visual pathway: light ray → cornea → aqueous humor → pupil → lens → vitreous humor → retina (rods and cones) → optic nerve fibers → optic chiasma → thalamus → cerebral cortex
4. Auditory sense: receptors located in the ears; mechanoreceptors (see Figure 2-23)
5. Ear: found on both sides of the head
  a. External ear
    1) Auricle (pinna): fleshy part visible on sides of head; collects sound waves and directs them toward the auditory meatus
    2) External auditory meatus: short tube that extends from the auricle to the tympanic membrane; lined with glands that produce cerumen (earwax) to protect and lubricate

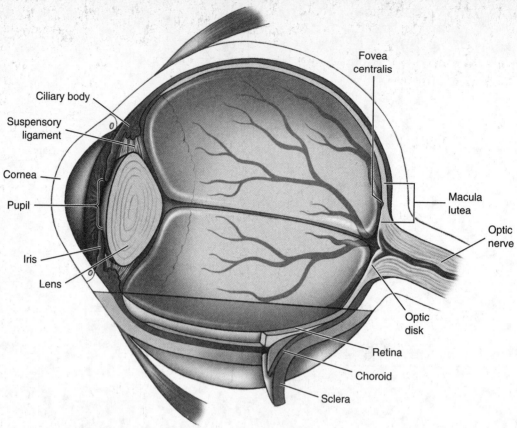

FIGURE 2-22. Structure of the eyeball. (Herlihy B, Maebius N: *The human body in health and illness,* ed 2, Philadelphia, 2003, Saunders.)

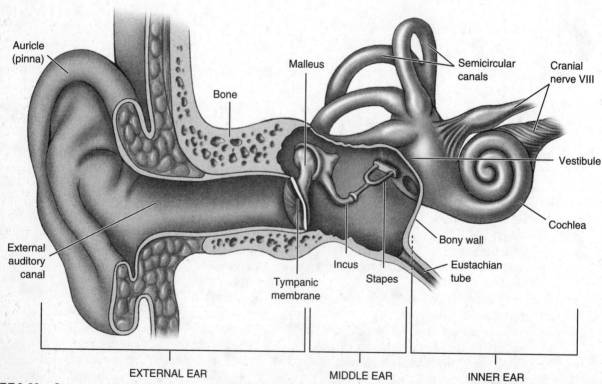

FIGURE 2-23. Structure of the ear and its three divisions. (Herlihy B, Maebius N: *The human body in health and illness,* ed 2, Philadelphia, 2003, Saunders.)

b. Middle ear: found in the temporal bone
1) Tympanic membrane: eardrum
2) Auditory tube: eustachian tube; extends from the middle ear to the throat; equalizes pressure between the outside air and the middle ear cavity
3) Ossicles: three tiny bones of the middle ear
   a) Malleus: attached to the tympanic membrane
   b) Incus: connects the malleus to the stapes
   c) Stapes: attached to the incus and oval window
4) Oval window: membrane covering the opening into the vestibule
c. Inner ear
   a) Bony labyrinth
      ■ Series of interconnecting chambers in the temporal bone
      ■ Contains membranous labyrinth filled with fluid (endolymph)
      ■ Space between the bony and membranous labyrinth; filled with fluid (perilymph)
      ■ Divided into three sections:
         (1) Vestibule: involved with balance
         (2) Semicircular canals: involved with equilibrium
         (3) Cochlea: snail-shaped structure involved with hearing; contains the organ of Corti, which contains receptors for sound
   b) Auditory pathway: sound wave → pinna → external auditory meatus → tympanic membrane → malleus → incus → stapes → oval window → cochlea → perilymph → auditory nerve fibers → cerebral cortex

D. DISEASES AND DISORDERS
1. Astigmatism: irregular focusing of light rays caused by a nonspheroid cornea
2. Blepharitis: inflammation of the eyelids
3. Cataract: opaqueness, cloudiness of the lens of the eye
4. Conjunctivitis: *"pinkeye"*; inflammation of the conjunctiva
5. Deafness: inability to hear
6. Diplopia: double vision
7. Glaucoma: accumulation of fluid in the eye: increases pressure that can cause damage to the retina and the optic nerve
8. Hordeolum: *"stye"*; infection of the sebaceous gland of eye
9. Hyperopia: farsightedness; ability to clearly see far objects but not near objects
10. Impacted cerumen: solidified earwax compacted within the ear canal
11. Keratitis: inflammation of the eyelids
12. Macular degeneration: degenerative disease in the center of the field of vision (macular lutea); affects central vision, not peripheral

13. Meniere's disease: chronic disease of the inner ear; characterized by vertigo, tinnitus, progressive hearing loss, and sensation of fullness, pressure, in the ear
14. Myopia: nearsightedness; ability to clearly see near objects but not far objects
15. Nystagmus: repetitive involuntary movement of the eye
16. Otitis media: inflammation of the middle ear
17. Otosclerosis: bone formation around the oval window and stapes; causes partial to complete deafness
18. Presbyopia: inability to focus quickly; caused by loss of lens elasticity caused by aging
19. Retinal detachment: partial or complete separation of the retina from the choroid; results in blindness
20. Ruptured tympanic membrane: an opening in the eardrum caused by middle ear inflammation caused by sharp objects in the canal or a blow to the ear; major risk is infection developing in the middle ear
21. Strabismus: *"lazy eye"*; inability of both eyes to focus on the same thing
22. Tinnitus: ringing in ears
23. Vertigo: dizziness

IX. Blood

A. GENERAL
1. Primary transport medium of the body
2. Pumped by the heart through a closed system of vessels
3. Classified as connective tissue (cells and matrix)
4. Approximately 5 liters in adult
5. 8% of body weight

B. FUNCTIONS
1. Transportation
   a. Carries O_2 and nutrients to cells
   b. Carries CO_2 and wastes from the tissues to the lungs and kidneys for removal
   c. Carries hormones from the endocrine glands to other parts of the body
2. Regulation
   a. Regulates body temperature by removing heat from active areas and transporting that heat to skin for dissipation
   b. Helps regulate fluid and electrolyte balance
   c. Regulates pH through buffers
3. Protection
   a. Provides clotting mechanism to prevent fluid loss when vessels are damaged
   b. White blood cells engulf and destroy invading microorganisms
   c. Antibodies react with the offending agents

C. COMPOSITION OF BLOOD (see Figure 2-24)
1. Plasma
   a. Liquid portion of circulating blood
   b. 55% of total blood volume

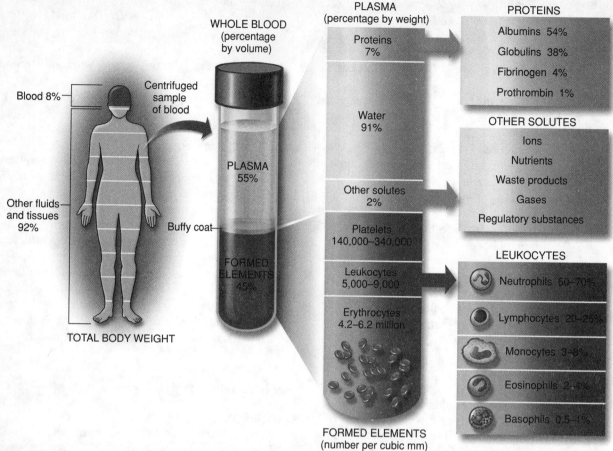

FIGURE 2-24. Components of blood. (Barbara Cousins, from Thibodeau GA, Patton KT: *The human body in health and disease,* ed 4, St. Louis, 2005, Mosby.)

c. 90% water

d. Continuously changing caused by dissolved solutes

e. Contains plasma proteins

  1) Albumin: maintains osmotic pressure

  2) Globulin: functions in lipid transport and immune reaction

  3) Fibrinogen: formation of blood clots

f. Also contains amino acids, urea, uric acids, nutrients, hormones, O_2, CO_2, antibodies, and electrolytes

2. Formed elements: produced by hemopoiesis (red blood cells in red bone marrow; white blood cells in lymphoid tissue); all types develop from stem cell (hematocytoblast)

a. Erythrocytes (red blood cells [RBCs])

  1) Most numerous of formed elements

  2) Normal range: 4.5 to 6 million per cubic millimeter of blood

  3) Biconcave disks (thin in the middle and thick around the edge)

  4) Mature cells have no nucleus

  5) Primary function: to carry O_2 to all body cells; O_2 combines with hemoglobin and is transported

  6) Formation regulated by hormone erythropoietin

  7) Iron, vitamin B-12, and folic acid are essential to RBC production

  8) Live approximately 120 days; are then destroyed by spleen and liver

b. Leukocytes (white blood cells [WBCs])

  1) Larger in size than RBCs, but fewer in number

  2) Normal range: 5000 to 10,000 per cubic millimeter of blood

  3) Each contains a nucleus

  4) Able to move through capillary walls into tissue

  5) Primary function: to provide defense against invading microorganisms and to promote or inhibit inflammatory response

  6) Types:

    a) Granulocytes: contains granules in cytoplasm

     ■ Neutrophil: most common; have multilobed nucleus; responds first to tissue damage; number increases in acute infection

     ■ Eosinophil: two-lobed nucleus; large granules in cytoplasm; neutralize histamine; numbers increase during allergic reaction and parasitic infections

     ■ Basophil: least numerous of WBCs; has large U-shaped nucleus; can leave blood and enter tissue, where they release histamine and heparin

b) Agranulocytes: granules absent in cytoplasm

▪ Lymphocytes: large round nucleus surrounded by small amount of cytoplasm; role in body's defense system

(1) T-lymphocytes: directly attacks microorganisms

(2) B-lymphocytes: produce antibodies

▪ Monocytes: largest in size of all WBCs; can enter the tissue (macrophage); finish the cleanup process of the neutrophils

c. Thrombocytes (platelets): small fragments of very large cells (megakaryocytes)

1) Normal range: 250,000 to 500,000 per cubic millimeter of blood

2) Initiates formation of blood clots

D. HEMOSTASIS

1. Stoppage of bleeding
2. Can be caused by either an injured vessel or stasis of blood flow
3. Includes three processes (see Figure 2-25):
   a. Vascular constriction: reduces flow of blood through torn vessel
   b. Platelet plug formation: platelets become sticky and adhere to each other
   c. Coagulation: complex series of steps that results in clot formation; requires calcium and vitamin K

E. BLOOD TYPING

1. Based on specific antigens and antibodies related to RBCs; blood type antigens are found on RBCs; antibodies in plasma
2. Main blood groups, ABO blood groups; blood types *must* match in transfusions:
   a. Type A: has A antigens on RBCs; has anti-B antibodies

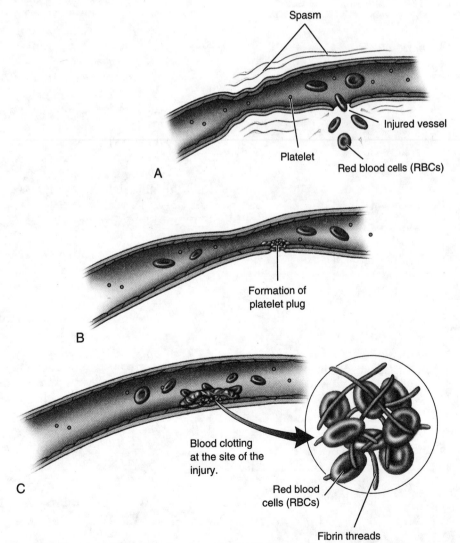

FIGURE 2-25. The steps of hemostasis: **A,** Vascular constriction. **B,** Formation of the platelet plug. **C,** Blood clotting (coagulation). (Herlihy B, Maebius N: *The human body in health and illness*, ed 2, Philadelphia, 2003, Saunders.)

b. Type B: has B antigens on RBCs; has anti-A antibodies

c. Type AB: has A and B antigens on RBCs; has no antibodies

d. Type O: has neither A nor B antigens on RBCs; has both anti-A and anti-B antibodies

3. Rh factor: Rh+ has Rh antigen on RBCs; Rh-has no antigens; neither has anti-Rh in plasma; hemolytic disease of the newborn may develop when Rh-mother has Rh+ fetus

F. DISEASES AND DISORDERS

1. Anemia: abnormal decrease in hemoglobin, RBC count, or hematocrit
2. Leukemia: malignant neoplasm of blood-forming organs; usually involves one specific type of blood cell
3. Polycythemia: abnormal increase in hemoglobin, RBC count, or hematocrit
4. Thrombocytopenia: decrease in thrombocytes; results in decrease in clotting capabilities

X. Lymphatic System

A. GENERAL

1. Part of the circulatory system
2. Transports a fluid (lymph) through lymphatic vessels and empties it into venous blood
3. Major role in the body's defense system

B. FUNCTIONS

1. Returns excess interstitial fluid to blood
2. Absorbs fats and fat-soluble vitamins from the digestive system
3. Provides defense against disease

C. ORGANS OF THE LYMPHATIC SYSTEM (see Figure 2-26)

1. Lymph
   a. Similar in composition to blood plasma
   b. Picked up from interstitial fluid and returned to blood plasma
2. Lymphatic vessels
   a. Found in tissue spaces
   b. Carry fluid away from the tissues
   c. Vessels empty into the lymphatic ducts
      1) Right lymphatic duct: drains lymph from upper right quadrant of the body
      2) Thoracic duct: drains the remainder of the body
3. Lymphatic organs
   a. Lymph nodes
      1) Located along the lymphatic vessels
      2) Superficial nodes found in the groin, axilla, and neck
      3) Filter and cleanse the lymph before it enters the blood
   b. Tonsils
      1) Provide protection against pathogens that may enter through the mouth or nose

2) Three groups:
   a) Pharyngeal tonsils: located near the opening of the nose into the pharynx; adenoids
   b) Palatine tonsils: *the tonsils*; located near the opening of the oral cavity into the pharynx
   c) Lingual tonsils: posterior surface of the tongue
4. Spleen: located in the upper left abdomen beneath the diaphragm, posterior to the stomach; filters blood; acts as a reservoir for the blood
5. Thymus: located posterior to the sternum; large in infants, atrophies after puberty; produces thymosin (stimulates the maturation of lymphocytes in the lymphatic organs)

D. RESISTANCE TO DISEASE

1. Resistance is the body's ability to counteract pathogens
2. Susceptibility is the lack of resistance
3. Resistance is accomplished through defense mechanisms
   a. Nonspecific defense mechanisms: directed against all pathogens and foreign substances; provides first line of defense against invasion (see Figure 2-27)
      1) Barriers
         a) Mechanical (e.g., skin)
         b) Chemical (e.g., hydrochloric acid in stomach)
      2) Chemical action
         a) Complement: promotes phagocytosis and inflammation
         b) Interferon: produced by virus-infected cells to provide protection for neighboring cells
      3) Phagocytosis: neutrophils and macrophages
      4) Inflammation: characterized by redness, warmth, swelling, and pain
   b. Specific defense mechanisms: programmed to be selective (specificity); ability to remember invading agent (memory); invading agent called antigen; B-lymphocytes produce antibodies that react with the antigen (see Figure 2-28)
      1) Acquired immunity
         a) Active natural immunity: results when a person has a disease
         b) Active artificial immunity: results when a specific antigen is deliberately introduced into a person (immunization)
         c) Passive natural immunity: results when antibodies are transferred from one person to another (as mother to child)
         d) Passive artificial immunity: results when antibodies that developed in another person or animal are injected into a person
      2) Natural immunity: acquired through normal activities

E. DISEASES AND DISORDERS OF THE LYMPHATIC SYSTEM

1. Acquired immunodeficiency syndrome (AIDS): suppression or deficiency of immune system caused by the human immunodeficiency virus (HIV)

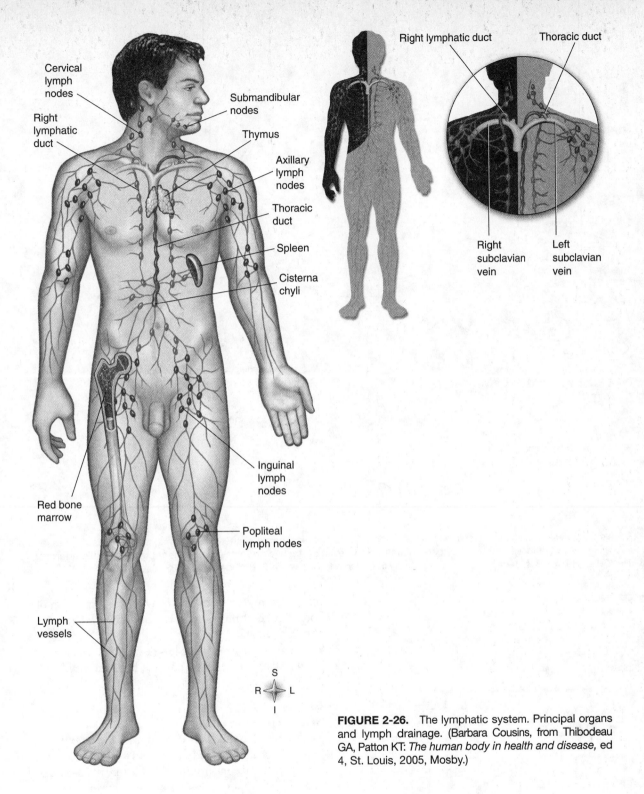

FIGURE 2-26. The lymphatic system. Principal organs and lymph drainage. (Barbara Cousins, from Thibodeau GA, Patton KT: *The human body in health and disease,* ed 4, St. Louis, 2005, Mosby.)

2. Hodgkin's disease: malignant condition of lymphatic tissue in spleen and nodes
3. Lymphedema: abnormal accumulation of lymph caused by obstruction of vessels; occurs in the extremities
4. Mononucleosis: acute infectious disease caused by Epstein-Barr virus by direct oral contact
5. Non-Hodgkin's lymphoma: malignant disease of lymphatic system

XI. Cardiovascular System

A. GENERAL
1. Closed, sterile system
2. Consists of heart and blood vessels

B. FUNCTIONS
1. Transportation: carries important elements throughout the body

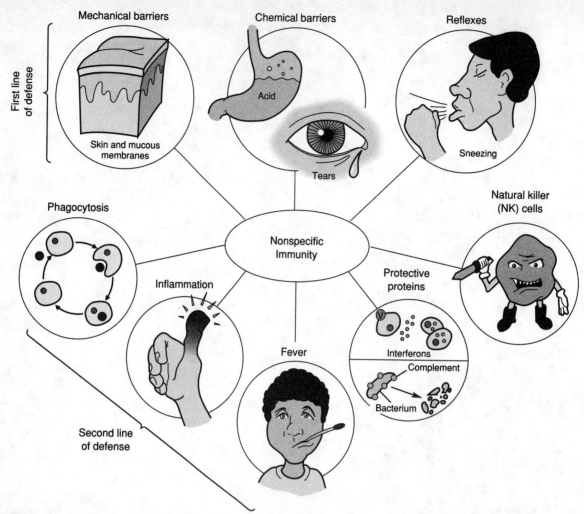

FIGURE 2-27. Nonspecific immunity. The first line of defense includes mechanical barriers, chemical barriers, and reflexes. Processes involved in the second line of defense are phagocytosis, inflammation, fever, protective proteins (complement proteins and interferons) and natural killer cells. (Herlihy B, Maebius N: *The human body in health and illness,* ed 2, Philadelphia, 2003, Saunders.)

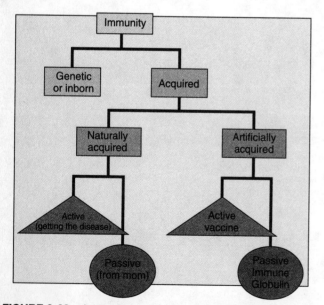

FIGURE 2-28. Immunity is either genetic or acquired. Immunity is acquired either naturally or artificially. Naturally acquired immunity can be either active *(triangles)* or passive *(circles).* (Herlihy B, Maebius N: *The human body in health and illness,* ed 2, Philadelphia, 2003, Saunders)

2. Temperature regulation: helps with the regulation of body temperature through dilation and constriction of blood vessels
3. Waste removal: assists the lungs, kidneys, and liver
4. Fluid balance: maintains balance between fluid loss and fluid retention

C. ORGANS
1. Heart (see Figure 2-29)
   a. Hollow, muscular, cone-shaped organ about the size of a fist; located slightly to the left of midline in the mediastinum; protected by the sternum and ribs; upper end is base; lower end is pointed and is the apex (apical pulse)
   b. Made up of three layers
      1) Epicardium: outer layer
      2) Myocardium: thick, middle muscular layer
      3) Endocardium: inner layer
   c. Covered by pericardium (double-layered sac that decreases friction and protects the heart)
   d. Contains four chambers
      1) Atria: (singular: *atrium*); two upper chambers; receive blood from veins

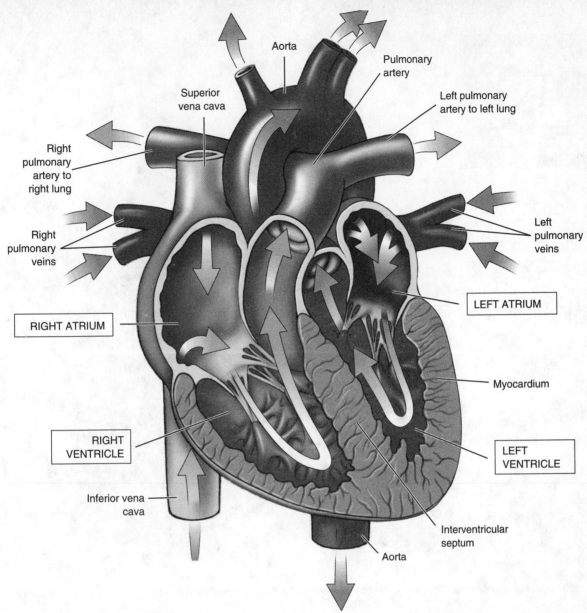

FIGURE 2-29. Chambers of the heart and the large vessels; blood flow through the heart. (Herlihy B, Maebius N: *The human body in health and illness,* ed 2, Philadelphia, 2003, Saunders.)

2) Ventricles: two lower chambers; receive blood from atria and pump it into the body
3) Septum: divides chambers into right and left
4) Valves: structures that allow one-way flow of blood throughout the heart
   a) Tricuspid valve: permits blood to flow from right atrium to right ventricle; composed of three flaps of tissue
   b) Bicuspid valve: (mitral valve); made up of two flaps of tissue; permits blood to flow from left atrium to left ventricle
   c) Pulmonary valve: located at the entrance of the pulmonary artery; prevents backflow of blood into the right ventricle; semilunar (half-moon shaped)
   d) Aortic valve: located at the entrance of the aorta; prevents backflow of blood into the left ventricle; semilunar:
   e) Blood enters right atrium → right ventricle → pulmonary artery → pulmonary capillaries (exchange of gases) → pulmonary vein → left atrium → left ventricle → aorta → capillaries in body tissues (exchange of gases) → superior and inferior vena cavae → right atrium
e. Electrical conduction system: initiates and maintains the rhythmic heart contractions (see Figure 2-30)
   1) Sinoatrial (SA) node: pacemaker of the heart; located in the right atrial wall near the superior vena cava; initiates heartbeat and sets its pace

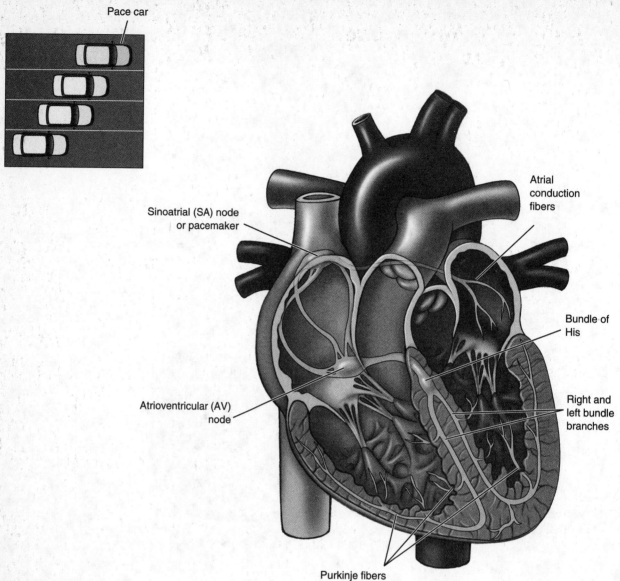

FIGURE 2-30.   Conduction system of the heart. (Herlihy B, Maebius N: *The human body in health and illness,* ed 2, Philadelphia, 2003, Saunders.)

2) Atrioventricular (AV) node: located in lower right atrial septum; causes the atria to contract
3) Bundle of His: located in ventricular septum
4) Bundle branches: two branches extending from bundle of His
5) Purkinje fibers: extend from the bundle branches; causes ventricles to contract

   f. Cardiac cycle: complete heartbeat; consists of contraction (systole) and relaxation (diastole) of both atria and ventricles; complete cycle lasts for 0.8 second (75 bpm); sounds associated with heartbeat described as *lubb-dupp*

2. Vessels

   a. Artery: vessels that carry blood away from the heart
1) Composed of three layers

a) Tunica adventitia: outermost layer of tough fibrous connective tissue
b) Tunica media: middle layer of smooth muscle tissue allowing for contraction and dilation
c) Tunica intima: innermost layer
2) Arteriole: small arteries

   b. Veins: vessels that carry blood toward the heart
1) Same layers as arteries, except tunica adventitia is thicker and tunica intima has valves to prevent backflow
2) Venules: small veins

   c. Capillaries: microscopic vessels, one cell-layer thick
1) Connects arterioles and venules
2) Exchange of substances takes place here

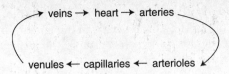

b. Aorta: largest artery in the body; comes from the heart; divided into ascending aorta, aortic arch, descending aorta, and abdominal aorta

c. Coronary: right and left branches off the ascending aorta; supplies the heart with blood

3. Major arteries (see Figure 2-31)

   a. Pulmonary: comes from the right ventricle; transports deoxygenated blood to lungs

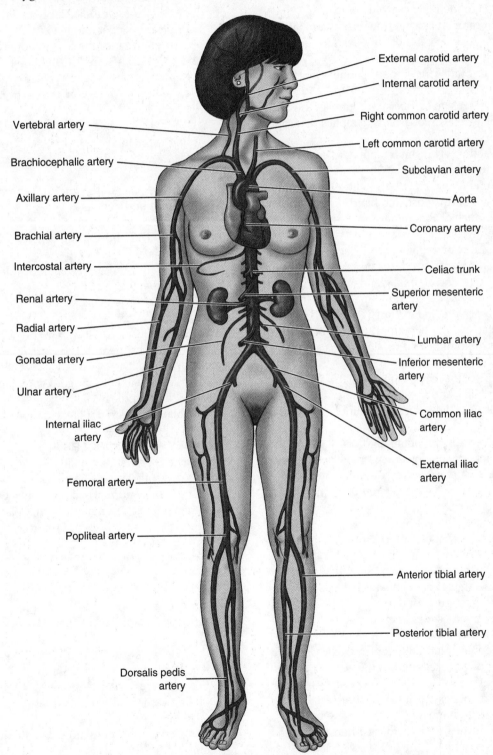

FIGURE 2-31. Major arteries of the body. (Herlihy B, Maebius N: *The human body in health and illness*, ed 2, Philadelphia, 2003, Saunders.)

d. Brachiocephalic: one of three major branches off the aortic arch; supplies blood to the neck, head, axilla, and upper arm
e. Subclavian: supplies arms and vertebrae
 1) Left subclavian branches from aortic arch
 2) Right subclavian branches from brachiocephalic
f. Carotid: supplies neck and head
 1) Left carotid branches from aortic arch
 2) Right carotid branches from brachiocephalic
g. Facial: branch of carotid; supplies face and cranium
h. Occipital: branch of carotid; supplies neck and cranium
i. Axillary: extension of subclavian; supplies the axilla
j. Brachial: extension of axillary; supplies the upper arm
k. Radial: branch of brachial; supplies forearm, wrist, and hand
l. Ulnar: branch of brachial on little finger side; supplies forearm, wrist, and hand
m. Celiac: branch of abdominal aorta; supplies upper abdomen and organs
n. Splenic: functions similarly to celiac
o. Renal: branch of abdominal aorta; supplies kidneys, ureters, and adrenal glands
p. Mesenteric: branch of abdominal aorta; supplies intestines, colon, and rectum
q. Iliac: extension of abdominal aorta; branches and supplies abdominal and pelvic regions and lower limbs
r. Femoral: extension of iliac; supplies abdominal wall, genitalia, and upper leg
s. Popliteal: extension of femoral; supplies knee and calf
t. Tibial: extension of popliteal
 1) Anterior supplies lower leg, ankle, and foot
 2) Posterior supplies lower leg, foot, and heel
u. Dorsalis pedis: extension of anterior tibial; supplies foot

4. Major veins (see Figure 2-32)
a. Pulmonary: transports blood from lungs to left atrium
b. Coronary: drains blood from the right atrium
c. Vena cava: largest vein in the body; leads from the body into the right atrium
 1) Superior vena cava: drains upper body
 2) Inferior vena cava: drains the lower body
d. Brachiocephalic: left and right branches go into the superior vena cava; drains the head, neck, and upper extremities
e. Jugular: branches go into the brachiocephalic; drains the head and neck
f. Facial: branches go into the jugular; drains the face and cranium
g. Occipital: branches go into the jugular; drains the cranium

h. Axillary: branches go into the brachiocephalic; drains the axillary area and the upper arm
i. Subclavian: branches go into the axillary; drains the upper arm
j. Cephalic: goes into the axillary; drains the upper and lower arm
k. Radial: goes into the axillary; drains the thumb side of the forearm and wrist
l. Basilic: goes into axillary on little finger side; drains the upper and lower arm
m. Ulnar: goes into the axillary; drains the little finger side of the forearm and wrist
n. Gastric, cholecystic, and splenic: goes into portal hepatic vein; drains the stomach, gallbladder, and spleen
o. Mesenteric: goes into the hepatic portal vein; drains the intestines, colon, and rectum
p. Hepatic: goes into the inferior vena cava; drains the liver
q. Renal: goes into the inferior vena cava; drains the kidneys and gonads
r. Iliac: extension of the inferior vena cava; drains the abdominal, pelvic, and lower limb regions
s. Femoral: extension of right and left iliac; drains the upper leg
t. Popliteal: extension of femoral; drains the knee and calf
u. Saphenous: longest vein in the body
 1) Great saphenous goes into femoral; drains the medial leg
 2) Small saphenous goes into popliteal; drains the lower leg
v. Tibial: goes into popliteal; drains the lower leg

D. DISEASES AND DISORDERS
1. Angina pectoris: chest pain; usually caused by a lack of blood supply to the heart
2. Aneurysm: abnormal ballooning of a vessel wall
3. Atherosclerosis: formation of fatty plaques along the vessel walls, causing them to narrow; can be the cause of arteriosclerosis
4. Arteriosclerosis: hardening of the arteries; walls of vessels become thick and lose elasticity
5. Bradycardia: abnormally slow heart rate (<60 bpm)
6. Cardiac arrest: unexpected stoppage of the heart function; may follow myocardial infarction (MI)
7. Congestive heart failure (CHF): characterized by the inability of the heart to keep blood circulating; results in generalized edema
8. Embolism: a blood clot, air, fat globule, or piece of tissue that has broken loose and entered the circulation
9. Endocarditis: inflammation of endocardium, including valves
10. Hypertension (HTN): high blood pressure (>140/90 mm Hg)

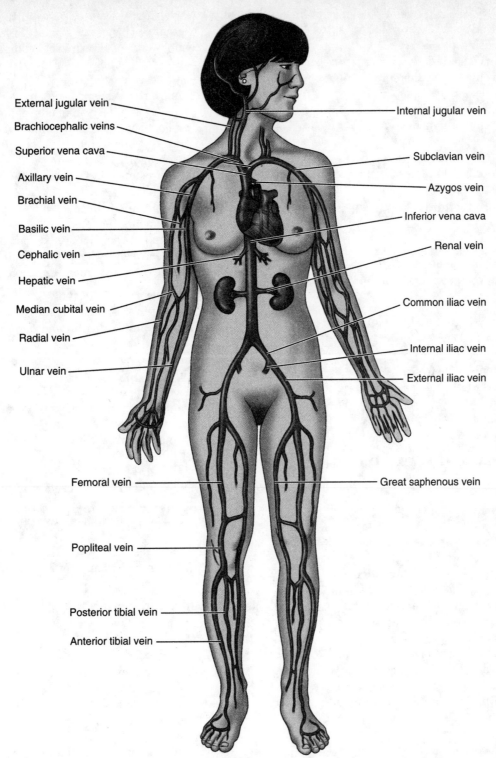

External jugular vein

Brachiocephalic veins

Superior vena cava

Axillary vein

Brachial vein

Basilic vein

Cephalic vein

Hepatic vein

Median cubital vein

Radial vein

Ulnar vein

Internal jugular vein

Subclavian vein

Azygos vein

Inferior vena cava

Renal vein

Common iliac vein

Internal iliac vein

External iliac vein

Femoral vein

Popliteal vein

Posterior tibial vein

Anterior tibial vein

Great saphenous vein

FIGURE 2-32. Major veins of the body. (Herlihy B, Maebius N: *The human body in health and illness,* ed 2, Philadelphia, 2003, Saunders.)

11. Mitral stenosis: narrowing of mitral valve that prevents normal flow of blood from the atrium to the ventricle

12. Myocardial infarction (MI): heart attack; caused by occlusion of coronary vessels that decreases the blood supply to the heart; tissue without blood supply necroses

13. Patent ductus arteriosus: abnormal opening between the aorta and the pulmonary artery

14. Rheumatic heart disease: can be caused by streptococci; causes inflammation of the heart and scarring of the valves; can be the result of rheumatic fever or MI

15. Tachycardia: abnormally rapid heart rate (>100 bpm)

16. Tetralogy of Fallot: congenital heart abnormality; characterized by four abnormalities:
    a. Ventricular septal defect
    b. Pulmonary stenosis
    c. Displacement of the aorta to the right
    d. Ventricular enlargement
17. Thrombophlebitis: inflammation of a vein accompanied by clot formation
18. Thrombus: blood clot
19. Varicosity (varicose veins): large, twisted, superficial vein; can occur in lower legs, rectum, esophagus

XII. Respiratory System

A. GENERAL
1. Supplies continuous supply of O_2 to the body
2. Works with the circulatory system to bring O_2 to the entire body and to remove waste products

B. FUNCTIONS
1. Air exchange and distribution: O_2 carried to tissues and CO_2 carried away
2. Filtration: small hairs in nasal cavity trap substances before air enters the trachea
3. Sound production: enhances sounds produced during speech
4. Sense of smell: located in the nose
5. pH regulation: regulates the pH of blood

C. ORGANS: DIVIDED INTO TWO SECTIONS (see Figure 2-33):
1. Upper respiratory tract: organs outside of thoracic cavity
    a. Nose
        1) External nose: nasal bones and cartilage; forms nostrils (nares)
        2) Internal nose: nasal cavity; found over roof of mouth; divided into two halves by the nasal septum; functions to warm, filter, and humidify air
    b. Pharynx;
        1) Throat
        2) Has three divisions
            a) Nasopharynx: nearest to nasal cavity; contains adenoids
            b) Oropharynx: behind the mouth; contains the tonsils
            c) Laryngopharynx: leads to trachea and esophagus
    c. Larynx: voice box; made up of cartilage with ciliated mucous membrane; contains vocal cords; carries air from pharynx to trachea
2. Lower respiratory tract: organs within the thorax
    a. Trachea: windpipe; made up of 16 to 20 C-shaped rings of cartilage that extend from larynx to the bronchi
    b. Bronchi: end of the trachea; divided into right and left bronchi; enters lungs and further divides into secondary bronchi that further branch into bronchioles; branches end in alveolar ducts
    c. Alveoli: air sacs; functional units of respiration; resemble clusters of grapes; these form the terminal end of bronchioles; composed of single layers of epithelium surrounded by capillaries; gases exchanged here
    d. Lungs: cone-shaped organs located in thoracic cavity; each contains approximately 300 million alveoli; responsible for air distribution and exchange; bottom portion (base) rests on diaphragm
        1) Left lung divided into two lobes (eight segments)
        2) Right lung divided into three lobes (10 segments)
    e. Covered by double-layered membrane (pleura); fluid between layers (pleural fluid) lubricates and reduces friction during respiration

D. RESPIRATION
1. Controlled by respiratory control center of medulla
2. Medulla controls rhythm and depth of inspiration and expiration
3. Monitors O_2, CO_2, and pH of blood, which triggers breathing
4. Involves two processes
    a. Pulmonary ventilation: carries out breathing by means of pressure gradient; has two phases
        1) Inspiration: air drawn into lungs by contraction of diaphragm (makes thoracic cavity larger)
        2) Expiration: air expelled from lungs by relaxation of diaphragm
    b. Cellular respiration; has two phases:
        1) External: exchange of gases between alveoli and capillaries
        2) Internal: exchange of gases between capillaries and body cells

E. DISEASES AND DISORDERS
1. Anoxia: lack of O_2
2. Apnea: lack of breathing
3. Asphyxia: decrease in O_2 intake
4. Asthma: spasms of bronchus; results in dyspnea and wheezing
5. Atelectasis: partial or complete collapse of alveoli
6. Bronchitis: inflammation of bronchi; may be chronic or acute
7. Carcinoma: malignant tumor of lung and/or respiratory system
8. Cheyne-Stokes respiration: alternating episodes of tachypnea and apnea; usually precedes death
9. Chronic obstructive pulmonary disease (COPD) and chronic obstructive lung disease (COLD): a group of disorders characterized by progressive, irreversible obstruction of airflow; major disorders observed include chronic bronchitis, emphysema, and asthma
10. Croup: acute viral infection characterized by bark-like cough

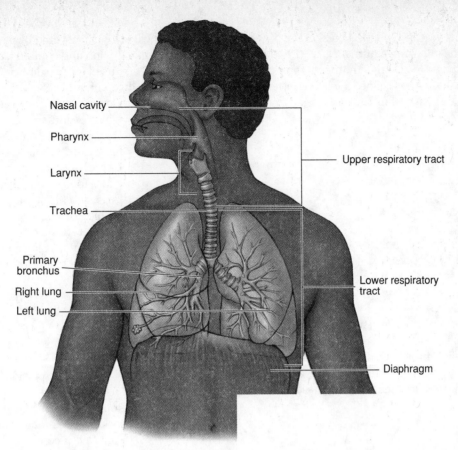

Nasal cavity

Pharynx

Larynx

Trachea

Primary bronchus

Right lung

Left lung

Upper respiratory tract

Lower respiratory tract

Diaphragm

FIGURE 2-33. Organs of the upper and lower respiratory tract. (Herlihy B, Maebius N: *The human body in health and illness,* ed 2, Philadelphia, 2003, Saunders.)

11. Dyspnea: painful or difficult breathing
12. Emphysema: loss of elasticity and enlargement of alveoli
13. Epistaxis: nosebleed
14. Hyperpnea: increase in the volume of breathing
15. Hypoxia: decrease in O_2
16. Infectious mononucleosis: mono; acute viral infection caused by Epstein-Barr virus; may include upper respiratory symptoms
17. Laryngitis: inflammation of larynx, causes loss of voice
18. Orthopnea: breathing facilitated by an upright position
19. Pertussis: whooping cough; lung disease caused by *Bordetella pertussis* bacterium; characterized by *"whoop"*-sounding cough
20. Pharyngitis: inflammation of throat
21. Pleurisy: inflammation of the pleural membranes
22. Pneumonia: inflammation of bronchioles and alveoli; can be viral or bacterial
23. Pneumothorax: collection of air in the pleural cavity; may cause the lung to collapse
24. Pulmonary edema: accumulation of fluid in lung tissue
25. Pulmonary embolism: clot located in the pulmonary artery or one of its branches; restricts blood flow to the lungs
26. Rales: crackling sounds on inspiration

27. Respiratory acidosis: decreased pH level of body caused by inadequate removal of CO_2 by the lungs; can progress to tissues outside of the lungs
28. Respiratory alkalosis: increased pH levels caused by excessive removal of CO_2 by the lungs
29. Sinusitis: inflammation of paranasal sinuses
30. Stridor: high-pitched sounds on inspiration caused by obstruction
31. Suffocation: prevention of breathing by external causes
32. Tachypnea: abnormal, rapid breathing
33. Tuberculosis (TB): communicable lung disease caused by *Mycobacterium tuberculosis;* characterized by tubercles in the tissue
34. Upper respiratory infection (URI): acute inflammatory process affecting mucous membranes that line the upper respiratory tract

XIII. Digestive System

A. GENERAL

1. Includes the digestive tract (gastrointestinal [GI] tract, alimentary canal) and accessory organs
2. Digestive tract: long, continuous tube that starts at the mouth and ends at the anus
3. Processes food into molecules small enough to be utilized by the body

B. FUNCTIONS

1. Digestion: physical and chemical breakdown of complex foodstuffs into simple nutrients
2. Absorption: passage of simple nutrients through the walls of the small intestine into the blood or lymph
3. Elimination: excretion of indigestible waste from the body in the form of feces

C. ORGANS (see Figure 2-34)

1. Mouth (oral cavity)
   a. Receives food by ingestion
   b. Breaks down food into small particles by mastication (chewing)
   c. Mixes food with saliva
   d. Lips and cheeks help hold food in place for chewing
   e. Also helps with speech
      1) Palate: separates oral cavity from nasal cavity
         a) Anterior portion (hard palate): supported by bone
         b) Posterior portion (soft palate): made of muscle and connective tissue; ends in finger-like projection (uvula); uvula and soft palate move upward during swallowing to keep food from entering the nasal cavity

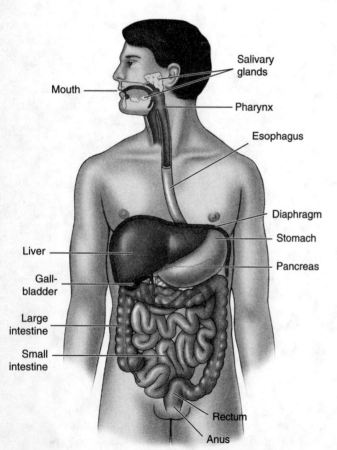

FIGURE 2-34. The digestive system. (Herlihy B, Maebius N: *The human body in health and illness,* ed 2, Philadelphia, 2003, Saunders.)

2) Tongue: moves food around in mouth; helps with speech; covered by papillae; papillae provide friction and contain taste buds
3) Teeth: used for mastication
   a) Two different sets develop:
      ▪ Deciduous *(baby teeth):* first 20 teeth, which eventually fall out
      ▪ Permanent: set of 32 adult teeth, which replace deciduous teeth
   b) Shape of tooth corresponds to the way it handles food
      ▪ Incisors: chisel-shaped and sharp edges for biting foods
      ▪ Cuspids (canines): conical-shaped with points for grasping and tearing foods
      ▪ Bicuspids: flat surfaces for crushing and grinding
      ▪ Molars: also have flat surfaces for crushing and grinding
   c) Tooth is divided into:
      ▪ Crown: exposed portion; covered with enamel (hardest surface in the body)
      ▪ Neck: narrow portion below crown, protected by gums
      ▪ Root: end portion of neck that fits into socket in mandible and maxilla
      ▪ Pulp cavity: central core of tooth; contains pulp, which consists of connective tissue, blood vessels, and nerves; surrounded by dentin
4) Salivary glands
   a) Produce saliva, which contains water, mucus, and enzyme amylase; moistens food; begins chemical digestion
   b) Three pairs of exocrine glands secrete saliva into the mouth:
      ▪ Parotid: largest pair; located in front of the ears (mumps)
      ▪ Submandibular: located in the floor of the mouth
      ▪ Sublingual: smallest pair; located under the tongue
2. Pharynx (throat): passageway that transports food to esophagus
3. Esophagus: muscular tube that carries food from pharynx to stomach
4. Stomach: located in the left upper quadrant of abdomen
   a. Can hold up to 1.5 liters
   b. Temporarily stores and partially breaks down food
   c. Secretes substances (mucus, hydrochloric acid (HCl), gastrin, pepsinogen) that aid in digestion
   d. Destroys bacteria that enters the digestive tract
   e. Three regions:
      1) Superior region (fundus); opening guarded by the cardiac sphincter
      2) Main portion (body)

3) Lower portion (pylorus); connects to small intestines; opening to the small intestines guarded by the pyloric sphincter

f. Wall of the stomach has three layers made up of smooth muscle; the innermost layer has folds (rugae), which allow for expansion

5. Small intestines

a. Coiled tubular structure approximately 6 meters in length and approximately 2.5 centimeters in diameter

b. Fills most of the abdominal cavity

c. Completes chemical digestion

d. Primary site for absorption of nutrients

e. Has three divisions:

1) Duodenum: upper portion

2) Jejunum: middle portion

3) Ileum: end portion

f. Suspended from the abdominal wall by a fold of peritoneum (mesentery)

g. Lining contains fingerlike projections (villi); villi contain capillaries and lacteals, which rise off of the surface area and absorb nutrients

6. Large intestines

a. Folded tube approximately 1.5 meters in length and 6 centimeters in diameter

b. Absorbs fluid and electrolytes; eliminates waste products

c. Produces vitamin K (necessary for blood clotting)

d. Divided into:

1) Cecum: first division connected to ileum of small intestine; contains ileocecal valve; vermiform appendix attached to cecum

2) Ascending colon: vertical length of colon that runs along the right side of the abdominal cavity

3) Transverse colon: horizontal length of colon that runs across the abdominal cavity

4) Descending colon: vertical length of colon that runs along the left side of the abdominal cavity

5) Sigmoid colon: S-shaped length of colon that connects to the rectum

6) Rectum: continues to the anal canal; thick muscular wall

7) Anal canal: continues from the rectum to outside (anus); guarded by two sphincter muscles

7. Peritoneum: serous membrane that covers most of the abdominal organs and holds them in place

a. Mesentery: holds intestines in coils

b. Transverse mesocolon: binds transverse colon to posterior abdominal wall

c. Omentum: sheet of serous membrane that contains fat; protects the abdominal organs

8. Accessory organs

a. Liver

1) Accessory organ of digestion

2) "Can't live without a liver"

3) Largest gland in the body

4) Located in the right upper quadrant

5) Divided into right and left lobes

6) Filters and destroys wastes and toxic substances

7) Produces bile, which breaks down (emulsifies) fats

8) Stores iron, glycogen, and vitamins A, B-12, D, E, and K

9) Produces clotting factors

10) Recycles iron and hemoglobin from worn-out red blood cells

11) Controls carbohydrate and lipid metabolism

b. Gallbladder

1) Pear-shaped sac attached to inferior surface of liver by cystic duct

2) Stores, concentrates, and sends bile into the duodenum through the common bile duct (the cystic duct joins the hepatic duct from the liver to form the common bile duct)

c. Pancreas

1) Located behind stomach

2) Endocrine and exocrine functions

a) Endocrine: beta cells of the islets of Langerhans secrete insulin, which lowers blood glucose levels; alpha cells of the islets of Langerhans secrete glucagon (which raises blood glucose levels)

b) Exocrine: acinar cells secrete digestive enzymes (amylase, trypsin, peptidase, and lipase)

D. DIGESTION

1. Breakdown of foodstuffs; has two processes:

a. Mechanical digestion: breaks down food, moves it along the canal, and eliminates the waste from the body;

1) Begins with mastication (chewing), which reduces the size of food and mixes the food with saliva to form a bolus

2) Bolus is swallowed (deglutition)

3) Wavelike motion of GI tract (peristalsis) moves food along the digestive tract

4) Food is churned in stomach to mix with gastric juices to form chyme

5) Chyme is pushed into the duodenum approximately every 20 seconds until empty

6) Chyme mixes with pancreatic liver and intestinal juices

7) Chyme leaves the jejunum approximately 5 hours after entering the small intestine

8) Residue not absorbed enters the large intestine, where excess water is absorbed and waste (feces) is formed and expelled from the body

b. Chemical digestion: breaks down large complex molecules into smaller molecules for absorption; accomplished by hydrolysis and enzymes

1) Carbohydrates: initially broken down by amylase; final breakdown by sucrase, lactase, and maltase

    2) Proteins: broken down into amino acids by proteases: pepsin (stomach), trypsin (pancreas), and peptidase (intestines)

    3) Fats: first emulsified by bile in small intestine; finally digested by pancreatic lipase

E. ABSORPTION

1. Process of transporting nutrients from small intestinal mucosa to blood or lymph
2. Most absorption occurs in small intestine
3. Nutrients travel to the liver through portal system

F. ELIMINATION

1. Solid waste expelled from body by process of defecation
2. Defecation is triggered by stimulation of receptors caused by full rectum
3. Controlled by internal sphincter (involuntary) and external sphincter (voluntary)

G. DISEASES AND DISORDERS

1. Anorexia: lack of appetite
2. Appendicitis: inflammation of appendix
3. Caries: dental cavities
4. Celiac sprue: malabsorption syndrome; characterized by intolerance to gluten and damage to intestinal mucosa
5. Cholelithiasis: (gallstones); caused by collection of solid cholesterol or calcium in the gallbladder or bile ducts
6. Cirrhosis: degenerative disease of the liver
7. Colitis: inflammation of the colon
8. Constipation: hard stools resulting in difficulty in defecating
9. Crohn's disease: common chronic inflammatory disease of the GI tract; walls of the bowel become edematous and inflamed
10. Diarrhea: loose, watery stools
11. Diverticulitis: inflammation of pouches (diverticula) in the colon
12. Emesis: vomiting
13. Gastritis: inflammation of the stomach
14. Gastroenteritis: inflammation of stomach and intestines
15. Gingivitis: inflammation of the gums
16. Hemorrhoids: inflammation and dilation of surface veins in the rectum and anus
17. Hepatitis: inflammation of the liver; can be acute or chronic
18. Hernia: protrusion of a part of the intestine into an adjacent area or cavity
19. Intussusception: telescoping of one part of the intestine onto another part just below it
20. Irritable bowel syndrome (IBS): collection of symptoms with no organic cause; characterized by abdominal pain, constipation, and diarrhea

21. Malabsorption syndrome: disease process that inhibits absorption of nutrients
22. Mumps: inflammation of parotid salivary glands
23. Pancreatitis: inflammation of the pancreas
24. Stomatitis: inflammation of mouth
25. Thrush: yeast infection of the mouth; caused by *Candida albicans*
26. Ulcer: lesion in the mucosa of the stomach or intestine
27. Vincent's angina: (trench mouth); ulcerations of the mucosa of the mouth

XIV. Urinary System

A. GENERAL

1. Produces and excretes urine from the body
2. Kidneys clean blood of waste products
3. Plays vital role in electrolyte, water, and acid-base balance

B. FUNCTIONS

1. Waste elimination: excretes nitrogen-containing liquid waste (urine) from the body
2. Regulation of blood volume: balances water loss and gain
3. Regulation of pH: balances gain and loss of bicarbonate and hydrogen ions
4. Regulations of electrolytes: balances levels through excretion and reabsorption
5. Detoxification: assists liver in neutralizing substances

C. ORGANS (see Figure 2-35)

1. Kidney: two bean-shaped organs located retroperitoneal; surrounded by a cushion of fat; two layers
   a. Cortex: outer layer
   b. Medulla: inner layer; contains renal pyramids
      1) Triangle-shaped wedges that contain the nephron
      2) Points of pyramids come together into a cup-like structure (calyx [singular])
      3) Calyces (plural) join together to form renal pelvis where urine is collected
      4) Nephron: microscopic functional unit of kidneys; filters blood and produces urine; made up of:
        a) Bowman's capsule: cup-shaped structure in renal cortex; holds the glomerulus
        b) Glomerulus: ball-shaped cluster of capillaries that sits in Bowman's capsule; Bowman's capsule and glomerulus make up the renal corpuscle
        c) Proximal convoluted tubule: extension of Bowman's capsule; makes up first part of the renal tubule
        d) Loop of Henle: extends from proximal convoluted tubule
        e) Distal convoluted tubule: extends from the loop of Henle

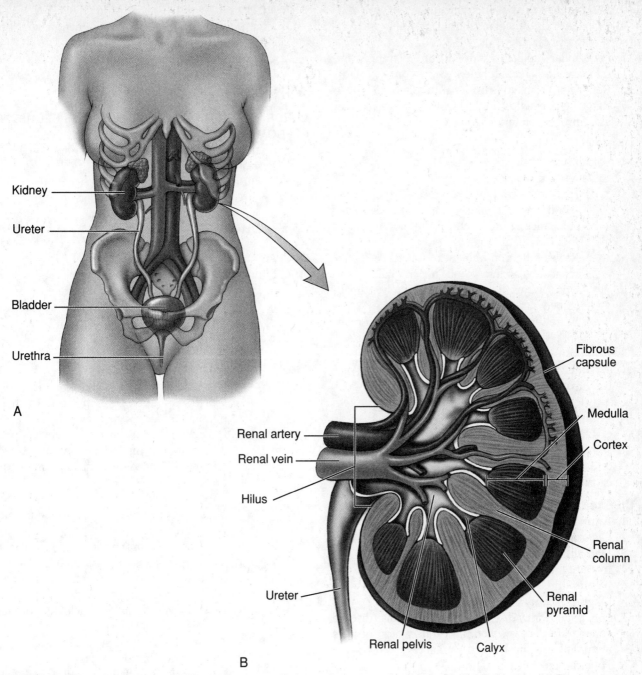

FIGURE 2-35. The urinary system. **A,** The major organs. **B,** Internal structure of a kidney. (Herlihy B, Maebius N: *The human body in health and illness,* ed 2, Philadelphia, 2003, Saunders.)

f) Collecting tubule: tubule formed by union of distal convoluted tubules; convoluted tubules join to form one renal pyramid; pyramids join to form calyx

2. Ureter
   a. Tube that runs from kidneys into urinary bladder
   b. Renal pelvis narrows as it leaves kidney to form ureter

3. Urinary bladder
   a. Muscular sac located behind symphysis pubis
   b. Capable of great expansion caused by folds (rugae) in its inner lining
   c. Serves as temporary storage place for urine

4. Urethra
   a. Tube that carries urine from the bladder to the outside of the body
   b. Opening to outside is urinary meatus

D. BLOOD FLOW TO KIDNEYS

1. Renal artery: enters kidney at hilum
2. Afferent arteriole: enters Bowman's capsule

3. Glomerulus: network of capillaries
4. Efferent arteriole: comes from glomerulus and exits Bowman's capsule
5. Peritubular capillaries: extend from efferent arteriole; surrounds renal tubule
6. Renal venule: extends from peritubular capillaries
7. Renal vein: extends from renal venule; exits kidney at hilum; joins inferior vena cava

E. URINE

1. Formation
   a. Series of three processes:
      1) Filtration: continuous process; glomerular blood pressure causes water and dissolved substances to filter out of the glomeruli and into Bowman's capsule
      2) Reabsorption: movement of substances out of renal tubules into blood in peritubular capillaries; water, nutrients, and electrolytes reabsorbed
      3) Secretion: movement of substances not reabsorbed into urine into collecting tubules
2. Composition
   a. Water: 95% of urine
   b. Nitrogenous waste products: urea, ammonia, uric acid, and creatinine (end products of protein metabolism)
   c. Electrolytes: sodium, potassium, phosphate, sulfates, ammonium, bicarbonate, and chloride
   d. Toxins
   e. Pigment: urochrome

F. DISEASES AND DISORDERS

1. Anuria: no urine produced
2. Glycosuria: glucose in the urine
3. Hematuria: blood in the urine
4. Incontinence: voiding urine involuntarily
5. Nephrolithiasis (renal calculi): kidney stones
6. Oliguria: scanty urine output
7. Polycystic kidney disease: collecting tubular disease characterized by swollen, fluid-filled sacs; tubules are unable to empty into the renal pelvis
8. Polyuria: excessive urination
9. Proteinuria: protein in the urine
10. Renal failure: kidneys fail to function; may be chronic or acute
11. Urinary tract infection (UTI): mostly caused by gram-negative bacteria; can occur in any organ in the tract

XV. Endocrine System

A. GENERAL

1. Body's slower-acting control system
2. Made up of glands that secrete substances (hormones)
3. Hormones travel through the bloodstream to target organs and cells

B. FUNCTIONS

1. Control: regulates internal body functions and processes
2. Communication: complements the nervous system; directs communication among the body systems for optimum functioning

C. HORMONES: CHEMICAL SUBSTANCES SECRETED FROM ENDOCRINE GLANDS

1. Tropic hormones: stimulate other endocrine glands to secrete their hormones
2. Sex hormones: stimulate reproductive tissue
3. Anabolic hormones: stimulate cells to grow and repair
4. Prostaglandins: tissue hormones that regulate cellular activity

D. GLANDS (see Figure 2-36)

1. Pituitary gland: master gland; hypophysis
   a. Located on inferior surface of the brain
   b. Connected to hypothalamus by stalk (infundibulum)
   c. Divided into two sections:
      1) Anterior hypophysis (adenohypophysis) (see Figure 2-37); secretes:
         a) Growth hormones (GH): promotes tissue growth; stimulates fat metabolism; helps maintain blood glucose levels
         b) Prolactin (PRL): promotes development of breast and milk secretion; works with luteinizing hormone during menstrual cycle
         c) Thyroid-stimulating hormone (TSH): stimulates development and hormone production of thyroid gland
         d) Adrenocorticotropic hormone (ACTH): stimulates development and hormone production of adrenal cortex
         e) Follicle-stimulating hormone (FSH)
            ▪ In female: stimulates follicle development and secretion of estrogen
            ▪ In male: stimulates sperm production
         f) Luteinizing hormone (LH)
            ▪ In female: stimulates secretion of estrogen and progesterone
            ▪ In male: stimulates secretion of testosterone
         g) Melanocyte-stimulating hormone (MSH): regulates normal color of skin; helps regulate adrenal gland's response to ACTH
      2) Posterior pituitary (neurohypophysis):
         a) Does not manufacture hormones
         b) Stores and releases hormones made in hypothalamus
            ▪ Antidiuretic hormone (ADH): prevents excessive formation of urine
            ▪ Oxytocin: stimulates the uterus to contract during childbirth; causes letdown of milk

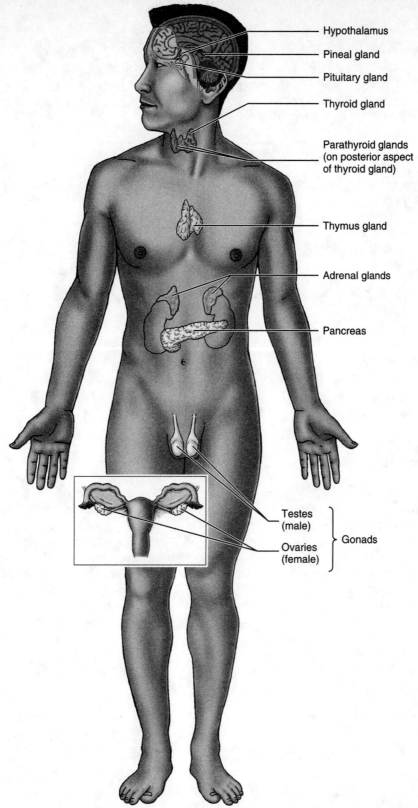

FIGURE 2-36.   Major endocrine glands of the body. (Herlihy B, Maebius N: *The human body in health and illness,* ed 2, Philadelphia, 2003, Saunders.)

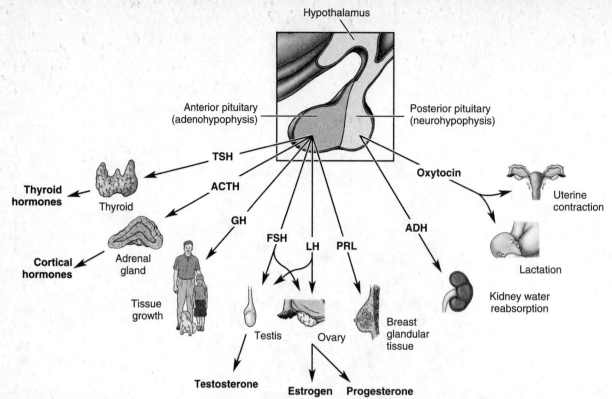

FIGURE 2-37. Pituitary gland. Hormones secreted by the anterior and posterior pituitary glands; also shows the target organs. (Herlihy B, Maebius N: *The human body in health and illness,* ed 2, Philadelphia, 2003, Saunders.)

2. Pineal gland
   a. Pinecone-shaped gland located behind the hypothalamus
   b. Produces melatonin that regulates the body's *"biological clock"*
3. Thyroid gland
   a. Butterfly-shaped gland located in the neck, lateral and anterior to the trachea
   b. Secretes two hormones:
      1) Thyroxine (tetraiodothyronine [T-4]) and triiodothyronine (T-3); regulates metabolism of the body; needs iodine for synthesis
      2) Calcitonin: stimulates movement of calcium from the blood to the bone
4. Parathyroid gland
   a. Four pea-shaped glands embedded in the thyroid gland
   b. Secretes parathormone (PTH), which causes calcium to leave bone and enter the bloodstream
5. Adrenal glands
   a. Located on top of each kidney
   b. Composed of two regions:
      1) Adrenal cortex: outer region: secretes corticosteroids
         a) Aldosterone: regulates mineral salts
         b) Cortisol: regulates blood pressure
         c) Androgen and estrogen: minor sex hormones

      2) Adrenal medulla: inner region: secretes hormones that are important in the sympathetic and parasympathetic nervous system
         a) Epinephrine
         b) Norepinephrine
6. Pancreas
   a. Elongated gland that extends posterior to stomach
   b. Produces glucagon; from alpha cells; stimulates conversion of glycogen to glucose in liver
   c. Produces insulin; from beta cells; decreases glucose levels in blood
   d. Produces somatostatin; from delta cells; regulates other pancreatic cells
7. Gonads
   a. Testes in male: secrete testosterone, which stimulates the development of male sex characteristics
   b. Ovaries in female
      1) Secrete estrogen: from follicles; stimulates development of female sex characteristics
      2) Secrete progesterone: from corpus luteum; maintains a pregnancy
8. Thymus
   a. Located in mediastinum below sternum
   b. Largest in children; atrophies during adolescence
   c. Produces thymosin; stimulates T-lymphocytes for immunity
9. Placenta: produces human chorionic gonadotropin (HCG) during pregnancy

E. DISEASES AND DISORDERS

1. Acromegaly: hypersecretion of GH after puberty
2. Addison's disease: hyposecretion of cortisol; characterized by hypotension and increased skin pigmentation
3. Cretinism: hypothyroidism caused by hyposecretion of thyroxine during infancy; characterized by slow growth, impaired intelligence, and delayed development of secondary sex characteristics
4. Cushing's syndrome: hypersecretion of cortisol; characterized by *"moon face"*, acne, fatty deposits on upper back
5. Diabetes insipidus: hyposecretion of ADH; characterized by polyuria and polydipsia
6. Diabetes mellitus: hyperglycemia; hyposecretion of insulin; characterized by polyuria, polyphagia, and polydipsia
7. Dwarfism: hyposecretion of GH; characterized by abnormally small size
8. Giantism: hypersecretion of GH; characterized by abnormally large size
9. Goiter: enlargement of thyroid gland; caused by iodine deficiency
10. Grave's disease: hyperthyroidism caused by hypersecretion of thyroxine; characterized by weight loss, exophthalmia, nervousness, diaphoresis, and heat intolerance
11. Myxedema: hyposecretion of thyroxine later in life; characterized by fatigue, weight gain, and cold intolerance

XVI. Reproductive System

A. GENERAL

1. Produces offspring for the survival of the species

B. FUNCTIONS

1. Production of egg and sperm cells
2. Nurturing of developing offspring
3. Production of hormones

C. ORGANS AND STRUCTURES OF THE MALE SYSTEM (see Figure 2-38)

1. Testes
   a. Essential organs (gonads)
   b. Produces sperm (male gamete)
   c. Glandular structures located outside of the body in the scrotum
   d. Made up of seminiferous tubules (sperm development) and interstitial cells (produces testosterone)
2. Epididymis
   a. Continuation of seminiferous tubules
   b. Lies on the superior surface of the testes
   c. Secretes part of seminal fluid
3. Vas deferens
   a. Extension of the epididymis
   b. Passes through the inguinal canal into the abdominal cavity; arches over the bladder and joins the seminal vesicles

c. Site of male sterilization (vasectomy)
4. Seminal vesicles
   a. Bilateral pouches behind the urinary bladder
   b. Secrete a nutrient-rich fluid that nourishes sperm
5. Ejaculatory duct
   a. Formed by the union of the vas deferens and seminal vesicles
   b. Passes through the prostate gland and enters the urethra
   c. Propels sperm and seminal fluid into the urethra during orgasm
6. Prostate gland
   a. Doughnut-shaped gland that encircles the base of the urethra on the posterior surface of the bladder
   b. Secretes an alkaline fluid that protects the sperm from the acidity of the vagina
7. Bulbourethral gland (Cowper's gland)
   a. Pea-shaped glands located on both sides of the urethra
   b. Secretes lubrication during intercourse
8. Scrotum
   a. Pouch of skin suspended from the perineal area
   b. Holds the testes and epididymis
   c. Keeps the testes away from the body; body temperature is too high for sperm production
9. Penis
   a. External male genitalia
   b. Composed of three cylinders of erectile tissue
   c. During sexual arousal, erectile tissue fills with blood and becomes erect
   d. Contains the urethra
   e. Distal end covered by the prepuce (foreskin), which is removed by circumcision

D. ORGANS AND STRUCTURES OF THE FEMALE SYSTEM (see Figure 2-39)

1. Ovaries
   a. Essential organs (gonads)
   b. Produce ova (female gamete)
   c. Almond-shaped glands located in the pelvic cavity
   d. Contain ovarian (Graafian) follicles where ova develop
   e. Produce estrogen and progesterone
2. Uterus
   a. Pear-shaped muscular organ located in the pelvic cavity between the bladder and rectum
   b. Three divisions:
      1) Fundus: upper region
      2) Body: large central region
      3) Cervix: lower neck region; opens to vagina
   c. Three layers:
      1) Endometrium: inner layer; the fertilized ovum implants and grows here; shed monthly (menstruation; menses)
      2) Myometrium: middle muscular layer
      3) Perimetrium (epimetrium): outer layer
   d. Contracts to deliver the fetus

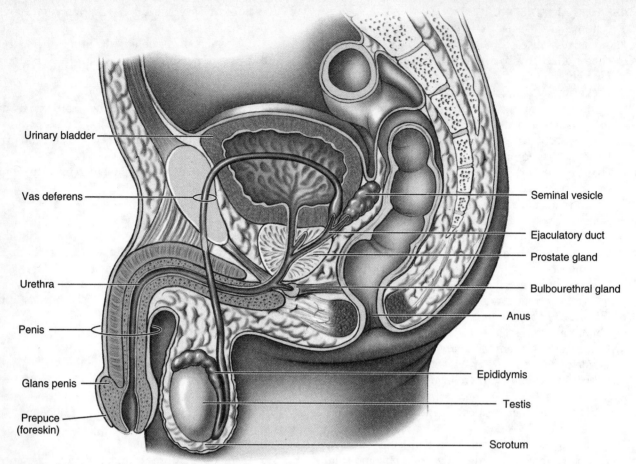

FIGURE 2-38.   Male reproductive organs. (Herlihy B, Maebius N: *The human body in health and illness,* ed 2, Philadelphia, 2003, Saunders.)

3. Fallopian tubes (oviducts)
   a. Attached to the upper, outer sides of uterus
   b. Serve as the site of fertilization; the fertilized ovum travels through the tube into the uterus for implantation
   c. Distal ends contain finger-like structures (fimbriae); gentle movement of fimbriae draws the ovum into the tube after release from the ovary
   d. Site of female sterilization (tubal ligation)
4. Vagina
   a. Tubular structure that extends from cervix to the outside
   b. Located between the rectum and urethra
   c. Capable of great expansion
   d. Serves as the birth canal and means of shedding menstrual tissues
5. Vulva
   a. External genitalia
   b. Includes:
      1) Mons pubis: fat pad that covers the symphysis pubis
      2) Labia majora: two large folds of skin extending from the mons pubis to the anus
      3) Labia minora: two small folds of skin medial to the labia majora
      4) Clitoris: small nodule of erectile tissue superior to the labia majora; plays a role in sexual arousal
      5) Bartholin glands: located at the entrance to the vagina; secretes lubricating fluid during intercourse
6. Perineum: region between the vaginal opening and the rectum; may be cut or torn during childbirth (episiotomy)
7. Breasts
   a. Mammary glands
   b. Fatty tissue and milk glands that overlie the pectoral muscles
   c. Produces milk (lactation) for offspring
   d. Nipple is protrusion for delivery of milk
   e. Areola is dark area that surrounds nipple

E. REPRODUCTIVE CYCLE
1. Ovarian cycle: ovum develops and matures in the ovary
2. Menstrual cycle
   a. Menses: days 1 to 5; if the ovum is not fertilized, the endometrium is shed
   b. Postmenstrual: days 6 to 13; the endometrium thickens as the ovum matures in the ovary; estrogen levels increase

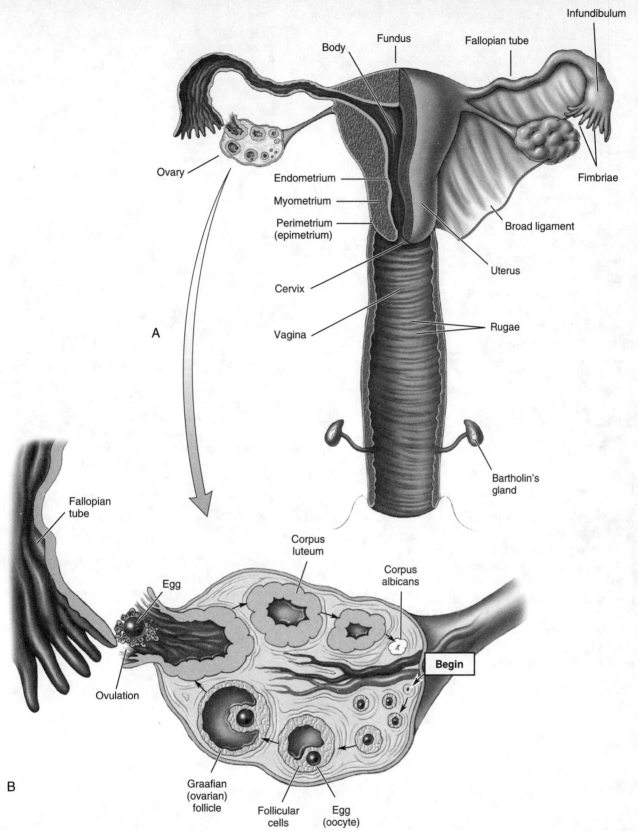

FIGURE 2-39. **A,** Female reproductive organs. **B,** Maturation of the ovarian follicle. (Herlihy B, Maebius N: *The human body in health and illness,* ed 2, Philadelphia, 2003, Saunders.)

c. Ovulation: day 14; the mature ovum is released from the ovary

d. Premenstrual: days 15 to 28; the corpus luteum develops on the ovary where the ovum was released and secretes progesterone; endometrium thickens in preparation for a fertilized ovum

F. PREGNANCY

1. Ovulation: release of ovum
2. Insemination: sperm are released into the vagina and travel through the cervix and uterus into the Fallopian tube
3. Conception: union of sperm and egg; occurs in the Fallopian tube; results in a zygote with 46 chromosomes (23 from ovum, 23 from sperm)
4. Zygote divides and implants in the uterine wall; becomes an embryo at the third week of development until the end of the eighth week; becomes a fetus at the ninth week until birth
5. Placenta: highly vascular disk-shaped organ; develops from embryonic and maternal tissues; attaches the developing fetus to the uterus; performs nutrition, excretory, and respiratory functions; excretes HCG for continued pregnancy
6. Gestation: lasts approximately 40 weeks; three 3-month trimesters
7. Parturition: childbirth; occurs in three stages:
   a. Onset of contractions to cervical dilation (10 centimeters)
   b. Dilation to birth of the fetus
   c. Expulsion of the placenta

G. DISEASES AND DISORDERS

1. Abortion: termination of a pregnancy; can be spontaneous (miscarriage) or therapeutic
2. Abruptio placenta: placenta prematurely separates from uterine wall
3. Amenorrhea: absence of menstruation
4. Benign prostatic hypertrophy (BPH): abnormal growth of prostatic cells causing enlargement of gland
5. Cryptorchism: undescended testes; testes remain in abdomen
6. Dysmenorrhea: painful menstruation
7. Dyspareunia: painful intercourse
8. Eclampsia (toxemia): serious condition of pregnancy characterized by hypertension, edema, and proteinuria; if untreated, may result in seizures and coma
9. Ectopic pregnancy: implantation of fertilized ovum outside of uterus; usually in the Fallopian tube
10. Endometriosis: growth of endometrial tissue outside of the uterus, usually within the pelvic cavity
11. Hydrocele: accumulation of fluid in the scrotum
12. Hyperemesis gravidarum: excessive vomiting during pregnancy
13. Hypospadias: abnormal congenital opening of the urethra on the underside of the penis
14. Impotence: inability to develop or sustain an erection
15. Orchitis: inflammation of the testes
16. Ovarian cyst: solid or fluid-filled cyst found on the ovary
17. Pelvic inflammatory disease (PID): acute or chronic infection of the female reproductive tract
18. Placenta previa: placenta implants over the cervix
19. Premenstrual syndrome (PMS): various symptoms that occur before the menstrual period; can include fatigue, irritability, depression, swollen and tender breasts, edema, and/or cramping
20. Prostatitis: inflammation of the prostate
21. Sexually transmitted disease (STD)
    a. Trichomoniasis: parasitic infection caused by *Trichomonas vaginalis*
    b. Gonorrhea: bacterial infection caused by *Neisseria gonorrhea*
    c. Syphilis: bacterial infection caused by *Treponema pallidum*
    d. Genital herpes: viral infection caused by herpes simplex virus type 2
    e. Genital warts: growths caused by human papillomavirus
    f. Chlamydia: bacterial infection caused by *Chlamydia trachomatis*

Law and Ethics 3

I. Introduction to the Law

A. DEFINITION OF LAW
1. System by which society gives order to our lives

B. FUNCTIONS OF LAW
1. Regulate: controls rules and standards
2. Punish: enforce penalties for infractions of rules and standards
3. Remedy: make wrongs that are committed right
4. Benefit: help society

C. SOURCES OF LAW
1. Common law: derived from the customs of society and court decisions
2. Administrative law: derived from agencies that enact state and federal law
3. Constitutional law: derived from the U.S. Constitution
4. Statutory law: derived from state and federal legislation

D. TYPES OF LAW
1. Civil law: a wrong, or perceived wrong, committed against a person or to property; civil law that affects the practice of medicine include:
   a. Contract law: governs enforceable promises
   b. Tort law: governs intentional or accidental acts that bring harm to a person or that damage property
   c. Administrative law: governs regulations set forth by governmental agencies
2. Criminal law: a wrong committed against a person or to property in violation of a statute or ordinance; criminal laws that may affect the practice of medicine include:
   a. Infraction: a minor offense that usually results only in a fine
   b. Misdemeanor: violation of a law that includes as punishment a maximum imprisonment of no more than 1 year
   c. Felony: a major crime that includes as punishment imprisonment of more than 1 year

II. Licensure, Registration, Certification

A. LICENSURE
1. Strongest form of administrative regulation
2. Mandatory credential to practice medicine
3. Granted by a state board; verifies that the person holding the license has met minimum standards; for physicians, defined by the Medical Practice Act; for licensed nurses, defined and governed by the Nurse Practice Act
   a. State statute that defines what is included in the practice of medicine within that state
   b. Governs the methods and requirements of licensure and establishes grounds for suspension and revocation of the license
4. Physicians can be licensed through:
   a. Examination: passing a written and/or oral examination
   b. Endorsement: acceptance of a national examination score
   c. Reciprocity: one state accepts another state's license
5. Licenses may be revoked or suspended for:
   a. Conviction of a misdemeanor or a felony
   b. Unprofessional conduct
   c. Personal or professional incapacity
6. License must be periodically renewed (if not renewed, will be suspended from practice)

B. REGISTRATION
1. Medical assistants can be registered
2. Voluntary process
3. Professional listed on a state or national registry
4. Process similar to certification
5. Usually accomplished by a written examination

C. CERTIFICATION
1. Medical assistants can be certified
2. Voluntary process

3. Identifies a professional as meeting minimum standards to be able to practice
4. Usually accomplished by written examination
5. Governed by a professional organization

III. Regulating Issues for the Medical Office

A. CLIA '88
1. Clinical Laboratory Improvement Acts of 1988
2. Identifies standards for laboratory testing
3. Any facility performing laboratory testing is subject to CLIA regulations

B. CON
1. Certificate of need
2. Process of acquiring approval, based on need to the community, to expand service

C. JCAHO
1. Joint Commission on Accreditation of Healthcare Organizations
2. Accreditation of health care facilities

D. OSHA
1. Occupational Safety and Health Administration
2. Regulation of safety in the workplace

E. ADA
1. Americans with Disabilities Act
2. Sets up rules protecting people with physical or mental disability from being discriminated against

F. HIPAA
1. Health Insurance Portability and Accountability Act
2. Standards for privacy of individually identifiable health information
3. Allows the flow of health information while protecting the privacy of patients

IV. Consent

A. DEFINITION OF CONSENT
1. Voluntary permission given by a capable person to receive medical care

B. TYPES
1. Express: oral or written expression of consent
2. Implied: actions or behavior that can be reasonably presumed to express consent

C. INFORMED CONSENT
1. Physician, or other caregiver, has an affirmative duty to explain to the patient information necessary to allow the patient to evaluate the medical care and make decisions on that information before having the medical care performed; implies an understanding of:
   a. What procedure is to be done
   b. Why the procedure should be done
   c. The risks involved in performing the procedure

d. The expected benefits of having the procedure performed
   e. Any alternative treatments that can be performed
   f. The risks involved in performing the alternative treatment

D. WHO MAY AND MAY NOT GIVE CONSENT
1. Persons who are mentally competent and of the age of majority can give consent
2. A parent, legal guardian, or someone legally charged with standing in place of the parent or guardian, can give consent for a minor (a minor is a person not yet of legal age, which is often 18); consent can legally be given by a minor under the following circumstances:
   a. Minor serving in the armed forces
   b. Emancipated minor
   c. Testing for sexually transmitted diseases
   d. Seeking contraception or abortion
3. Living will
   a. Also known as an *advanced directive*
   b. Authorizes in advance the withholding of artificial life-support methods in case of terminal illness or accident
   c. Encouraged by the Patient Self-Determination Act of 1990
4. Uniform Anatomical Gift Act of 1968: allows for competent adults to give their body or body parts in the event of their death for research, transplantation, or placement in a tissue bank
5. Persons who are *non compos mentis* ("not of sound mind") cannot give consent, and these persons require some form of guardianship to give consent
6. In emergencies, consent to treatment is implied only as long as the emergency exists; the Good Samaritan Act provides immunity from liability to non-negligent volunteers at the scene of an accident
7. Mentally competent persons have the right to refuse medical treatment (refused consent)
   a. Patient's refusal must be documented
   b. Patient must sign a document *(release)* absolving the caregiver of liability for not giving treatment
   c. Patient's *refused consent* can be overruled by a court of competent jurisdiction
8. Consent obtained by fraudulent means or misrepresentations is not binding
9. Without proper consent for treatment, a caregiver may be charged with:
   a. Assault: intentional, unlawful attempt of bodily injury to another by force
   b. Battery: willful and unlawful use of force or violence (or touching) on another person

V. Contracts

A. GENERAL
1. An agreement creating an obligation
2. Can be oral or written, expressed or implied

B. EXPRESS CONTRACT

1. Agreement between two or more parties
2. Contains the explicit terms of the agreement either orally or in writing

C. IMPLIED CONTRACT

1. Conclusion drawn from the actions of two or more parties
2. Patient-physician contract is implied

D. NECESSARY ELEMENTS OF A CONTRACT

1. Offer: one party makes an offer
2. Acceptance: another party agrees to the offer made
3. Consideration: mutual exchange of something of value between the parties
4. Capacity: all parties must be legally able to make the offer and to accept the terms
5. Legality: legal in nature and not against public policy

E. PATIENT AND PHYSICIAN CONTRACT MAY BE TERMINATED BY:

1. Patient: circumstances need to be fully documented in chart
2. Physician
   a. Must give patient notice (abandonment)
   b. Physician writes a certified letter with return receipt; copy in patient's record
   c. Letter should include:
      1) Reasons why care is being discontinued
      2) Assurance that physician will turn over patient records as directed
      3) Notice that patient should seek alternative care as soon as possible

VI. Torts

A. DEFINITION OF A TORT

1. An act, intentional or accidental, that brings harm against another person or damage to another person's property

B. NEGLIGENCE

1. Unintentional (accidental) tort
2. Characterized by commission of an act that an ordinary, reasonable, and prudent person would not have done or omission of an act that an ordinary, reasonable, and prudent person, would have done:
   a. Forms of negligence:
      1) Nonfeasance: failure to act when there was a duty to act causing or resulting in harm
      2) Misfeasance: improper performance of an act causing or resulting in harm
      3) Malfeasance: performance of an improper or unlawful act causing or resulting in harm
      4) Malpractice: negligence of a professional person, with the action or inaction compared with an ordinary, reasonable, and prudent professional

   b. *Four Ds* of negligence
      1) Duty: exists when a patient-physician relationship has been established
      2) Derelict: neglect of professional obligation
      3) Direct cause: injury was directly caused by the physician's poor actions or by the physician's failure to act
      4) Damages: harm resulting to the patient—three types:
         a) Nominal: the damage exists in name only; token compensation
         b) Compensatory: actual damages suffered by the patient because of the physician's negligence
         c) Punitive: damages above the actual damage suffered by the patient; to punish the physician for the negligent act

C. *RES IPSA LOQUITUR*

1. Meaning: "the thing speaks for itself"
2. Describes a situation in which the nature of the injury implicates negligence

D. INTENTIONAL TORTS

1. Assault: deliberate threat to make bodily contact
2. Battery: intentional physical contact
3. Abandonment: one-sided termination of the patient-physician relationship by the physician without proper notice to the patient
4. Invasion of privacy: giving out patient information without patient consent
5. Defamation: injury to a person's reputation caused by a false statement by another person
6. Libel: false or malicious writing against another person
7. Slander: false or malicious oral statement against another person
8. False imprisonment: unlawful restraint, or holding, of an individual against his or her will
9. Fraud: intentional misrepresentation that might cause harm

E. PRODUCT LIABILITY

1. Liability of a manufacturer of products for injuries caused by defect of those products

F. VICARIOUS LIABILITY

1. *Respondeat superior* (meaning: "let the master answer")
2. Employers are liable for the conduct of their employees while the employees are performing within the scope of their employment

VII. Business Law

A. EMPLOYMENT PRACTICES

1. National Labor Relations Act of 1935 (NLRA): defines unfair labor practices land provides hearing or mediation of complaints

2. Fair Labor Standards Act of 1938 (FLSA): defines minimum wage, equal pay for equal work, and child labor restrictions
3. Equal Pay Act of 1963 (EPA): amendment of FLSA that addresses wage disparities based on sex
4. Equal Employment Opportunity Act of 1972 (EEOA): prohibits employment discrimination based on age, race, color, religion, sex, or national origin
5. Age Discrimination in Employment Act of 1967 (ADEA): prohibits discrimination based on age
6. Americans with Disabilities Act of 1990 (ADA): prohibits discrimination against persons with physical or mental disabilities
7. Workers' compensation laws: state-mandated programs to provide wage continuation and medical treatment compensation for persons with work-related injuries and/or illnesses

B. SEXUAL HARASSMENT
1. *Quid pro quo* ("something for something"); conditions of employment (raise, promotion) are based on a person's acceptance or rejection of unwelcome sexual conduct
2. Hostile work environment: creation of an intimidating, offensive, or hostile workplace resulting from unwelcome sexual conduct; interferes with a person's ability to perform job functions

C. PAYROLL
1. FLSA requires all employee records of hours worked to be continuously maintained
2. Federal Insurance Contributions Act (FICA): Social Security Tax; applied toward old-age benefits
3. Federal Unemployment Tax Act (FUTA): tax to provide income during unemployment
4. Payroll reports and forms
    a. Form 944: Employer's Quarterly Federal Tax Return; filed each 3 months, with payment of quarterly tax due
    b. Form 8109: Federal Tax Deposit Book; used to pay FICA and federal income tax
    c. Form W-2: Wage and Tax Statement; given to employees yearly, itemizing the wages earned and all taxes deducted from wages for that year
    d. Form W-3: Transmittal of Income and Tax Statement; submitted to Social Security Administration; compares W-2 forms with Form 941
    e. Form W-4: Employee's Withholding Allowance Certificate; employee decides the number of withholding allowances for the company to take out of wages earned, based on the number of dependents claimed

VIII. Public Health Duties

A. GENERAL
1. States require physicians to report certain information

2. Reported information helps to provide for the health, safety, and welfare of the public

B. BIRTHS
1. Birth certificate completed by birth attendant

C. DEATHS
1. Death certificate completed by physician in attendance
2. Medical examiner must be called in cases of:
    a. Violent or criminal activity death
    b. Death without a physician present
    c. Death from undetermined cause
    d. Death within 24 hours of admission to a hospital or health care facility
    e. Death without prior medical care

D. COMMUNICABLE DISEASES
1. Communicated to county health department
2. Includes smallpox, scarlet fever, rubella, measles, tuberculosis, plague, cholera, and sexually transmitted diseases

E. NATIONAL CHILDHOOD VACCINE INJURY ACT
1. Requires providers who administer vaccines to report the following information to public health agencies:
    a. Date the vaccine was administered
    b. Lot number and manufacturer of vaccine
    c. Any adverse reactions to the vaccine
    d. Name, title, and address of the person administering the vaccine

F. NEWBORN DISEASES
1. Inborn errors of metabolism (e.g., phenylketonuria [PKU])

G. ABUSE
1. If suspected by the provider, the provider has the legal duty to report suspected abuse to the authorities
2. Medical assistants are also considered *mandatory reporters*
3. Types of abuse to be reported:
    a. Child abuse
    b. Spouse or domestic abuse
    c. Elder abuse
    d. Drug abuse
    e. Patient abuse in hospital and nursing homes

H. CRIMINAL ACTS
1. When identified by the provider, the provider has the legal duty to report suspected criminal acts to authorities
2. Types of criminal acts to be reported:
    a. Injuries by weapons
    b. Assault
    c. Attempted suicide
    d. Rape (may require a release by the victim because of confidentiality)

IX. Introduction to Ethics

A. GENERAL
1. A set of moral principles or values
2. Concerns the thoughts, judgments, and actions on issues that have greater implications of moral right and wrong

B. DUTIES
1. Obligations and/or committments to act in certain ways
2. Includes:
   a. Nonmalfeasance: not doing any harm
   b. Beneficence: acting to create good
   c. Fidelity: meeting the patient's expectations through respect, competence, adherence to laws, and honoring agreements
   d. Veracity: telling the truth
   e. Justice: sharing of benefits and burdens

C. RIGHTS
1. Claims made on a person or society
2. Correlated with duties

D. VIRTUES
1. Character traits that make a person act in a certain way
2. Principles are written in the form of a Code of Ethics

X. American Association of Medical Assistants (AAMA) Code of Ethics

A. GENERAL
1. As agent of physician, the medical assistant is governed by ethical standards
2. Decisions made in practice should be based on the professional nature of the professional and scope of practice
3. Code of Ethics is standard for all medical assistants to honor
4. Patterned after the American Medical Association (AMA) Code of Ethics
5. *Never* practice medicine; do not identify themselves as a "nurse"

XI. AMA Code of Ethics

A. GENERAL
1. Written code of conduct for medical practice
2. Includes four components:
   a. Principles of medical ethics
   b. Fundamental elements of the patient-physician relationship
   c. Current opinions with annotation
   d. Reports of the Council of Ethical and Judicial Affairs; includes opinions on:
      1) Abortion: not prohibited by ethical standards
      2) Abuse: legal and ethical requirement to report
      3) Allocation of health resources: the physician must remain a patient advocate and allow institutional procedures to determine allocation
      4) Artificial insemination: requires informed consent; deals with who has parental rights
      5) Clinical investigation: the patient-physician relationship does not exist in clinical investigation
      6) Cost: quality of patient care should be the physician's first consideration, not cost
      7) Provision of adequate health care: an adequate level of health care for all persons
      8) Genetic counseling: concerns for the quality of life
      9) Organ donation: the donor should not receive payment for organ donation; involves protection of the right to privacy for both donor and recipient
      10) Quality of life: primary consideration of what is best for the patient
      11) Withholding or withdrawing life-prolonging treatment: the physician must be committed to saving life and relieving suffering; the patient may have his or her wishes known
      12) Euthanasia: incompatible with the physician's role

XII. Professional Relationships

A. HOSPITAL RELATIONS
1. Privileges granted based on competence and experience, not fees

B. ADVERTISING
1. Only restrictions are those that protect the public from deceptive practices; physicians can advertise fees, identification of educational background, and specialty, but physicians cannot include any statements as to the quality of their services

C. COMMUNICATION WITH THE MEDIA
1. Physician may not discuss a patient's condition with the press (unless a release has been granted); may release only authorized information that is in the public domain (births, deaths, accidents, and police cases)

D. COMPUTERS
1. The AMA has developed guidelines for the use and sharing of computerized information

E. FEES AND CHARGES
1. Physician may not split patient fees with another physician for patient referral (fee splitting)
2. Physician's staff should assist in completing insurance forms without charge
3. Physician may request that the patient make payment at the time treatment is rendered
4. Insurance co-payments may be waived or written off if access of care is threatened by inability to pay the co-payment
5. Professional courtesy is a tradition

F. PHYSICIAN'S RECORDS

1. Physician owns the notes prepared by him or her while treating a patient
2. Original medical records may not be released; records can be reproduced only on the physician's death, retirement, or sale of the physician's practice

XIII. Professional Rights and Responsibilities

A. DISCIPLINE

1. Physician should expose dishonest, corrupt, incompetent, or unethical colleagues

B. FREE CHOICE

1. Physician in private practice may decline to accept any individual as a patient

C. PATENT

1. Physicians may patent any device that he or she discovers or invents

D. PATIENT–PHYSICIAN RELATIONSHIP

1. Both parties are free to enter into, or decline to enter into, the relationship

E. INFECTIOUS DISEASE

1. Physician who is infected with an infectious disease should not engage in any patient contact or activity that may create a risk for the patient

F. SUBSTANCE ABUSE

1. Physician should not practice under the influence of any controlled substance, of alcohol, or of chemical agents that impair the ability to render treatment

HIPAA 4

I. Definition

A. HEALTH INSURANCE PORTABILITY AND ACCOUNTABILITY ACT (HIPAA)

1. Involved with privacy, security, and claims issues in the health care system
2. Issues identified by state and federal agencies
3. Failure to comply with mandates can lead to sanctions and fines
4. Enacted in 1996
5. Two provisions:
   a. Title I : Insurance Reform
   b. Title II : Administrative Simplification
6. Long-term benefits of HIPAA include:
   a. Lower administrative costs
   b. Increased accuracy of data
   c. Increased patient and customer satisfaction

II. Title I: Health Insurance Reform

A. GENERAL

1. Provision of continuous insurance coverage for workers and their insured when the worker changes or loses a job
2. Limits use of preexisting condition exclusions
3. Prohibits discrimination for past or present poor health
4. Guarantees individuals the right to purchase gap health insurance coverage after losing a job
5. Allows renewal of health insurance coverage regardless of an individual's health condition

III. Title II: Administrative Simplification

A. GENERAL

1. Focuses on the health care setting
2. Intended to reduce administrative costs
3. Accomplished by standardizing the exchange of health care data
4. Includes provisions to ensure the privacy and security of an individual's health data

5. Standardization of electronic transmissions will reduce the number of forms and methods used in claims processing
6. Two parts to this provision include:
   a. Development and implementation of standardized electronic transactions using common sets of descriptors (code sets)
   b. Implementation of privacy and security procedures to prevent the misuse of health information and ensure confidentiality

IV. Roles and Relationships

A. GENERAL

1. Department of Health and Human Services (HHS): establishes and implements standards
2. Centers for Medicare and Medicaid (CMS): enforces insurance portability and code set requirements of HIPAA
3. Office of Civil Rights (OCR): enforces privacy standards
4. Covered entity: may be a health plan (e.g., Blue Cross/Blue Shield), health care clearinghouse, or health care provider
5. Electronic media: mode of electronic transmission; may include the Internet, extranet, telephone lines, fax modems, or disks or magnetic tape
6. Transaction: transmission of information between two parties; can include:
   a. Health care claims
   b. Health care payments
   c. Coordination of benefits
   d. Claim status
   e. Enrollment and disenrollment in a health plan
   f. Eligibility for a health plan
   g. Premium payments
   h. Referral certification or authorization
   i. First report of injury

V. Privacy Rule

A. GENERAL

1. Privacy: condition of being secluded from the view or presence of others
2. Confidentiality: use of discretion in keeping information private
3. Disclosure: release, transfer, access to, and/or divulgence of information
4. Individually identifiable health information (IIHI): any part of an individual's health information collected from an individual (e.g., demographic information, date of birth)
5. Protected health information (PHI): IIHI that is transmitted by electronic media, maintained in electronic form, or transmitted or maintained in any other form or medium; all patient information is protected regardless of the way it is maintained; includes paper records, computerized practice management or billing systems, spoken words, and x-ray films
6. Use: sharing, application, use, examination, or analysis of IHII; PHI is protected both inside and outside of the organization unless the use is specifically required or permitted

VI. Patient Rights Under HIPAA

A. RIGHT TO NOTICE OF PRIVACY PRACTICES

1. Patients are entitled to receive written notice of privacy practices (NPP) from the provider at the first appointment
2. NPP outlines patient's rights
3. Must be written in plain language; staff should obtain signature acknowledging receipt
4. Can be done at front desk

B. RIGHT TO REQUEST RESTRICTIONS ON CERTAIN USES AND DISCLOSURES OF PHI

1. Patient has right to ask for restrictions on how the office will use and disclose PHI
2. Restrictions must be agreed on by the office; if agreed, restrictions must be documented and followed
3. Practice may disclose confidential information without written authorization, such as communicable diseases, victims of abuse, and law enforcement purposes
4. Patient may identify any other person whom information may be disclosed or not disclosed

C. RIGHT TO REQUEST CONFIDENTIAL COMMUNICATION

1. Patient can request to receive confidential communication by alternative means or alternative location (call patient at work instead of home; test results sent in writing instead of over the telephone)
2. Office must accommodate reasonable requests
3. Requests may be required in writing

D. RIGHT TO ACCESS PHI

1. Patient has the right to access, inspect, and obtain a copy of his or her PHI
2. Request must be made in writing
3. Request must be acted on within 30 days
4. Reasonable fee for copies and postage may be applied
5. Patients do not have the right to access psychotherapy notes, information compiled for use in legal proceedings, or information exempted under the Clinical Laboratory Improvement Acts of 1988 (CLIA)
6. If health care provider has determined that the patient may be endangered by accessing information, access may be denied
7. State law may take precedence

E. RIGHT TO REQUEST AMENDMENT OF PHI

1. Patient has the right to request that their PHI be changed
2. Request should be made in writing
3. Must be done in a timely manner

F. RIGHT TO RECEIVE AN ACCOUNTING OF DISCLOSURES OF PHI

1. Providers should keep a log of disclosures
2. Patients may request an accounting or tracking of their disclosures once a year without charge; additional accountings may be charged a fee

VII. Organization and Staff Responsibilities

A. GENERAL

1. Organization must implement written policies and procedures
2. Guidelines tailored to each practice
3. Documentation must be maintained in written or electronic form and maintained for 6 years

B. VERIFICATION OF IDENTITY

1. Office must verify identity of person requesting PHI
2. Identification may be by date of birth, social security number, or password

C. VALIDATION OF PATIENT PERMISSION

1. Office must have appropriate permission
2. Permission is maintained in practice management system or patient chart

D. TRAINING

1. Office must train all members
2. Must include practice's policies and procedures that deal with PHI
3. Each person's role should be addressed

E. SAFEGUARDS

1. Ensure that information is secure
2. Include administrative, technical, and physical measures that will safeguard PHI from any disclosure, intentional or accidental

F. COMPLAINTS

1. Process must be in place for complaints
2. Staff members are subject to appropriate sanctions for failure to comply (warning to termination)

VIII. Code Set Regulations

A. GENERAL

1. Transaction and code set (TCS): developed to streamline electronic data transactions
2. Makes data processing transactions more efficient and reduces costs
3. Single standard similar to a bank's automatic teller machine or grocery self-checkout
4. Can be used by anyone to enter into a specific space on a form
5. Electronic, not paper
6. Documents why patients are seen (diagnosis, *International Classification of Diseases*, ninth edition, Clinical Modification [ICD-9-CM]) and what is done to them at the encounter (procedure, *Current Procedural Terminology*, fourth edition [CPT-4], Health Care Financing Administration Common Procedure Coding System [HCPCS])

IX. Guidelines for HIPAA Privacy Compliance

A. REASONABLE AND APPROPRIATE SAFEGUARDS MUST BE TAKEN TO ENSURE THAT ALL CONFIDENTIAL INFORMATION IS PROTECTED

1. Conversations can be overheard; consider privacy glass at the front desk and moving conversations away from populated settings; move dictation stations away from patient areas; telephone conversations in front of patients should be avoided
2. Check medical record to see if any special instructions for contacting the patient are noted
3. Limit the information (reason for visit) on patient sign-in sheets; change them throughout the day
4. Patient must sign a form acknowledging the receipt of the NPP
5. Formal policies for transferring and accepting PHI must be in place; these include couriers, billing services transcription services, and e-mail
6. Computers should be turned so the screen is not visible to others; screensavers may be used; computer should automatically log off a user after a period of being idle
7. Keep user names and passwords confidential, and change them often
8. Safeguard the work area by keeping confidential information from patient view; keep PHI from cleaning services that may have access after business hours
9. Medical records should be placed face down at reception area; when placing medical record on the door of the examination room, turn the chart so the identifying information faces the door
10. Do not post the provider's daily schedule in areas accessible to patients
11. Fax machines should not be placed in patient rooms or reception area where incoming documents may be viewed
12. Direct mail and telephone calls to the appropriate persons
13. For coding and billing purposes, recognize, learn, and use HIPAA TCS
14. Send all privacy-related concerns and questions to the appropriate staff member
15. Immediately report any suspected or known improper behavior to supervisor

5 | *Psychology and Stages of Human Growth and Development*

I. Major Theorists

A. SIGMUND FREUD

1. Provided the foundation from which all other psychological theories developed
2. Believed that infancy and childhood are the critical periods for psychological development
3. Psychoanalytical theory: theory of personality development that includes:
   a. Levels of awareness
      1) Conscious: experiences within one's immediate awareness; reality-based
      2) Subconscious: stores memories, thoughts, and feelings
      3) Unconscious: closed to one's awareness
   b. Components of the personality
      1) Id: body's basic primitive urges
      2) Ego: closely related to reality
      3) Superego: further development of ego; makes judgments; controls and punishes
   c. Psychosexual stages of development
      1) Oral stage: birth to end of first year of life; mouth is the source of all comfort and pleasure
      2) Anal stage: end of first year of life to third year; elimination gives pleasure and satisfaction
      3) Phallic stage: ages 3 to 6; associates pleasure and conflict with genital organs; Oedipus complex (boy's unconscious sexual attraction to his mother) and Electra complex (girl's unconscious sexual attraction to her father) develop
      4) Latency stage: ages 6 through 12; sexual urges are dormant; peer relationships develop with the same sex
      5) Genital stage: begins at puberty; body is preparing for reproduction; sexual attraction and heterosexual relationships begin

B. ERIK ERIKSON

1. Broadened Freud's theory of personality development
2. Psychosocial theory: eight stages

   a. Trust versus mistrust: birth to 18 months; to develop a basic trust in the mothering figure and to be able to generalize it to others
   b. Autonomy versus shame and doubt: 18 months to 3 years; to gain self-control and independence within the environment
   c. Initiative versus guilt: 3 to 6 years; to develop a sense of purpose and the ability to initiate and direct the individual's own activities
   d. Industry versus inferiority: 6 to 11 years; to achieve a sense of self-confidence by learning, competing, performing successfully, and receiving recognition from others
   e. Identity versus role confusion: 12 to 20 years; to integrate the tasks mastered in the previous stages into a secure sense of self
   f. Intimacy versus isolation: 20 to 30 years; to form an intense, lasting relationship or a commitment to another person, cause, institution, or creative effort
   g. Generativity versus stagnation: age 30 to 65; to achieve the life goals established for oneself while considering the welfare of future generations
   h. Ego integrity versus despair: age 65 to death; to review the individual's life and derive meaning from both positive and negative events while achieving a positive sense of self-worth

C. JEAN PIAGET

1. Cognitive development
2. Concerned with acquisition of intellect and development of thought processes
3. Believed that the child's cognitive abilities progress through four stages:
   a. Sensorimotor stage: birth to 2 years; acquires knowledge through exploration of the environment; attaches meaning and recognition of things
   b. Preoperational stage: 2 to 6 years; develops language; child sees him or herself as the center of the universe

c. Concrete operational stage: 6 to 12 years; begins to solve problems and to think logically; becomes less egocentric and more social
d. Formal operational stage: 12 to 15 years; ability to think logically in hypothetical and abstract terms; cognitive maturity achieved

D. ABRAHAM MASLOW

1. Described human behavior as being motivated by needs that are ordered in a hierarchy
2. Believed people must meet their most basic needs before they can move up the hierarchy to any higher level
3. Hierarchy begins at the bottom with basic survival needs and moves to the top with more complex needs
   a. Physiologic needs: basic fundamental needs; includes food, water, elimination, air, sleep, exercise, shelter, and sexual expression
   b. Safety and security: these needs are for avoiding harm and maintaining comfort, order, structure, physical safety, protection, and freedom from fear
   c. Love and belonging: needs for giving and receiving affection, companionship, satisfactory interpersonal relationships, and identification with a group
   d. Self-esteem: seeks self-respect and respect from others, works to achieve success and recognition within the group, and desires prestige from accomplishments
   e. Self-actualization: possesses a feeling of self-fulfillment and the realization of the person's highest potential

E. LAWRENCE KOHLBERG

1. Introduced a theory of moral development
2. Expanded on Piaget's theory
3. Believed that the child progressively develops moral reasoning as he or she gains the ability to think logically
4. Identified three levels of moral development, subdivided into six stages of acquired moral reasoning:
   a. Level 1: preconventional thinking; ages 4 to 10; the child learns reasoning through parents' demands for obedience; begins to recognize right from wrong
      1) Stage 1: obedience and punishment orientation
      2) Stage 2: instrumental relativist orientation
   b. Level 2: conventional thinking; ages 10 to 13; the child begins to seek approval from society; influenced by external forces such as peers and environment
      1) Stage 3: interpersonal concordance orientation
      2) Stage 4: law and order orientation
   c. Level 3: postconventional thinking; postadolescence; develop our own moral code based on our own principles

1) Stage 5: social contract legalistic orientation
2) Stage 6: universal ethical principle orientation

F. ELISABETH KÜBLER-ROSS

1. Identified stages of dying
2. Can also apply to the grieving process
3. Stages:
   a. Denial: direct denial and/or periods of disbelief
   b. Anger: realization of what is happening; may display rage
   c. Bargaining: attempts to make deals with a deity
   d. Depression: may show signs and symptoms such as withdrawal, lethargy, and periods of crying
   e. Acceptance: comes to accept the facts and fate

G. CARL JUNG

1. Understanding of psyche through examination of dreams, art, mythology, religion, and philosophy
2. Pioneer in field of dream analysis; studied with Freud
3. Concepts:
   a. Archetype: reconciliation between the individual and the broader world through symbolic language (art, dreams, drama, and religion)
   b. Collective unconscious: humans have a shared psychological predisposition; revealed through examination of symbolic communication (art, dreams, religion, and myth)
   c. Anima (female) and animus (male): components of both sexes
   d. Introvert (finding meaning within) and extrovert (finding meaning in the outside world)
   e. Family systems theory: family members who are *type-alike* form allies; persons who are unlike are naturally in conflict; children who have preference different from parents may be coerced into a false personality; the child may resist, and conflict may occur

II. Stages of Life Cycle

A. NEWBORN TO 1 YEAR

1. Physical characteristics:
   a. Head is larger in proportion to the rest of the body at birth; fontanelles close between 12 and 18 months
   b. Birth weight doubles by 5 to 6 months and triples by the first year
   c. Teething begins at approximately 5 to 6 months
   d. Senses are present at birth and develop more fully during the first year
   e. Blood pressure increases, and pulse and respiration decrease as the child ages
2. Developmental milestones:
   a. Gross motor skills (involve large muscles of the arms and legs)
      1) 2 months: controls head
      2) 3 months: sits without support

   3) 7 months: sits alone
   4) 10 months: creeps
   5) 9 to 11 months: stands without support
   6) 12 to 15 months: walks alone
 b. Fine motor skills (refined use of hands and fingers)
 c. Psychosocial (Erikson's stages of growth and development)
 d. Cognitive (mostly sensorimotor; heightened use of touch, taste, sight, hearing, and smell)

B. TODDLERHOOD (1 TO 3 YEARS)

1. Physical characteristics:
   a. Grows up to 3 inches each year
   b. Gains 4 to 6 pounds each year
   c. Extremities grow faster than the trunk
   d. Face and jaw grow bigger to permit room for more teeth
   e. Bones begin to ossify
   f. Visual acuity developing; hearing is fully developed
2. Developmental milestones:
   a. Gross motor skills
      1) Depends on growth and maturation of muscles, bones and nerves
      2) Can usually run, and walk up steps using both feet
   b. Fine motor skills
      1) Puts simple puzzles together
      2) Can turn knobs and open jar lids
   c. Psychosocial
      1) Attached to mother; tolerates short separation
      2) Dresses and undresses self
      3) Nearly toilet trained
   d. Cognitive
      1) Searches for and finds toys
      2) Locates body parts
      3) Gives full name on request
   e. Language
      1) Uses words and gestures to indicate needs
      2) Uses two-word sentences
      3) Initiates sounds and words
      4) Can sing simple songs
      5) Vocabulary of approximately 1000 words

C. PRESCHOOL (3 TO 6 YEARS)

1. Physical characteristics:
   a. Trunk and body lengthen in proportion to rest of body
   b. Gains 5 to 7 pounds each year
   c. Grows 2½ to 3 inches each year
   d. Deciduous teeth may begin to fall out; dental health is important
   e. Visual acuity improves to 20/20; frequent ear infections
2. Developmental milestones:
   a. Gross motor skills
      1) Able to walk and run on tiptoes

   2) Able to hop and to balance on one foot
   3) May begin certain sports such as soccer, baseball, skating, and dance
 b. Fine motor skills
   1) Manages self-care activities
   2) Manipulates clothing and clothing fasteners with ease
   3) Handles eating utensils; can begin to learn table manners
   4) Can draw faces, copy letters, and print own name
 c. Psychosocial
   1) Learns to trust
   2) Aware of genital organs and sexual identity
   3) Needs discipline and limits
 d. Cognitive
   1) Longer attention span than as toddler
   2) Develops memory
   3) Can pretend
 e. Language
   1) Becomes talkative
   2) May show some difficulty with pronunciation
   3) Can recite full name, address, and telephone number
   4) Imitates others

D. SCHOOL AGE (6 TO 11 YEARS)

1. Physical characteristics:
   a. Growth is steady but slows
   b. Permanent teeth appear
   c. Weight increases by 4½ to 6½ pounds each year
   d. Height increases by 2 to 3 inches each year
   e. Visual maturity achieved; peripheral vision and depth perception improve
   f. Immune system matures
2. Developmental milestones:
   a. Gross motor skills
      1) Increase in muscle mass improves skills
      2) Gender differences exist in motor skills
   b. Fine motor skills
      1) Can print and begins to master script writing
      2) Can throw and catch
      3) Can begin to learn to play musical instruments
   c. Psychosocial
      1) Outgoing, talkative, and enthusiastic
      2) Fearlessness puts child at risk for injury
      3) Sexual curiosity continues
      4) Initiates a task and able to see it through to completion
      5) Sibling rivalry can occur
      6) Peers are more important than family
      7) Privacy becomes important
      8) Emotions have wide range of expression
   d. Cognitive
      1) Has collections of stickers, books, and sports cards

      2) Breaks things down into small parts and reassembles them

      3) Takes views of others into consideration

      4) Understands concepts of time, space, and dimension

      5) Starts and continues formal education

  e. Language

      1) Use of language and communication techniques improve

      2) Language becomes important for socialization

      3) Can use proper parts of speech, proper tense of words

E. ADOLESCENCE (11 TO 19 YEARS)

1. Puberty (ages 11 to 14); puberty ends and adolescence begins with the onset of menses (menarche) in girls and sperm production in boys
   a. Rapid physical growth
   b. Changes in body proportions; trunk and limbs grow swiftly
   c. Development of primary sexual characteristics
   d. Development of secondary sexual characteristics
2. Physical characteristics:
   a. Puberty is the period of the greatest amount of rapid growth; growth slows after puberty
   b. Muscular strength increases greatly
   c. Epiphyseal line closes in long bones; growth nearly complete
   d. Trunk broadens at the hips and shoulders
   e. Posture may be poor from the fast growth; slouching
   f. Sexual growth and development are completed
   g. Shows great concern about one's changing body
   h. Sebaceous glands produce more oil and become larger
   i. Changes in fat distribution
3. Developmental milestones:
   a. Motor development
      1) Comparable to adult
      2) Hand-eye coordination improves
   b. Sexual development
      1) Heightened emotions
      2) Increased worries
      3) Lack of self-confidence
      4) Sex is given high priority; girls set limits on interactions
      5) Good sex education enables responsible choices
   c. Psychosocial
      1) Rebelliousness, argumentative, and/or rude
      2) Egocentric
      3) Need for privacy
      4) Dishonesty
      5) Responsibility
      6) Curfews
      7) Friends
      8) Self-absorbed

      9) Society places many demands

      10) Discipline is important

  d. Cognitive

      1) Maturation of central nervous system leads to formal operational thought processes (logical thought)

      2) School is at the center of development

      3) Moral reasoning and spiritual awareness develop

  e. Communication

      1) Vocabulary increases

      2) Verbal communication allows thoughts and beliefs to be known

      3) Development of common language typical to a group, time, and culture (slang)

F. EARLY ADULTHOOD (20 TO 40 YEARS)

1. Physical characteristics:
   a. Physical growth is completed
   b. Men usually have more muscle mass
   c. Wisdom teeth erupt; may need to be removed
   d. Other body systems begin to decline at the end of this period
2. Developmental milestones:
   a. Major milestones include choosing and establishing a career, fulfilling sexual needs, establishing a family and a home, expanding social circles, and developing maturity
      1) Motor development
         a) Peak physical efficiency reached
         b) Physical efficiency declines toward the end of this period
      2) Sexual development
         a) Sexuality established
         b) Ability to experience and share love
      3) Psychosocial development
         a) Strong sense of identity
         b) Sharing of innermost thoughts
         c) Career and work roles understood
      4) Cognitive development
         a) No longer egocentric, as a rule
         b) Can solve problems and process information
         c) Attends college or vocational school
      5) Health concerns
         a) Pap smear
         b) Mammography and breast self-examination
         c) Testicular self-examination
         d) Cholesterol
         e) Obesity
         f) Stress
         g) Family planning

G. MIDDLE ADULTHOOD (MID-40S TO EARLY 60S)

1. Physical characteristics:
   a. May lose height
   b. Body contour changes; higher percentage of body fat

    c. Visual and aural acuity decline

    d. Skin becomes less elastic; wrinkles form

    e. Gradual loss of taste

  2. Developmental milestones:

    a. Sexual development

      1) Menopause and loss of reproductive capacity

      2) Options, opportunities, and means of sexual expression may change

    b. Psychosocial development

      1) Achievement of goals

      2) Desire to serve the larger community

      3) Family roles may change from child-centered to couple-centered roles

      4) Grandparenting

      5) Change in relationship with parents

      6) Peak earning capacity

    c. Cognitive development: capable of thinking in a concrete manner

H. LATE ADULTHOOD (AGE 65 TO DEATH)

  1. Physical characteristics:

    a. Quality of life depends on the person's ability to perform activities of daily living (ADL)

    b. Formation and composition of body changes

    c. Body systems begin to decline

    d. Sensory systems become less efficient

    e. Problems with memory loss and learning difficulty develop

  2. Developmental milestones:

    a. Motor development

      1) Movement slows

      2) Fine motor skills affected by stiffening of the joints

    b. Sexual development: capable of enjoying a satisfying sexual relationship

    c. Psychosocial development

      1) Ego integrity achieved

      2) Life review reassures about accomplishments and worth

      3) Body image changes

      4) Fear of loss of independence

      5) Death of a spouse produces change of roles

      6) Work and leisure activities change

      7) Concept of death takes on a different meaning

    d. Cognitive development

      1) Healthy persons retain cognitive abilities

      2) Memory changes; short-term stores less than long-term

III. The Sick Role

A. GENERAL

  1. Illness and/or injury forces the patient to adopt the *sick role*; includes duties and rights (Parsons, 1951)

  2. Duties include:

    a. Duty 1: make every effort to get well

    b. Duty 2: seek professional help, and cooperate to get well

  3. Rights include:

    a. Right 1: exempt from responsibility for injury or illness

    b. Right 2: exempt from normal social obligations

B. SICK ROLE MAY BRING BENEFITS

  1. Financial protection: disability, workers' compensation

  2. Social gain: sympathy and attention

C. SICK ROLE MAY BRING DETRIMENT

  1. Uncertainty about the future

  2. May create social stigmas

  3. Loss of independence

  4. Loss of privacy

  5. Loss of income

  6. Loss of body image and self-esteem

  7. Loss of social role

D. TERMINALLY ILL OR DYING PATIENT HAS SPECIAL NEEDS

  1. Kübler-Ross' stages of dying

  2. Excessive stress

IV. The Provider Role

A. MAIN ROLE IS TO EMPOWER THE PATIENT, NOT TO UNDERMINE THE PATIENT'S PARTICIPATION IN CARE

B. PROVIDER–PATIENT RELATIONSHIP IS UNEQUAL

C. PROVIDER IS RESPONSIBLE FOR:

  1. Concern for the patient's well being

  2. Carrying out ethical duties

  3. Respect for each patient as an individual

  4. Knowing what is important to the patient

  5. Assisting patient in adapting to the sick role

  6. Assuming cooperation from the patient

  7. Displaying confidence

  8. Promoting and encouraging proper patient behavior

D. DIFFICULTIES IN PROVIDER–PATIENT RELATIONSHIP CAN OCCUR

  1. May be the result of:

    a. Personal bias: describes a person's feelings toward a patient or a thing

    b. Prejudice: strong adverse attitude toward a patient because of that patient's association with a particular group

    c. Overidentification: "I know how you feel"; difficulty seeing the patient as an individual

    d. Countertransference: response to the patient in a personal manner, such as a child or sibling

    e. Transference: overdependence by the patient on the provider

E. CULTURAL DIFFERENCES ARE IMPORTANT

  1. The medical assistant needs to be aware of various cultural norms for optimum care and optimal patient comfort

F. PROVIDER AND MEDICAL ASSISTANT NEED TO BE AWARE OF *DISTANCE* AND *PERSONAL SPACE* WHEN GIVING CARE
1. Intimate space: actual physical contact
2. Personal space: 1 to 4 feet
3. Social space: 4 to 12 feet
4. Public space: 12 to 25 feet
5. Distance and personal space can be cultural

6 | Communication

I. Communication

A. DEFINITION OF COMMUNICATION
1. The process of sharing meaning

B. COMMUNICATION PROCESS
1. Source
   a. Sender of the message
   b. Can be a person, a group, or a company
   c. What is sent varies and is affected by the sender's experiences
2. Message
   a. What is sent by the source
   b. Message has three parts:
      1) Meaning: usually ideas or feelings
      2) Symbols: words or actions that represent the meaning; the process of turning words or actions into symbols is *encoding*
      3) Organization or form: syntax and grammar of the message; putting the symbols in order
3. Channel
   a. Which symbols are given
   b. Can be visual, audio, print, or touch
4. Receiver
   a. Where the message is being sent
   b. Receiver processes into meaning (decoding)
5. Feedback
   a. Response of the receiver
   b. Can be verbal or nonverbal
   c. Tells the source if the message was heard, seen, or understood
6. Noise
   a. Anything that interferes with the communication process
   b. Can be:
      1) External: stimuli that draws attention away from the message
      2) Internal: personal thoughts and feelings that draw a person away from the message

   3) Semantic: message symbols that prevent the meaning from being understood (accents, dialect, grammar)

C. THERAPEUTIC COMMUNICATION
1. Process of relaying information from health care provider to patient
2. Can be through verbal disclosure, touch, or gesture
3. Techniques include:
   a. Acknowledgment: emphasizes the importance of the patient in the communication process
   b. Establishing guidelines: helps the patient know what is expected of him or her
   c. Focusing: directs the communication toward important topics
   d. Listening: communicates interest in the topics raised by the patient
   e. Open-ended comments: helps the patient to decide what is relevant; encourages discussion ("Describe what you think is going to happen.")
   f. Reflecting: shows the importance of the patient's ideas and feelings
   g. Restating: lets the patient know how the health care provider interpreted the message the patient sent ("I hear you saying…")
   h. Clarification: demonstrates the desire to understand what the patient is communicating (may ask who, what, where, when)
   i. Silence: communicates acceptance
4. Ineffective techniques include:
   a. Advising: telling what the patient should do
   b. Minimizing: health care provider making light of the patient's situation
   c. Defending: health care provider protecting self from criticism
   d. Stereotyping: health care provider using clichés when responding
   e. Probing: health care provider discussing, or trying to discuss, topics the patient does not want to discuss

f. Approval and disapproval: health care provider overly approving or disapproving of the patient's behavior

g. Agreeing and disagreeing: health care provider overly agreeing or disagreeing with the patient's perceptions, thoughts, or feelings

5. Barriers to communication
   a. Embarrassment: patient may be in awe of the health care provider, thereby being embarrassed to ask questions of the health care provider
   b. Discomfort: patient may be uncomfortable or ashamed to discuss patient's private body parts or symptoms
   c. Communication difficulties: patient can see disabilities as making the patient intellectually inferior
   d. Withdrawal: patient does not respond to health care provider's communication
   e. Ineffective techniques (see previous discussion) by health care provider may raise barriers

D. NONVERBAL COMMUNICATION

1. Messages conveyed without the use of words
2. Body language
3. Involves the health care provider's grooming, dress, eye contact, facial expressions, hand gestures, space, tone of voice, and posture

II. Patient Relationships

A. GENERAL

1. Medical assistant needs to understand the patient's concerns, needs, and reactions
2. Stress and anxiety are common patient responses

B. UNCONSCIOUS DEFENSE MECHANISMS

1. Compensation: overemphasizing a trait to make up for a failure
2. Denial: avoiding reality
3. Displacement: shifting an impulse from a threatening to a nonthreatening one
4. Dissociation: disconnecting the significance from an event
5. Identification: mimicking the behavior of another
6. Introjection: adopting the feelings of others
7. Projection: assigning the person's own feelings to another as if these feelings had originated with the other person
8. Rationalization: justifying the person's thoughts, feelings, or behavior
9. Regression: returning to a former behavior or more immature behavior
10. Repression: putting unpleasant thoughts or events out of the person's mind
11. Sublimation: diverting unacceptable thoughts or feelings into acceptable behaviors
12. Substitution: making up for a deficiency by concentrating on another

13. Suppression: deliberately forgetting or avoiding dealing with an unpleasantness

C. INTERACTION WITH PATIENTS

1. Interaction is a therapeutic relationship
2. Assists patients to resolve problems and achieve goals
3. Maximizes patient comfort
   a. Children
      1) Establish a friendly relationship
      2) Be aware of your own feelings toward children in general
      3) Speak in quiet tones; speak at the child's physical level (not looking down at the child)
      4) Use language appropriate for the child's age
      5) Allow the child to assist in his or her treatment
      6) Keep the child patient from experiencing long waits
      7) Understand that the child may regress when ill
      8) Be truthful with the child, which fosters trust
      9) Offer rewards for proper behavior
      10) Allow the child to play with the health care provider's equipment if doing so is safe and appropriate
      11) Infants should be held and comforted before any treatment procedures
   b. Adolescents
      1) Patient demands independence yet requires comfort
      2) Permit patient's privacy
      3) Health care provider must allow examinations with the patient's parent present
      4) Treat the patient with respect and dignity
      5) Set fair limits for the patient
      6) Answer the patient's questions openly and honestly
      7) Explain the procedures to the patient in terms he or she will understand
   c. Elderly patient
      1) Allow additional time with the patient; this circumstance may be a social interaction for a lonely patient
      2) Keep the patient physically and environmentally comfortable
      3) Patient may find comfort in a health care provider's routine
      4) Allow as much independence as possible
      5) Do not overprotect or be overattentive
      6) Speak slowly and precisely, but do not patronize
   d. Terminally ill patient
      1) Help both the patient and the patient's family adjust to the patient's loss in strength, sensation, mobility, and endurance

2) Give support to the patient's family members
3) Be willing to listen
4) Patient will likely experience some, or all, of the stages of dying

e. Angry patient
   1) Patient's anger may be caused by the patient's medical condition
   2) Health care provider's goal is to calm the patient
   3) Health care provider must remain calm, firm, and direct
   4) Health care provider must not take the anger personally
   5) Health care provider must listen closely to the patient's concerns
   6) Health care provider must keep speaking tone calm and in control
   7) Keep the angry patient out of public areas of the office; escort the angry patient to a private room

f. Sensory-impaired patient
   1) Patient may need an interpreter (if hearing impaired or if speaks only a foreign language) to assist in communication
   2) Health care provider should be positioned directly in front of the patient and should speak slowly
   3) For the sight-impaired patient, the health care provider should ask how best to assist the patient
   4) Health care provider should be flexible, open, and supportive

g. Frightened patient
   1) A frightened patient may be uncooperative
   2) Health care provider should recognize fear and assist the patient in dealing with the fright
   3) Health care provider should maintain control of the situation

h. Depressed patient
   1) The depressed patient will experience feelings of gloom, hopelessness, and dread and may have feelings of no self-worth
   2) Health care provider should provide sympathy, support, and a friendly ear
   3) Health care provider should demonstrate an interest in the patient's needs
   4) Health care provider should keep the environment secure and nonthreatening

i. Suicidal patient
   1) Suicidal feelings can be the patient's final response to his or her depression
   2) Suicidal patient may disclose intentions to the health care provider
   3) All suicidal threats or attempts must be taken seriously
   4) Health care provider must listen closely to the suicidal patient
   5) Health care provider should demonstrate empathy
   6) Health care provider should seek professional advice and/or actions for the suicidal patient

j. Mentally impaired patient
   1) Patient may be confused and disoriented
   2) By correcting the patient's confusion, the health care provider may make the patient less frightened
   3) Health care provider must treat the patient kindly but must not be condescending

k. Abused patient
   1) Health care provider must treat the abused patient's physical injuries first
   2) Health care provider must focus on the patient as a victim; health care provider should express assurances of the patient's self-worth
   3) Refer the abused patient to existing social agencies

l. Drug-dependent patient
   1) Health care provider should not belittle the patient for the patient's behavior
   2) Health care provider should be compassionate, empathetic, and patient
   3) Health care provider should involve the patient's family in the patient's treatment

m. Significant others
   1) Part of the patient's emotional support group
   2) Health care provider should respect the wishes of the patient concerning the patient's loved ones
   3) Health care provider should keep any waiting relatives notified of progress and keep them informed of any delays
   4) Health care provider should address the concerns of the patient's family and friends
   5) Health care provider must be aware of confidentiality issues

Patient Reception 7

I. Reception

A. GENERAL
1. Patient's first impression of the health care provider's office
2. Influences patient's perception of the office
3. Receptionist's attitude and appearance are important to set the tone of the office

II. Reception Area

A. GENERAL
1. Place to receive patients
2. Planned for patient comfort
3. Should be clean and uncluttered
4. Receptionist should be behind a counter that is high enough for health care provider privacy (of hard records, of patient information on computer screens, and of patient financial records)
5. Colors should be calming and restful
6. Lighting should be adequate for reading and safety
7. Adequate ventilation is essential
8. Temperature should be regulated for patients' comfort
9. Play area for children, if appropriate
10. Spacious coat rack to store patients' outerwear
11. Furniture arranged for patients' comfort, movement, and safety
12. Periodicals should be up to date and appropriate

III. Receptionist

A. GENERAL
1. First professional person with whom the patient comes in contact, either in person or by telephone
2. Medical assistant should display pride in him or herself and the job
3. Communication skills should demonstrate competence and a positive attitude
4. Clothing, hair, and makeup should be appropriate; follow office policies
5. Should have friendly, cheerful, caring, courteous, and respectful demeanor
6. Should be professional at all times
7. Greet every patient on arrival by name (using correct pronunciation)
8. A friendly farewell can show caring and courtesy
9. Duties may include:
   a. Answering telephones
   b. Scheduling appointments
   c. Registering patient and taking history
   d. Handling complaints
   e. Preparing charts
   f. Handling nonpatient visitors (vendors, sales representatives, pharmaceutical representatives)

IV. Telephone Techniques

A. GENERAL
1. Majority of receptionist's communication occurs through the telephone
2. Telephone is the critical component of a successful health care provider's practice
3. Communication and listening skills are important
4. Incoming telephone calls may be from:
   a. Established patients calling for appointments or advice
   b. Patient emergencies
   c. Other physicians making patient referrals
   d. Laboratories reporting information regarding health care provider's patient
   e. New patients making a first contact
5. Telecommunication devices for the deaf (TDD)

B. EQUIPMENT
1. Six-button key set
   a. Several incoming lines
   b. Office intercom line

   c. Hold button
   d. Lights flash slowly for incoming calls, flash rapidly for reminder of call on hold
2. Two-line speakerphone
   a. Allows conversation without using the handset
   b. Last number redial
   c. Volume control
   d. Speed-dial and memory for frequent calls
   e. Intercom paging
   f. May have liquid crystal display (LCD) screen
3. Headset
   a. Lightweight plastic earphone and microphone combination
   b. Allows hands-free telephone use
4. Cellular telephone
   a. Mobile, transportable telephone
   b. Permits communication outside an office or within a vehicle
5. Pager
   a. Activated by calling the pager's number
   b. Can leave a voice message or digital message
6. Facsimile (fax) machine
   a. Transmits print material over telephone lines to other facilities that have fax capability
   b. Can send and receive copies of printed documents
   c. If sending sensitive patient information, call ahead to ensure that only the appropriate person receives the fax
7. Directories
   a. White pages: alphabetical listing by last name, includes last name, first name, sometimes middle initial, address, and telephone number
   b. Yellow pages: alphabetical listing by category of commercial business; in each category, alphabetical listing by company name (or businessperson's last name), includes company name (or businessperson's name), company address, and company telephone number or numbers
   c. Personal office directory: collection of frequently called telephone numbers within that office; can be stored in a Rolodex or in a 3 × 5 index card file

C. INCOMING CALLS

1. Answer promptly (ideally on the first ring, always by the third ring)
2. Hold the telephone instrument correctly (with the mouthpiece approximately 1 inch from your mouth)
3. Develop a pleasing telephone voice
4. Identify the health care provider's office; identify yourself
5. Gain the identity of the caller (ask to whom you are speaking if the caller does not first identify him or herself)
6. Offer assistance (using proper words and proper tone)
7. Screen incoming calls (follow any office policies about how incoming calls are to be handled and categorized)
8. Minimize caller waiting time (caller should experience no more than 1 minute without voice contact of some type)
9. When answering a second call, ask the first caller to please hold, transfer to the second incoming line, identify the second caller, ask the second caller to please hold, and return to the first caller
10. End each call pleasantly and graciously (say "thank you" and some form of "good-bye")

D. TELEPHONE MESSAGES

1. May be recorded on message sheet or in an office telephone log
2. Message should include the following information:
   a. Name of the person to whom the call is directed
   b. Name of the person calling
   c. Caller's daytime telephone number (include pager and/or cellular telephone numbers)
   d. Reason for the call
   e. Action to be taken by the recipient
   f. Date and time the call was received
   g. Initials of the person taking the call

E. OUTGOING TELEPHONE CALLS

1. Know what needs to be said, how it is to be said, and have all pertinent information on hand before placing the call
2. Voice should convey warmth, friendliness, confidence, and intelligence
3. Address the person by name
4. Use "please" and "thank you"
5. Do not rush the call
6. Use discretion when conveying personal or confidential patient or medical information
7. Long distance (check with office manager to verify this procedure because different long-distance carriers have different calling requirements)
   a. Direct dial: 1 + area code + seven-digit telephone number
   b. Long-distance directory assistance: 1 + area code + 555-1212
   c. Operator assisted: 0 + area code + seven-digit telephone number
      1) Person-to-person (operator will not connect the line until the person to whom you requested answers the telephone)
      2) Station-to-station (operator will connect the line as soon as anyone at the receiving telephone number answers the telephone)
      3) Collect call (operator will not connect the line until a recipient agrees to be billed for the long-distance telephone call)
      4) Bill to third party (operator verifies that a third party [someone not a party to this long-distance

telephone call] will accept the charges for the phone call)

    5) Request for time and charges (the operator, if asked before connecting the long-distance line, will call you back after the call is ended and will tell you the time of the long-distance call, as well as the cost of the long-distance call; you will then be able to verify the long-distance charge against the next telephone bill)

  d. Time zones
    1) Pacific Time: 1:00 (WA, OR, NV, CA)
    2) Mountain Time: 2:00 (MT, UT, ID, WY, CO, NM, AZ; parts of ND, SD, NE, KS)
    3) Central Time: 3:00 (MN, WI, IA, MO, AR, OK, TX, LA, MS, IL, AL; parts of TN, KY, ND, SD, NE, KS)
    4) Eastern Time: 4:00 (all other states, except for HI and AK)

  e. Wrong number dialed
    1) Verify the telephone number with the person answering
    2) Apologize
    3) If long distance, call the operator to credit the office account

F. ANSWERING SERVICES

Health care provider must be able to be contacted at all times in order to respond to emergencies (to prevent abandonment charges)

1. Answering services
  a. Provides coverage when the office is closed
  b. Answering services answer and screen incoming telephone calls
2. Electronic answering devices
  a. Recorded message that tells caller how to reach the health care provider (or health care provider's colleague) or invites the caller to leave a voice message
  b. Messages can be retrieved directly from the machine or can be remotely accessed
  c. Answering message may be changed as necessary
3. Voice mail: computerized system used to record, send, or retrieve voice message from the telephone system
4. Automatic routing
  a. Telephone calls answered by automated operator that announces a list of options from which the caller selects one
  b. This system is rather impersonal but may be good for the larger clinic

V. Appointment Scheduling

A. GENERAL

1. Process that determines which patients will be seen by the health care provider (*appointment*), the dates and times for the appointments, and the allotted time for each appointment
2. Allotted time for each appointment is based on the patient's complaint as compared with the health care provider's availability
3. Important factor in the success of health care provider's practice
4. Many approaches to scheduling

B. GUIDELINES

1. Understand the nature of the practice
2. Know the personalities and habits of the medical staff
3. Be aware of the time needed to assess each patient complaint type
4. Plan realistically

C. MATERIALS NEEDED

1. Appointment book (see Figure 7-1)
  a. May be for one or several health care providers
  b. May show day, week, or month per page
  c. May be blank or preprinted
  d. May be loose-leaf or spiral bound
  e. Each block of time must have sufficient space to record the patient's name, the patient's telephone numbers, and the purpose of patient's visit to the health care provider
  f. Entire book must fit comfortably on the receptionist's desk and be easily accessible to all who are responsible for scheduling; the book must always be left in place
  g. Appointment book is a legal document and must be preserved as such
2. Pen and/or pencil
  a. Appointments should be written in black ink (because it is a legal document)
  b. Must be corrected in the same manner as correcting the patient chart (no erasing, no scribbling, no White-Out® or correction fluid)
  c. Use of pencil is more practical than a pen in anticipation of any appointment changes or cancellations
  d. Occasional use of colored ink (or pencil) may denote new or special patient
3. Appointment card
  a. Given to each patient after the follow-up appointment is made in the office
  b. Often preprinted with the clinic name, address, and telephone number, space on the card for date, day and time of appointment, and patient name

D. METHODS OF SCHEDULING

1. Open-office hours
  a. Clinic is open only for specified time period
  b. Patients are seen in the order of their arrival in the clinic (patients sign into a log-book on arrival), with provision that emergency treatment is given priority
  c. Least efficient method of scheduling
  d. Common among urgent care centers

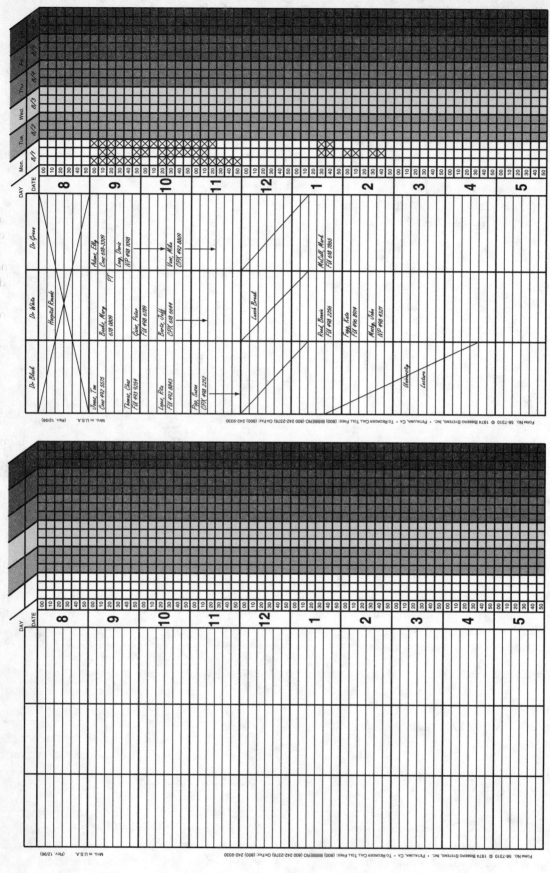

FIGURE 7-1. Sample appointment book. (Courtesy of Bibbero Systems, Inc., Petaluma, California 94954-1180, 800-242-2376; fax: 800-242-9330, *http://www.bibbero.com.*)

e. Triage: used to screen and classify sick or injured patients for priority
2. Flexible office hours
   a. Clinic is open at odd hours in addition to normal office hours (early morning or evening hours on certain days of the week)
   b. Accommodates various work schedules of patients
   c. Usually used in group practices
3. Time-specified hours
   a. Most common system
   b. Each patient is given a specific time on a specific day for the appointment
   c. Does not easily accommodate the unplanned illness or accident and does not allow any buffer time (unless one or two open appointments each day are kept for such use)
4. Wave
   a. Gives short-term flexibility within each hour
   b. Assumes that the average time needed for the appointments will average out over the course of the day
   c. Each hour is divided into the average time the health care provider should spend with each patient (hour divided into 10-minute, 15-minute, or 20-minute blocks)
   d. Patients are scheduled on the hour (6 per hour for 10-minute block, 4 per hour for 15-minute block, etc.) and are seen by the health care provider in the order in which they sign in with the receptionist
   e. This system allows for late arrivals, allows for the patient whose accident or illness needs more (or less) time than the average, allows for the failed appointment, and allows for unscheduled interruptions of the health care provider
   f. Variable waiting times may result from this method of scheduling
5. Modified wave: appointments are staggered throughout the health care provider hour
6. Double booking
   a. Scheduling two patients at the same time
   b. Not an efficient way to schedule
   c. Can be wavelike if two patients each needing 5 minutes are both scheduled in the same 15-minute block
7. Grouping
   a. Similar procedures (e.g., Pap smears, well-baby checks, complete physicals) are all scheduled at a specific time of a specific day of the week or at specific hours
   b. These like procedures can be color-coded for ease of view

E. SCHEDULING PROCEDURES
1. Establish a matrix
   a. Block out times the health care provider is not available for appointments
   b. Establish a buffer time both in the morning and in the afternoon for catch-up
2. Chief complaint
   a. Identify the reason for patient visit
   b. Identify the level of urgency of the patient visit
   c. Identify the health care provider resources available
3. Referral: determine whether the patient has been referred by another health care provider
4. Locate the first available time to see the patient, as well as one alternative time; offer the dates and times to the patient
5. Enter the patient's name, telephone numbers, and complaint in the appointment book in the corresponding date and time block agreed to by the patient
6. Explain the pertinent office policies and instructions to the patient
7. Repeat the date and time to the patient for double-check before ending the call

F. APPOINTMENT PROBLEMS
1. Patient habitually late: schedule this patient near the end of the day
2. Consecutive appointments: schedule at the same time and day (different dates) for ease of remembering
3. Cancellations: offer the patient an alternative appointment
4. Missed appointment and no-show
   a. Prevent with a reminder telephone call the day before the appointment
   b. Patient may legally be charged for the missed appointment
   c. Patient may be discharged from health care provider's care for habitual no-shows
   d. Note all missed appointments in both the patient's chart and the appointment book
5. Emergencies
   a. Follow office protocol
   b. Emergencies take precedence over all other appointments
   c. Call 911 if the emergency is outside of the office protocol
6. Acute needs
   a. Provide the first available appointment to patient
   b. Double booking may be necessary
7. Referrals
   a. Process of sending patient to another health care provider (a specialist) for diagnosis and treatment

b. Appointment may be made by the patient or by the referring health care provider

c. Make sure all appropriate documents are provided to the referred health care provider (necessary patient records, x-rays, insurance referral letter)

8. Delays

a. Attempt to call affected patients about health care provider delays, and request that they come later that day or reschedule for another date and time

b. Explain courteously if the health care provider is called out of the office on an emergency

c. Waiting patients should be given an explanation, an estimated time of the current delay, and the patients' option to wait on the health care provider or reschedule

Records Management | 8

I. The Medical Record

A. GENERAL
1. The "chart"
2. Chronological system used to annotate patient's medical care that the health care provider renders
3. Ensures competent and necessary (nonredundant) medical care
4. Legal document

B. PURPOSE
1. Establishes the patient database
2. Serves as a communication link between the health care provider and the staff
3. Helps with the planning of effective patient care
4. Provides evidence of care given to the patient
5. Can provide data for research or education

C. CONTENT
1. Specific as to the type of practice
2. Usually includes:
   a. Chief complaint (CC): main reason for the patient seeking care
   b. Past medical history (PH or PMH): gives information regarding usual childhood diseases (UCD), past illnesses, surgeries, and current health status; may be prepared by the patient, by the health care provider, or by the medical assistant
   c. Family history (FH): information regarding the patient's parents and siblings; may include health status, age, cause of death, and hereditary diseases
   d. Present illness (PI): expanded CC
   e. Social history (SH): information on patient's personal habits; may include exercise, sleep, diet, tobacco and/or alcohol use, drug use, sexual history, sexual preference, and hobbies
   f. Occupational history (OH): information regarding patient's employment
   g. Physical examination (PE): complete physical examination; gives information regarding each body system (review of systems [ROS]); may serve as a baseline against the future
   h. Test results: diagnostic and laboratory tests; arranged with the more recent on top of the older
   i. Consultations: reports on evaluations made by other health care providers as requested by this health care provider
   j. Past medical records: records from other health care providers that have bearing on present treatment
   k. Correspondence: all correspondence related to patient care
   l. Progress notes: notes written in the chart by the health care provider regarding the patient's care, diagnosis, and/or treatment

D. ORGANIZATION
1. Source-oriented record
   a. Observations and data are categorized according to their source (health care provider, laboratory, x-ray, nurse)
   b. Forms are filed in reverse chronological order (most recent on top)
   c. Information is filed in separate sections (laboratory reports section, x-ray reports section, progress notes section, etc.)
2. Problem-oriented medical record (POMR)
   a. Data is organized according to patient's disease or condition
   b. Divided into four parts:
      1) Database: includes CC, PI, PE findings, and laboratory results; each condition will have its own page
      2) Problem list: numbered and titled list of every problem complained of patient; may include physical, psychological, and social problems related to the patient's condition

3) Plan: diagnostic and treatment decisions for the condition; each plan is titled and numbered
4) Progress notes: structured notes that correspond to each problem number; uses the acronym SOAP
   a) S (subjective data): signs, symptoms, and feelings that the patient describes in the patient's own words
   b) O (objective data): clinical evidence that the health care provider determines
   c) A (assessment = S + O): describes the physical impression and finally diagnosis
   d) P (plan = S + O + A): action needed to solve the problem; may include treatment, medications, consultations, and surgery

E. DOCUMENTATION
1. Chart in black ink
2. All entries must be dated and initialed, or signed, by the health care provider making the entry
3. All patient visits and telephone calls must be documented
4. No-shows must be recorded
5. Patient's name should appear on each page
6. Corrections are made by using the SLIDE rule:
   a. SL: single line through the error
   b. I: initials of the person correcting the error
   c. D: date and correct the error
   d. E: write the word *error*
7. Correspondence sent to the patient requires a note in the chart
8. *"If it was not charted, it was not done"*

F. SIX "Cs" OF CHARTING
1. Current
2. Complete
3. Concise
4. Correct
5. Confidential
6. Clean

G. LEGALITIES AND THE MEDICAL RECORD
1. The chart is a legal document
2. The chart belongs to the health care provider or the clinic, but the patient owns the information found on the chart
3. Records that patients or third parties request may be released only if the health care provider and the patient give consent, usually by a medical records release form
4. Records can be withheld from patients if the information can reasonably be expected to cause harm to the patient (doctrine of professional discretion)
5. Patient information is confidential and privileged (this patient confidentiality can be waived in writing by the patient or overruled in a courtroom)

6. Release of confidential patient information without the patient's written consent could lead to a charge of invasion of privacy by the patient
7. Medical records must be kept up to date, complete, and accurate
8. Records are retained according to the requirements of each state's statutes; medical records are usually retained permanently, until the patient's death
9. Medical records are destroyed by shredding or burning
10. Entries into medical records should be type-written or written in black ink

II. Records Management

A. PURPOSE
1. To classify, arrange, and store documents in an efficient, orderly, and accessible manner
   a. Records to be stored include:
      1) Medical records (charts)
      2) Financial records
      3) Patient correspondence
      4) Business records
      5) Research records
   b. Records can be stored as:
      1) Hard, printed, copies of the records
      2) Computer documents
      3) Microfiche and microfilm

B. EQUIPMENT AND SUPPLIES FOR RECORDS MANAGEMENT
1. Storage cabinet
   a. Vertical: file cabinet style
   b. Lateral: chest of drawers style
   c. Shelf: open or closed storage
2. Guides
   a. Plastic or cardboard dividers; permit grouping of similar type files
   b. Outguide: guide used to replace a file taken from the cabinet; enables technician to replace the file in the proper place when ready
3. Folders
   a. Cardboard or plastic holders that contain the patients' medical records
   b. Have tabs within them for separating contents
4. Labels
   a. Small stickers placed onto folders to identify the contents or folder identity

C. PROCESS
1. Condition
   a. Check for damage and, if found, repair it before refiling the record
   b. Date your work on the record, if required
2. Inspect and release
   a. Documents cannot be filed until the responsible parties have seen the document and have taken action on the record

b. Release mark of some sort (office protocol) must be noted on the file
3. Index and code
   a. Determine where the document should be filed
   b. Identify the caption to be used in filing the document
4. Sort
   a. Arrange the documents according to the office protocol (system) used
5. Store
   a. Place the documents in the appropriate file folder and place in the filing cabinet

D. FILING METHODS
1. Alphabetical
   a. Used with names of persons, businesses, or organizations; oldest, simplest, and most commonly used method
   b. Rules include:
      1) Names are divided into units and filed left to right
      2) Surname is unit 1, given name is unit 2, middle name (initial) is unit 3, and so on
      3) Names are alphabetized according to first unit letter; second unit considered if first units are the same; third unit considered if first two units are the same
      4) Initials filed before complete names starting with the same letter
      5) Units having no name filed before those that do (nothing before something)
      6) Hyphenated name is considered a single unit; if business name, each name is a separate unit
      7) Apostrophes are disregarded
      8) Abbreviations are indexed as if written in full
      9) Numbers as part of a name are indexed as if written out
      10) Titles and degrees are indexed last
      11) Married women are indexed by their own given name (first name)
      12) If two names are identical, patient's address is used as an index unit
      13) For names of organizations:
         a) Index in order as written, except when organization name includes a person's name (surname first, then given name)
         b) Numbers are indexed as if written out
         c) Disregard punctuation
         d) Directional terms are indexed as separate units

      e) Articles, conjunctions, and prepositions are disregarded unless *the* is the first word (if so, *the* is indexed as the last unit)
2. Numerical
   a. Used when each patient is assigned a number that is used on the patient's chart
   b. Patient number is cross-referenced with the patient's name and filed alphabetically
   c. Numerical filing is used in large clinics, group practices, and hospitals
   d. Types include:
      1) Consecutive numeric system
         a) Simplest system
         b) Patients are assigned consecutive numbers in the order of the date of their first visit to the facility
      2) Terminal digit system
         a) Patients assigned consecutive numbers as they visit the facility
         b) Digits in the patient number are separated into groups of two or three
         c) Read in groups from right to left, instead of left to right, and filed backwards in groups
      3) Social Security Number
         a) Patient's Social Security Number is patient's filing number
         b) Not every patient has a Social Security Number
3. Subject
   a. Documents indexed by subject matter and then filed alphabetically, then filed numerically, or both
   b. Generally not used for medical records
4. Color coding
   a. Colored tabs are used to represent patient information at a glance
   b. Used on letters of the patient's surname
   c. Can help keep files from being misfiled
   d. Selection of colors and division of the alphabet are determined by the practice's needs
   e. Can be used as colored folders, adhesive labels, or a combination
   f. Can be filed alphabetically or numerically
5. Tickler file
   a. System that organizes items chronologically for follow-up
   b. Can be notations on the daily calendar, or a card file divided into months, with months divided into days
   c. Must be checked daily for effectiveness

9 | *Administrative Practices*

I. Computer Basics

A. GENERAL
1. Electronic device that accepts, processes, exports, and stores data
2. Classified according to size
   a. Mainframe: large computer that can handle many users at the same time
   b. Microcomputer: personal computer (PC)
   c. Laptop: portable PC

B. HARDWARE: COMPUTER EQUIPMENT
1. Central processing unit (CPU)
   a. Control unit: supervises data processing operations
   b. Arithmetic logic unit (ALU): carries out arithmetic and logic operations
   c. Primary storage unit: stores data and program instructions
      1) Random access memory (RAM): computer's temporary memory
      2) Read-only memory (ROM): computer's permanent memory
2. Input devices
   a. Allows communication between the user and the computer hardware
   b. Allows data to be entered into the computer
   c. Keyboard: the *typewriter*; allows input of alphanumeric data
   d. Mouse: handheld pointing device; contains a ball that is moved when the mouse is rolled on a flat surface; movement of the mouse and thus the ball, moves the cursor on the computer screen
   e. Scanner: device that *reads*, or converts, printed matter directly into a computer-readable format
   f. Voice recognition: device that reads voices and creates a computer-readable format
3. Output devices
   a. Allows data to be displayed or recorded
   b. Monitor: device that resembles a television set; displays computer-generated information
   c. Printer: device that records computer-generated information onto paper (hard copy)
4. Storage
   a. Methods of saving the information input for future reference or for printing
   b. Hard drive: part of the computer hardware inside the computer box; contains the computer-operating information
   c. Floppy disk: part of the computer software; *diskette*; thin disk of magnetic material that can be inserted into the computer's disk drive
   d. Compact disk (CD) ROM: allows the storage of data on a removable disk; holds more information than a diskette
   e. Disk drive: loads a program or data that is stored on a diskette into the computer; also can be used to transfer stored information from the computer onto a diskette for safekeeping; each microcomputer may have more than one drive
   f. Portable disk drives: ZIP® drive, flash drive; jump drive; attached externally to the computer; contains a very high storage capacity; usually used as backup; can be stored somewhere other than the facility

C. SOFTWARE
1. Typically referred to as a *program*; provides processing instructions to the computer
2. Systems software: manages the overall operations of the computer system; program instructions that control, interface with, and communicate between the applications software and the workstation
3. Applications software: mainly commercially prepared programs that perform specific data processing functions
4. Diskettes or CDs on which computer information may be stored

D. DATA PROCESSING

1. Transforms raw information (data) into useful information
2. The smallest piece of information processed is a *bit* (binary digit); an 8-bit unit is a *byte*
3. 1 byte is required to represent one character
4. 1 kilobyte (KB) equals 1024 bytes
5. 1 megabyte (MB) equals 1000 kilobytes
6. All data is processed in a cycle
7. Input: data is entered into the computer by an input device
8. Processing: data is manipulated
9. Output: processed information is accessed from an output device
10. Storage: information is stored for future use

II. Word Processing

A. GENERAL

1. Use of computer to produce documents
2. Software programs that allow the preparation of written documents

B. KEYBOARD KEYS

1. Alphanumeric: keys that represent letters, numbers, and symbols
2. Backspace: allows the cursor to be moved to the left; erases character over which it is backspaced
3. Caps Lock: keeps the alphabet keys in uppercase
4. Ctrl and Alt (control and alternate keys): used in combination with other keys to increase the number of functions on the keyboard
5. Cursor control arrows: allows the cursor (the blinking arrow [or dash] on the screen that identifies where the data will be placed on the screen) to be moved up, down, to the left, or to the right
6. Del (delete): erases characters to the right of the cursor
7. End: moves the cursor to the end of a line of printing
8. Enter (or Return): returns the cursor to the beginning of the next blank line
9. Esc (escape): allows the exit of a program or window
10. F1 through F12 (function keys): perform special program-directed moves
11. Home: moves the cursor to the upper, lower, left, or right margin
12. Page Up, Page Down: moves the cursor 1 page up or down
13. Print Screen: allows only the displayed screen to be printed (if allowed by the program)
14. Shift: places the alphabet key in uppercase when the Shift key is pressed simultaneously
15. Space bar: allows blank spaces to be placed between letters or words
16. Tab: moves the cursor a predetermined number of blank spaces; used to indent

C. FORMATTING

1. Determines the physical layout of the document
   a. Margins: the amount of blank space at the edges of the document
   b. Tab Set: sets a specific number of blank spaces to be used in each tab
   c. Line spacing: sets a specific number of blank lines between each line of input text (usually set for single or double spacing)
   d. Pitch: number of characters per inch of type
   e. Justification: alignment of text to the left and/or right margin
   f. Header and Footer: information to be included at the top (header) or bottom (footer) of each page
   g. Pagination: positions and prints the page numbers on each page
   h. Widows and Orphans: eliminates a last paragraph line that appears alone at the top of the next page (widow), or eliminates a first paragraph line that appears at the bottom of the previous page (orphan)
   i. Font: style and size of the print used

D. EDITING

1. Allows changes to be made within a document
   a. Highlight and Block: text can be highlighted for manipulation by using the cursor
   b. Delete: erases the highlighted text block
   c. Copy and Paste: copies the highlighted text block for placement (Paste) elsewhere in the document, at the new cursor location, without erasing
   d. Cut and Paste: takes (Cut) the highlighted text block and places (Paste) it elsewhere in the document, at the new cursor location, without erasing
   e. Print: allows the document to be recorded (Print) on paper (hard copy)
   f. Save: allows data to be placed in storage on a diskette, on a CD, or on the hard drive
   g. Retrieve (open): allows data that has been previously stored to be brought onto the screen

E. WORD PROCESSING TERMINOLOGY

1. Default: predefined settings automatically loaded by the program used, unless changed by the user
2. Directory: index of files on a floppy or hard drive
3. Grammar check: application that identifies input grammar and/or punctuation errors
4. Help screen: provides explanations and/or instructions about a particular task within a particular program
5. Menu: display on the screen that gives a list of options for word processing
6. Page break: places the beginning of a new page where the cursor is positioned
7. Prompt: a message displayed on the screen that gives the user helpful information and/or instructions
8. Reveal codes: normally invisible word processing codes are made visible for quick editing

9. Sort: organizes a list in alphabetical or numerical order
10. Spell check: application that checks for misspelled words (a medical spell check program is available for separate purchase)
11. Thesaurus: identifies synonyms and antonyms for the word on which the cursor sits
12. Window: an application that allows more than one program to be in use at the same time
13. Word wrap: automatically moves the beginning of a line to the next line without having to press Enter (or Return)

III. Written Communication Skills

A. TYPES OF WRITTEN COMMUNICATION WITHIN THE MEDICAL OFFICE
1. Transcription from machine dictation
2. Formal handwritten consultation and/or surgical reports
3. Composition of letters to patients, consulting physicians, and suppliers
4. Replies to inquiries
5. Responses to requests for information
6. Written collection letters
7. Supply orders
8. Documentation of treatment instructions for patients
9. Other types of office communication

B. LETTERS
1. Parts of a letter
   a. Heading
      1) Printed letterhead at the top of the page
      2) Dateline: three blank lines below the letterhead; name of the month written in full, followed by the day and year
   b. Opening
      1) Inside address
         a) Four blank lines below the dateline
         b) Title, name, and address of receiver
         c) Street, avenue, or boulevard; east, west, north, and south are all spelled out
         d) Street numbers 1 through 10 are spelled out
         e) Street numbers 11 and above are identified by numerals
         f) City is spelled out, followed by a comma
         g) State uses the standard two-letter abbreviation without any period
         h) Zip code uses the five, or nine if available, numerals one space after the state
      2) Attention line (optional)
         a) Placed two blank lines below the inside address
         b) Directs the letter to a particular department or person when the letter is addressed to an organization

      3) Salutation
         a) Opening greeting to the letter
         b) Two blank lines below the inside address
         c) Recipient's title and name followed by a colon (personal correspondence allows use of a comma)
         d) Use the courtesy title (Dr., Mr., Mrs., Ms.) when the letter is addressed to a specific individual
         e) Use the phrase *To Whom it May Concern:* or *Dear Sir or Madam:* when the letter is addressed to an unidentified individual within an organization
   c. Body
      1) Placed two blank lines below the salutation
      2) Contains the message of the letter
      3) Each line is single-spaced; a double space is placed between paragraphs
   d. Closing
      1) Complimentary closing
         a) Placed two blank lines below the body of the letter
         b) Only the first letter of the first word in the closing is capitalized
         c) Comma follows the complimentary closing
         d) May be formal (*Truly yours,* or *Very truly yours,*) or common (*Sincerely,* or *Sincerely yours,*)
      2) Signature line
         a) Placed four or five blank lines below the complimentary closing
         b) Typed name of the person authoring the letter
         c) Author's title follows author's name, separated by a comma
         d) Author signs name above the signature line
      3) Reference notation
         a) Placed two lines below the signature line
         b) Identifies the letter's author and the transcriber (*DH:lb* or *DH/lb*), with the author's initials in uppercase letters, the transcriber's initials in lowercase letters
         c) If the author types his or her own letter, then no reference notation is necessary
      4) Enclosure notation
         a) Placed one or two blank lines below the reference notation (or signature line)
         b) Identifies any printed material accompanying the correspondence (*Enc:, Enclosure:, Enclosures:*)
      5) Copy notation
         a) Placed one or two lines below enclosure notation
         b) Indicates that a copy of the correspondence, with any enclosures, was also forwarded to a third party (*cc: Rob David*)

c) If more than one third-party recipient exists, then the recipients are listed alphabetically or in order of authority

d) Blind carbon copy *(bcc: Rob David)* allows a short note to be typed on the copy to be sent to one third party; the short note is placed only on the one copy of the letter that is sent to the blind carbon copy recipient

6) Postscript

a) An afterthought

b) Places two lines below the last typed line *(P.S.:)*

2. Letter styles

a. Full block (see Figure 9-1)

1) All lines begin flush at the left margin

2) Most efficient style, although the least attractive on paper

b. Modified block (see Figure 9-2): all lines begin flush at the left margin except for the dateline and the complimentary close (these two lines begin at the center of the page)

c. Semiblock (see Figure 9-3): same as modified block, except the beginning of each new paragraph of the body of the letter is indented five blank spaces

d. Hanging indentation: same as the modified block, except that all lines of each new paragraph of the body of the letter are indented five blank spaces, except the first line of each paragraph

e. Simplified: same as the full block, except that no salutation and no complimentary close are inserted

3. Margins

a. Short letter (<100 words in the body): 2-inch margins

b. Medium letter (100–200 words): 1½-inch margins

c. Long letter (>200 words): 1-inch margins

4. Multiple pages

a. Use plain paper in same stock (weight) as letterhead

b. Type the recipient's name seven blank lines from the top of the page; type the page number one line below the recipient's name; type the current date one line below the page number

c. The body of the letter continues three blank lines below the page heading

d. The same page heading (with corresponding page number) on all subsequent pages

C. ENVELOPES

1. Sizes

a. #6¾: 6½ × 3⅝ inches

b. #10: 9½ × 4⅛ inches

2. Folding letters for insertion (see Figure 9-4)

a. #6¾ envelope

1) Fold the page in half, bottom up, and crease

2) Fold the right one third over the left, and crease

Elizabeth Blackwell, M.D.
223 Orange Avenue, N.W.
Cottonwood, UT 84121

January 26, 20—

Mr. Richard Fluege
3678 North Willow Avenue
Palm Beach, FL 33480

Dear Mr. Fluege:

Please send me full particulars on the professional suites you expect to offer for sale or rent in the Medical Arts Professional Annex.

In about six months, I will be ready to open my practice, and I am interested in locating to Florida. My preference is a street-level suite of approximately 2,000 square feet.

After I have had an opportunity to study the information you send me, I will write or telephone you if I have further questions.

Very truly yours,

Elizabeth Blackwell, M.D.

EB:mek

FIGURE 9-1. Block letter style. (Young AP, Kennedy DB: *Kinn's the medical assistant: an applied learning approach,* ed 9, Philadelphia, 2003, Saunders.)

MEDICAL ARTS PROFESSIONAL ANNEX
3678 North Willow Avenue
Palm Beach FL 33480

January 29, 20—

Elizabeth Blackwell, M.D.
223 Orange Avenue, N.W.
Cottonwood, UT 84121

Dear Doctor Blackwell:

We have two remaining street-level suites available for occupancy about July 1. These are marked on pages 3 and 4 of the enclosed descriptive brochure. If one of these suites appeals to you, we will be pleased to customize it for your practice.

Please feel free to call me collect at the number on the brochure for further discussion of your needs.

Sincerely yours,

Richard Fluege
Business Manager

RF:ab
Enclosure

FIGURE 9-2. Modified block letter style. (Young AP, Kennedy DB: *Kinn's the medical assistant: an applied learning approach,* ed 9, Philadelphia, 2003, Saunders.)

WILLIAM OSLER, M.D.
1000 South West Street
Park Ridge, NJ 07656

January 26, 20—

Robert Koch, M.D.
398 Main Street
Park Ridge, NJ 07656

Dear Doctor Koch:

Mrs. Elaine Norris

Thank you for referring your patient, Mrs. Elaine Norris, for consultation and care. She was examined in my office today.

FINDINGS: The patient complained of pain in the left lower quadrant and some abdominal tenderness. She had a temperature of 100.2 degrees.

RECOMMENDATION: The patient was placed on a soft, low-residue, bland diet, antibiotics, and bed rest for a few days. Upper and lower gastrointestinal x-rays will be performed next week.

TENTATIVE DIAGNOSIS: Diverticulitis of large bowel.

Mrs. Norris has been asked to return here for reevaluation in about ten days.

Sincerely yours,

William Osler, M.D.

WO:gm

FIGURE 9-3. Modified block letter style with indented paragraphs. (Young AP, Kennedy DB: *Kinn's the medical assistant: an applied learning approach,* ed 9, Philadelphia, 2003, Saunders.)

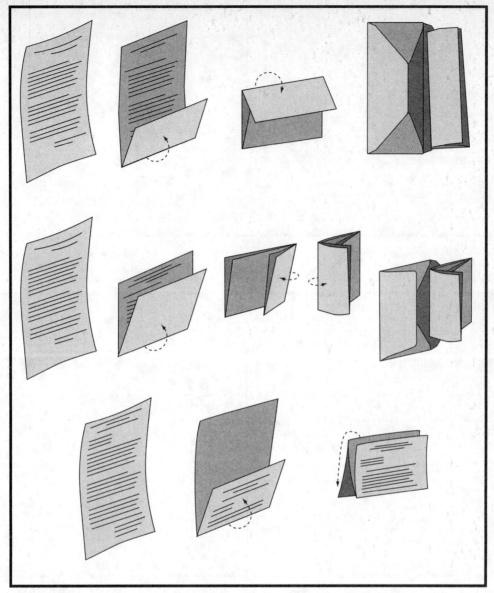

FIGURE 9-4. Correct methods of folding letters. (Young AP, Kennedy DB: *Kinn's the medical assistant: an applied learning approach,* ed 9, Philadelphia, 2003, Saunders.)

3) Fold the left one third over the right, and crease
4) Insert the last-creased edge into the envelope first
b. #10 envelope
1) Fold the bottom one third, bottom up, and crease
2) Fold the top one third, top down, and crease
3) Insert the last-creased edge into the envelope first
3. Return address
a. Placed three blank lines from the top edge, five spaces from the left edge (if the return address is not preprinted on the envelope)
b. Always place the complete return address on the envelope

4. Mailing address (see Figure 9-5)
a. #6¾ envelope: placed 2 inches down from the top edge and 2½ inches to the right of the left edge
b. #10 envelope: placed 2 inches down from the top edge and 4 inches to the right of the left edge
c. Type the address in block format; capitalize all letters; no punctuation used (copy the inside address from the letter to insert onto the envelope)
d. Use standard two-letter state abbreviation
5. Notations
a. Directed to the recipient (*Personal and Confidential*): types two blank lines below the return address
b. Directed to the post office (*Special Delivery* or *Certified Mail*): capitalize all letters in upper-right side, below the area of stamp placement

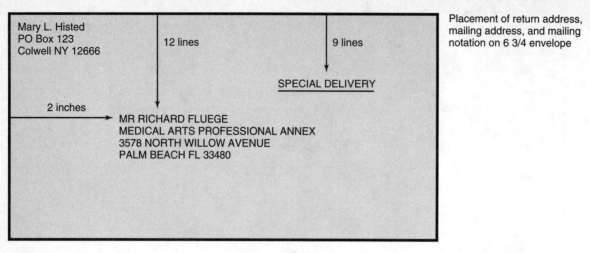

Mary L. Histed
PO Box 123
Colwell NY 12666

12 lines

9 lines

Placement of return address,
mailing address, and mailing
notation on 6 3/4 envelope

SPECIAL DELIVERY

2 inches

MR RICHARD FLUEGE
MEDICAL ARTS PROFESSIONAL ANNEX
3578 NORTH WILLOW AVENUE
PALM BEACH FL 33480

Placement of mailing address
and Personal notation on
No. 10 envelope

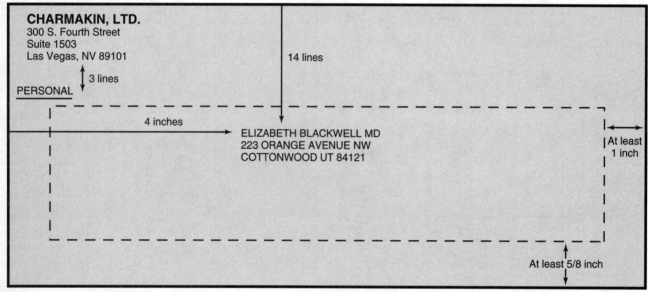

CHARMAKIN, LTD.
300 S. Fourth Street
Suite 1503
Las Vegas, NV 89101

14 lines

3 lines

PERSONAL

4 inches

ELIZABETH BLACKWELL MD
223 ORANGE AVENUE NW
COTTONWOOD UT 84121

At least
1 inch

At least 5/8 inch

FIGURE 9-5.   Addressing envelopes. (Young AP, Kennedy DB: *Kinn's the medical assistant: an applied learning approach*, ed 9, Philadelphia, 2003, Saunders.)

D. MEMORANDA (see Figure 9-6)
1. Written communication within an office or organization
2. Use headings, including Receiver, Sender, Date, and Subject of Memo; each office will have a template to be used in all memoranda
3. Information pertaining to the headings should be on the same line and two or three spaces after the heading, separated by a colon
4. Message should begin three blank lines below the last line of the headings
5. Can have a reference notation, and a copy notation (use the same format as for letters)

E. MANUSCRIPTS
1. Written document submitted for publication
2. Different professional organizations require different standard formats (template) for manuscript

preparation and submission (each will forward its template on request)
3. Includes:
   a. Title page
      1) Identifies the title or theme of the manuscript
      2) Title, author, and author's credentials are normally centered horizontally and vertically on the title page (can vary depending on the organization's shell)
   b. Acknowledgments
      1) Identifies persons who have assisted the author in research or preparation
      2) Placed on a separate page following the title page
   c. Abstract
      1) Summary of the manuscript, normally in 100 to 200 words
      2) Placed on the third page

INTEROFFICE MEMORANDUM

TO   All Staff

FROM   Office Manager

DATE   December 1

SUBJECT   Holiday Schedule

Our entire facility will be closed on December 24, December 25, December 31, and January 1. The office will be on reduced staff during the days of December 26, 27, 28, 29, and 30. Assignments will be based on seniority of staff members. Please submit your preferences as soon as possible.

A

MEMO TO: George Walker

FROM: Stanley Barr

DATE: February 8

SUBJECT: Office rental

We are experiencing unexpectedly rapid growth in our business office and will soon need additional space for our increased number of employees. Do you have a larger facility available in this building? If so, I would like to hear from you regarding the location, square footage, and anticipated rental costs.

B

FIGURE 9-6. Examples of memoranda. (Young AP, Kennedy DB: *Kinn's the medical assistant: an applied learning approach*, ed 9, Philadelphia, 2003, Saunders.)

---

   d. Text
     1) Title is typed, in capital letters, 13 lines from the top of page
     2) Body of the manuscript begins three blank lines below the title
     3) Text of the manuscript is double-spaced
   e. References
     1) Identifies published works of others referenced within the text
     2) In the final version, each reference is indicated by numerical superscripts or numbers in parentheses after each citation (depending on the style of the journal to which the manuscript is being submitted); references are listed in numerical order at the end of the manuscript
   f. Footnote: cites references and their explanations near the bottom of the page on which the referenced material is written
   g. Bibliography: list of reference books, manuscripts, articles, or other sources that were used to prepare the manuscript; listed in alphabetical order by name of document or by last name of document author
   h. Illustrations and tables: placed on separate sheets at the end of the manuscript and assigned consecutive numbers

IV. Processing Mail

A. MAIL CLASSIFICATIONS

   1. Express mail, next-day service
     a. Available 7 days a week, 365 days a year
     b. Cost is normally one standard price per item
   2. First class
     a. Sealed or unsealed material
     b. Includes letters, postcards, and business-reply mail
     c. Cost is based on weight (in 1-oz increments)
   3. Priority mail
     a. First class mail weighing more than 11 oz (maximum weight is 70 lb)
     b. Postage calculated on the combined basis of weight and destination
   4. Second class
     a. Regular rates
     b. Available to newspapers and periodicals preauthorized by the post office
   5. Third class
     a. Includes catalogs, circulars, books, photographs, and other preprinted materials
     b. Must be marked *Third Class*
   6. Fourth class: merchandise, books, and preprinted material (media mail) not included in First or Second Class and that weigh 16 oz or more

7. Registered mail
   a. First class mail additionally protected by registration
   b. Post office receives an additional fee for this service
   c. Post office verifies delivery of the material
   d. Recipient may be required to sign a form to acknowledge receipt, if the sender requests
   e. Registered mail request form must be filled out before mailing
8. Certified mail
   a. Delivery of mail requiring the recipient's signature as proof of delivery
   b. Certified mail request form must be filled out before mailing

B. EQUIPMENT AND SUPPLIES
1. Postage scale: used to weigh mail to determine the correct postage
2. Postage meter
   a. Machine used to print prepaid postage directly on the envelope or on an adhesive label, depending on the weight of the material
   b. The date and the amount of postage are set by pressing the appropriate buttons
3. Stationery
   a. Standard size and weight, as determined by the office manager
   b. Normally light-colored paper with darker imprinting
4. Rubber stamps
   a. Can indicate the date of receipt of mail
   b. Can be used to endorse checks for deposit

C. INCOMING MAIL
1. Schedule a set time during which to sort and distribute received mail
2. Date-stamp the front (or the back) of each piece of paper within each envelope, and date-stamp the envelope, depending on the office method (except for checks)
3. *Personal* or *personal and confidential* noted mailings are delivered directly to the addressee without being opened
4. Any mail that is opened by mistake must be resealed with tape and noted on the envelope that it was opened by mistake
5. All checks received must be endorsed immediately and forwarded to the accounts receivable clerk

V. Transcription

A. GENERAL
1. Process of listening to voice-recorded dictation and translating it into written form
2. Can also be the typing into standard format of consultation or surgical notes

3. Standard office formats and styles should be followed
4. Main requirements of the transcription are appearance, clarity, and legibility
5. Three definite stages within the transcription:
   a. Author speaks into a dictating (recording) unit
   b. Transcriptionist listens to (or deciphers what has been written) the recording
   c. Transcriptionist keyboards the text into a printed document, using the office-standard format and punctuation

B. EQUIPMENT
1. Audiocassettes: contain recorded notes
2. Transcriber: machine used by transcriptionist
3. Headphones: used to hear the recorded tapes
4. Foot pedal: allows the transcriptionist to manipulate the recorded tapes while keeping both hands free for keyboarding

C. FORMAT
1. Title of document
   a. Centered on first line of page
   b. All uppercase letters; underlining is optional to the office
2. Identifying information
   a. Patient name, patient record number, physician name, and date of admission and treatment
   b. Typed at the left margin; used as header titles
   c. Capitalize the first letter of each name; each different name or number is separated by a colon
   d. Each header should be double-spaced
   e. Narrative information begins two blank spaces after the colon
3. Headings
   a. Major headings, typed in all-capital letters, followed by colon
      1) History
      2) Chief Complaint
      3) History of Present Illness
      4) Family History
      5) Social History
      6) Past Medical History
      7) Review of Systems
      8) General
      9) Physical Exam
      10) Diagnosis (or Impression or Conclusion)
      11) Admitting Diagnosis
      12) Surgical Procedures
      13) Lab Data
   b. Secondary headings, typed in all-capital letters, followed by a colon
4. Format styles
   a. Full block
      1) All headings, except title, are flush with the left margin
      2) Headings are double-spaced from the last line of the previous narrative

3) Narrative begins two spaces after the colon following the heading
   b. Indented
   1) Subheadings are indented three to five spaces under the main headings
   2) Headings are double-spaced from the last line of the previous narrative
   3) Narrative begins on the same line as the heading, with the first two lines indented 23 to 27 spaces from the left margin
   4) Third and subsequent lines begin at the left margin
   c. Modified block
   1) All headings begin at the left margin
   2) All headings are double-spaced from the last line of the previous narrative
   3) Narrative begins on the same line as the headings
   4) Second and subsequent lines are 23 to 27 spaces from the left margin
   d. Run-on
   1) All headings begin at the left margin
   2) No double spaces between any headings
   3) The narrative begins on the same line as the headings
   4) Second and subsequent lines are flush with the left margin

5. Signature line
   a. Type solid line from the center page to the right margin, four to six blank lines following the end of the narrative
   b. Type the physician's full name immediately below the solid line

6. Notations and date
   a. Typed two lines below the physician's name at the left margin
   b. Identify the dictator and the transcriptionist
   c. Type the dictator's initials in all capital letters, followed by a colon, followed by transcriptionist's initials in all lowercase letters (e.g., *DH:gm*)
   d. Immediately below the initials, insert the date the report was dictated (use *D:* followed by two spaces and the relevant date)
   e. Immediately below the date, insert the date the report was transcribed (use *T:* followed by two spaces and the relevant date)

7. Multiple pages
   a. Type the word *(continued)* in parentheses two lines below the last line of the narrative on the page, at the left margin

   b. Begin the next page with patient's name, the reporting physician's name, the date of treatment, and the page number
   c. Do not begin a new page with only the physician's signature line; include at least two lines of narrative from the preceding page (this is a legal requirement)

8. Syntax
   a. Uses sentence fragments; type as dictated, and punctuate accordingly
   b. Follow the instructions stated by the dictator

D. STYLE (ACCORDING TO *AMERICAN MEDICAL ASSOCIATION MANUAL OF STYLE*)

1. Eponyms are capitalized
2. Drug product names are capitalized; generic names are not capitalized
3. Underline or italicize scientific names of organisms; genus is capitalized; species is not capitalized
4. Capitalize proper names of religions, languages, and races
5. Patient allergies are in all-capital letters and are underlined
6. Capitalize acronyms
7. Numbers from 1 to 10 are spelled out; use numerals for 11 and higher
8. Use numerals for numbers in measurements
9. Use numerals when using symbols with the numbers (e.g., 100%)
10. Numbers less than 1 expressed as a decimal must be preceded by *0* (e.g., 0.25)
11. Spell out ordinals except with a date (e.g., *second day*, but *May 2*)
12. Vertebrae are abbreviated (e.g., C1 to C7, T1 to T12, L1 to L5)
13. Cranial nerves are written as Roman numerals
14. Titers and ratios include a colon (e.g., 1:2)
15. Patient temperature readings include indication of *F* or *C*
16. Suture material is indicated as *2-0* or *00*
17. Use subscripts or superscripts, as noted by dictator
18. Use numbers for cancer grades, electrocardiographic leads, and military time
19. Abbreviate metric without a period
20. Pharmacologic abbreviations are written in lowercase without periods

10 | *Finances*

I. Accounting

A. GENERAL
1. Process of recording, classifying, summarizing, reporting, analyzing, and interpreting financial data
2. Provides financial information about the business operation

B. ACCOUNTING ELEMENTS
1. Asset
   a. Property owned or controlled by a business
   b. Includes:
      1) Land, buildings, fixtures, and furnishings
      2) Medical or office equipment
      3) Money
      4) Accounts receivable
      5) Stocks, bonds, and investments
2. Liability
   a. Debt obligation of the business
   b. Includes:
      1) Accounts payable
      2) Bank debts
3. Owner's equity
   a. Amount by which assets exceed liabilities; *net worth*
   b. Includes:
      1) Revenue (assets in)
      2) Expense (assets out)
      3) Drawing (personal use of assets)
4. Accounting equations
   a. Assets = Liabilities + Owner's Equity
   b. Liabilities = Assets − Owner's Equity
   c. Owner's Equity = Assets − Liabilities

II. Bookkeeping

A. SYSTEMS
1. Single-entry system
   a. Oldest and simplest method
   b. Simple to use, inexpensive, and requires little training

   c. Includes three basic records:
      1) Journal: also called the daily log, daybook, day sheet, or charge journal; records of charges and receipts are entered daily
      2) Cash payment journal: simple form of a checkbook
      3) Accounts receivable ledger: record of the amounts that patients owe the office; each patient has his or her own card; statements are prepared from these cards
2. Pegboard (write-it-once) system (see Figure 10-1)
   a. Most common manual method used in the physician's office
   b. All transactions are recorded at one time
   c. Uses the following materials:
      1) Pegboard
         a) Plastic board with pegs along the left edge
         b) Pegs hold perforated accounting entry pages
      2) Day sheet
         a) Page size of pegboard
         b) Keeps record of all daily charges and receipts
      3) Ledger card: record of all charges and payments for each patient
      4) Charge slip or charge receipt
         a) Form used to record a charge
         b) Serves as a bill or receipt if payment is made by the patient
         c) May be in the form of a *superbill* (a multipage, carbonless charge slip; one copy of the form is given to the patient, and one copy is kept by the office; one copy of the form is forwarded to the patient's insurance company)
   d. Day sheet is affixed to the pegboard (perforations on the sheet are placed over the pegs on the pegboard)
   e. Each patient ledger card is placed over the day sheet, hooked onto the pegs so that the columns and rows line up with the day sheet

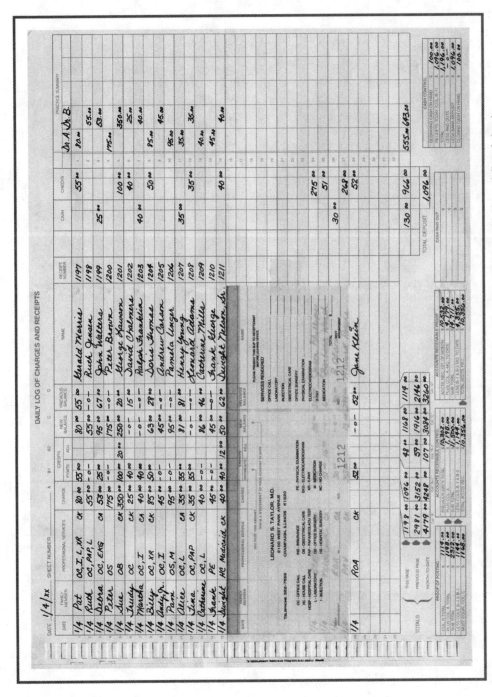

FIGURE 10-1. Sample day sheet for pegboard bookkeeping system, with deposit list of checks and optional business analysis summaries. (Courtesy of Patterson Office Supplies, a division of Patterson Companies, Inc., 1-800-637-1140.)

f. Charge slip or charge receipt is placed over the patient ledger card

g. Bookkeeping entries are made and recorded simultaneously on all forms on the pegboard

3. Double-entry system

a. Inexpensive method but requires some training

b. Transactions may be recorded manually or by computer

c. Each transaction is recorded in a way that keeps a balance of accounting equation

d. Each transaction affects two accounts: one is debited, the other is credited

B. ACCOUNTS RECEIVABLE

1. Fees that patients owe for services performed

2. Most receipts come from third-party payments (e.g., insurance carrier); payments might not be received for 30 to 90 days after service

3. Accounts are classified according to the amount of time that the balance remains unpaid (current, 30 days, 60 days, over 90 days, past due)

C. ACCOUNTS PAYABLE

1. Money owed to vendors

2. Payments to vendors for purchases and services

3. Invoice normally accompanies the purchase

4. Record of payments kept by making an entry into the appropriate accounts payable record

D. PETTY CASH

1. Cash kept within the office to cover minor purchases

2. Usual amount is $50.00

3. Eliminates the need to write a check for minor purchases

4. Fund is established by writing a check on the office account; this check is cashed by the bank, and the cash is placed in a safe place within the office

5. One person is designated to make disbursements from the petty cash fund

6. A voucher is normally required to draw cash out of the fund; the voucher should show the name of the person taking the cash, the amount of cash taken, and the purpose of the petty cash draw; this voucher is used to balance the account

7. A register should be maintained to track the vouchers

8. The petty cash fund is replenished by again writing and cashing a check

III. Billing

A. FEES

1. Should reflect the revenue necessary to maintain the financial stability of the practice

2. Influenced by the time to be spent and the degree of difficulty in providing the service

3. Set up by a schedule that includes code numbers, detailed description, and cost of each particular service rendered within the practice

4. The schedule must be available to all patients

a. Usual fee: fee most frequently charged for a particular service

b. Customary fee: range of usual fees charged for the particular service by practitioners of similar training and experience

c. Reasonable fee: fee assigned to an unusual service or a service that has complex features; meets the criteria of usual and customary fees

B. FORMS

1. Patient information form

a. Used to collect and maintain general information about the patient for billing purposes

b. Includes the patient's name, home address, home telephone number, occupation, business address, business telephone number, Social Security Number; name of the insured, insurance carrier, and policy number; the spouse's name, occupation, business address, and business telephone number; and an emergency contact telephone number

2. Release of information form

a. Used to request information gathered by other medical providers

b. Patient's signature authorizes a third party (e.g., insurance company) to be given information about the patient's treatment

3. Assignment of benefits form: patient's signature requests the insurance company to send insurance proceeds directly to the provider

C. BILLING METHODS

1. Time-of-service

a. Fee collected when the service is provided

b. Reduces collection costs

c. Increases cash flow

2. Monthly billing: a bill is sent to each patient on a monthly basis

3. Cycle billing: a bill is sent to certain segments of the patient population at a consistent time each month, with each segment being sent at a different time during the month

4. Billing service: the office may contract with an outside agency to prepare and send the bills to the patients

D. STATEMENTS

1. Typed: each patient bill is individually typed

2. Ledger cards: copies are made of the patient's ledger card entries and mailed to the patient

3. Superbill (see Figure 10-2)

a. Presented to the patient at each visit

b. Payment is made at the time of the office visit or mailed in at a later date

4. Computerized: data are keyed into an accounting computer program; statements are automatically generated by the accounting software

STATE LIC. # 123456789
SOC. SEC. # 000-11-0000
PIN # _____

TELEPHONE: (123) 234-5678

JOHN R. JOHNSON, M.D.
Family Practice
1000 MAIN STREET, SOME PLACE, USA 70000

☐ PRIVATE ☐ BLUECROSS ☐ IND. ☐ MEDICARE ☐ MEDI-CAL ☐ HMO ☐ PPO

PATIENT'S LAST NAME	FIRST	ACCOUNT #	BIRTHDATE / /	SEX ☐ MALE ☐ FEMALE	TODAY'S DATE / /
INSURANCE COMPANY	SUBSCRIBER		PLAN #	SUB. #	GROUP

ASSIGNMENT: I hereby assign my insurance benefits to be paid directly to the undersigned physician. I am financially responsible for non-covered services.
SIGNED: (Patient, or Parent, if Minor)   DATE: / /

RELEASE: I hereby authorize the physician to release to my insurance carrers any information required to process this claim.
SIGNED: (Patient, or Parent, if Minor)   DATE: / /

✔	DESCRIPTION	M/Care	CPT/Mod	DxRe	FEE	✔	DESCRIPTION	M/Care	CPT/Mod	DxRe	FEE	✔	DESCRIPTION	M/Care	CPT/Mod	DxRe	FEE
	OFFICE CARE						**PROCEDURES**						**INJECTIONS/IMMUNIZATIONS**				
	NEW PATIENT						Treadmill (In Office)		93015				Tetanus Toxoid		90703		
	Focused		99201				24 Hr. Holter Monitor		93224				Hypertet	J1670	90782		
	Expanded		99202				Recording Only		93225				Pneumococcal		90732		
	Detailed		99203				Interp. & Report		93227				Influenza		90724		
	Comprehensive-Mod.		99204				EKG w/Interpretation		93000				TB Skin Test (PPD)		86585		
	Comprehensive-High		99205				EKG (Medicare)		93005				Antigen Injection-Single		95115		
							Sigmoidoscopy		45300				Multiple		95117		
	ESTABLISHED PATIENT						Sigmoidoscopy, Flexible		45330				B12 Injection	J3420	90782		
	Minimal		99211				Sigmoidos., Flex. w/Bx.		45331				Injection, IM		90788		
	Focused		99212				Spirometry. FEV/FVC		94010				Compazine	J0780	90782		
	Expanded		99213				Spirometry, Post-Dilator		94060				Demerol	J2175	90782		
	Detailed		99214										Vistaril	J3410	90782		
	Comprehensive-Mod.		99215										Susphrine	J0170	90782		
	Comprehensive-High		99215				**LABORATORY**						Decadron	J0890	90782		
							Routine Venipuncture		36415				Estradiol	J1000	90782		
	CONSULTATION-OFFICE						Urinalysis, Chemical		81005				Testosterone	J1080	90782		
	Focused		99241				Throat Culture		87081				Lidocaine	J2000	90782		
	Expanded		99242				Occult Blood		82270				Solumedrol	J2920	90782		
	Detailed		99243				Pap Handling Charge		99000				Solucortef	J1720	90782		
	Comprehensive-Mod.		99244				Pap Life Guard		88150-90				Hydeltra	J1690	90782		
	Comprehensive-High		99245				Gram Stain		87205				Pen Procaine	J2510	90788		
	Dr.						Wet Mount		87210								
	Post-op Exam		99024				Urine Drug Screen		99000				**INJECTIONS - JOINT/BURSA**				
	EVALUATION/CASE MANAGEMENT												Arthrocentesis-Small Jt.		20600		
	Brief Eval.-30 Mins.		99361										Arthrocent.-Interm. Jts.		20605		
	Intermed. Eval.-60 Mins.		99362				**SUPPLIES**						Arthrocent.-Major Jts.		20610		
	Telephone-Brief		99371										Trigger Point Injection		20550		
	Telephone-Intermed.		99372										**MISCELLANEOUS**				
	Telephone-Complex		99272														

DIAGNOSIS:	ICD-9						
__ Abdominal Pain	789.0_	__ Gout	274.0	__ C.V.A. - Acute	436.	__ Electrolyte Dis.	276.9	__ Herpes Simplex	054.9
__ Abscess (Site)	682.9	__ Asthma	493.90	__ Cere. Vas. Accid. (Old)	438	__ Fatigue	780.7	__ Herpes Zoster	053.9
__ Adverse Drug Rx	995.2	__ Asthmatic Bronchitis	491.20	__ Cerumen	380.4	__ Fibrocys. Br. Dis	610.1	__ Hydrocele	603.9
__ Alcohol Detox	291.8	__ Atrial Fib.	427.31	__ Chestwall Pain	786.59	__ Fracture (Site)	829.0	__ Hyperlipidemia	272.4
__ Alcoholism	303.90	__ Atrial Tachycardia	427.89	__ Cholecystitis	575.0	__ Open/Close		__ Hypertension	401.9
__ Allergic Rhinitis	477.9	__ Bowel Obstruct.	560.9	__ Cholelithiasis	574.00	__ Fungal Infect. (Site)	117.9	__ Hyperthyroidism	242.9
__ Allergy	995.3	__ Breast Mass	611.72	__ COPD	496	__ Gastric Ulcer	531.90	__ Hypothyroidism	244.9
__ Alzheimer's Dis.	290.1_	__ Bronchitis, Acute	466.0	__ Cirrhosis	571.5	__ Gastritis	535.0	__ Labyrinthitis	386.30
__ Anemia	285.9	__ Bursitis	727.3	__ Cong. Heart Fail.	428.9	__ Gastroenteritis	558.9	__ Lipoma (Site)	214.9
__ Anemia - Pernicious	281.0	__ Cancer, Breast (Site)	174.9	__ Conjunctivitis	372.30	__ G.I. Bleeding	578.9	__ Lymphoma	202.8
__ Angina	413.9	__ Metastatic (Site)	198.2	__ Contusion (Site)	924.9	__ Glomerulonephritis	583.89	__ Mit. Valve Prolapse	424.0
__ Anxiety Synd.	300.00	__ Colon	153.9	__ Costochondritis	733.99	__ Headache	784.0	__ Myocard. Infarction (Area)	410.9
__ Appendicitis	541	__ Cancer, Rectal	154.1	__ Depression	311.	__ Headache, Tension	307.81	__ M.I., Old	412
__ Arterioscl. H.D.	414.0_	__ Lung (Site)	162.9	__ Dermatitis	692.9	__ Migraine (Type)	346.9	__ Myositis	729.1
__ Arthritis, Osteo.	715.90	__ Skin (Site)	173.9	__ Diabetes Mellitus	250.00	__ Hemorrhoids	455.6	__ Nausea/Vomiting	787.01
__ Rheumatoid	714.0	__ Card. Arrhythmia (Type)	427.9	__ Diabetic Ketosis	250.10	__ Hernia, Hiatal	553.3	__ Neuralgia	729.2
__ Lupus	710.0	__ Cardiomyopathy	425.4	__ Diverticulitis	562.11	__ Inguinal	550.9	__ Nevus (Site)	216.9
		__ Cellulitis (Site)	682.9	__ Diverticulosis	562.10	__ Hepatitis	573.3	__ Obesity	278.00

DIAGNOSIS: (IF NOT CHECKED ABOVE)

SERVICES PERFORMED AT: ☐ Office ☐ E.R. ☐ CLAIM CONTAINS NO ORDERED REFERRING SERVICE
☐   ☐

REFERRING PHYSICIAN & I.D. NUMBER

RETURN APPOINTMENT INFORMATION:
5 - 10 - 15 - 20 - 30 - 40 - 60
[DAYS] [WKS.] [MOS.] [PRN]

NEXT APPOINTMENT
M - T - W - TH - F - S
DATE / /   TIME:

ACCEPT ASSIGNMENT?
☐ YES
☐ NO
AM
PM

DOCTOR'S SIGNATURE

INSTRUCTIONS TO PATIENT FOR FILING INSURANCE CLAIMS:

1. Complete upper portion of this form, sign and date.
2. Attach this form to your own insurance company's form for direct reimbursement.

MEDICARE PATIENTS - DO NOT SEND THIS TO MEDICARE.
WE WILL SUBMIT THE CLAIM FOR YOU.

☐ CASH
☐ CHECK
    # _____
☐ VISA
☐ MC
☐ CO-PAY

TOTAL TODAY'S FEE	
OLD BALANCE	
TOTAL DUE	
AMOUNT REC'D. TODAY	

INSUR-A-BILL ® BIBBERO SYSTEMS, INC. • PETALUMA, CA • FORM #11-9999 © 6/94 (STOCK)

FIGURE 10-2. Superbill. (Courtesy of Bibbero Systems, Inc., Petaluma, California 94954-1180, 800-242-2376, fax 800-242-8330, *http://www.bibbero.com*.)

IV. Collections

A. GENERAL
1. Revenue from services rendered must be collected to cover expenses
2. Harassing debtors is illegal

B. TELEPHONE COLLECTIONS
1. Making threatening or abusive calls when attempting to collect a debt is illegal
2. Call between 8:00 AM and 8:00 PM and only to the patient's home telephone when attempting to collect a debt
3. Determine the identity of the person with whom you are discussing debt collection by using the debtor's full name
4. Be positive and assertive
5. State the purpose of your call
6. Attempt to obtain a commitment by the debtor before ending the debt-collection call; attempt to get the debtor to promise to deliver a certain sum by a certain date
7. After this initial debt collection contact, follow up with another confirmation call

C. MAILINGS
1. Use letters within opaque envelopes for debt collection, never postcards
2. Prepare correspondence to meet the situation (begin debt-collection process with a friendly tone, progressing to a more assertive tone as debt collection lags)
3. Debt-collection letters should be signed by the office manager
4. Inform the patient by Certified Mail or Return Receipt Requested of possible collection agency action or legal action to collect the debt

D. PROGRESSIVE COLLECTION PROCESS
1. Office should have developed a color-coded or written stage-by-stage process by which the office can keep track of debt collection efforts (with the process identified first by friendly tones, progressing to more assertive tones as debt collection lags)

E. COLLECTION AGENCY
1. Forward the past-due account to the collection agency once the account has been determined uncollectible by office personnel
2. Once the account is given to a collection agency, the clinic may not continue collection efforts on the debt
3. Patients should make payments on their debt only to the collection agency once the account has been turned over to the agency
4. The collection agency will keep a percentage of the amount collected as their fee

V. Payroll

A. GENERAL
1. Affected by federal and state laws and regulations
2. Income tax, Federal Insurance Contributions Act (FICA), and Federal Unemployment Tax Act (FUTA) amounts withheld from employee checks must be paid to the Internal Revenue Service (IRS) and to the state tax commissioner at regular intervals
3. Payroll procedures must be explained to all new employees

B. LAWS AND REGULATIONS
1. Detailed records must be kept in the office for each employee, including:
   a. Name, address, Social Security Number
   b. Amount and date of each wage payment and period covered by the payment
   c. Amount of wages subject to taxes
   d. Amount and type of taxes withheld from employee's pay
   e. Date when employee begins work; date when employee leaves the employment
2. Fair Labor Standards Act
   a. Sets minimum wage
   b. Requires employers to pay 1½ times employee's regular wage for time worked over 40 regular hours
3. Title VII, Civil Rights Act of 1964: prohibits discrimination based on employee's race, color, religion, or gender in hiring, firing, or promoting employees
4. Age Discrimination in Employment Act: prohibits unfair practices in employment decisions regarding people over 40 years of age
5. Americans with Disabilities Act: prohibits unfair practices in employment decisions (and in many other areas) regarding people with physical, mental, or medical disabilities
6. Family Medical Leave Act of 1993
   a. In the case of birth, adoption, sick or injured family member, an employee is entitled to unpaid leave to care for the child, spouse, parent, or for him or herself
   b. The employee is entitled to benefits and job protection while on leave

C. TAXES
1. Income tax
   a. Employers are required by law to withhold employee income tax
   b. Amount withheld from the employee's paycheck is based on a graduated rate table
2. FICA
   a. Social Security and Medicare Tax
   b. Employers are required to withhold (collect) these taxes from employee wages
   c. Employer submits amounts withheld to the IRS when the employer pays the employer's taxes

d. Taxes are deducted from the employee's earnings each pay period

e. Every dollar paid by the employee is matched, dollar for dollar, by the employer

3. FUTA
   a. Federal law requires employers to withhold tax to support the unemployment insurance programs
   b. Amount of tax withheld is computed on a graduated rate table based on employee earnings

D. FORMS AND REPORTS

1. Form SS-4
   a. Federal Tax Identification Number application form
   b. Required for employers who hire employees and who withhold taxes from employee pay
2. Form SS-5
   a. Social Security number application form
   b. All employees are required to have a Social Security number
3. Form W-2
   a. Wages and Tax Statement
   b. Given to all employees
   c. Lists the wages earned (by one employee) and taxes withheld on wages for the preceding year
   d. Used to prepare personal income tax return
   e. Must be provided to employees by January 31 of the following year
   f. Consists of six parts:
      1) Copy A: sent to the Social Security Administration
      2) Copy 1: sent to the state tax department
      3) Copy B: filed with the employee's federal tax return
      4) Copy C: kept by the employee
      5) Copy 2: filed with employee's state tax return
      6) Copy D: retained by the employer
4. Form W-3
   a. Transmittal of Income and Tax Statement
   b. Used to report the total amount of income and FICA tax withheld during the year
   c. Filed by the employer with the Social Security Administration
5. Form W-4
   a. Employee's Withholding Allowance Certificate
   b. Identifies the total number of withholding allowances claimed by the employee
6. Form 940: employer's annual federal unemployment tax return
7. Form 941
   a. Employer's quarterly federal tax return
   b. Filed quarterly to report FUTA and income tax amounts to the federal government
8. Form 8109
   a. Federal Tax Deposit Coupon Book
   b. Used to make quarterly federal income tax and FUTA payments
9. Form 1099
   a. IRS form to report income other than wages
   b. A physician-employer's honoraria from speaking engagements would be claimed on this form
10. Form I-9: confirms U.S. citizenship or legality of working papers if a foreign national

E. PAYROLL SYSTEMS

1. Manual
   a. Most common for smaller organizations
   b. Payroll is computed and processed by hand
2. Computerized
   a. Data is entered into accounting management computer program
   b. Payroll calculations automatically prepared by the software
   c. Detailed records and reports are automatically prepared by the software
3. Payroll services
   a. Payroll data is sent to the payroll service
   b. Service prepares the payroll and delivers detailed records, reports, and the payroll checks to the office

VI. Checking Accounts

A. GENERAL (see Figure 10-3)

1. The majority of money transactions out of the office are conducted by check
2. A check is a commercial paper drawn on funds deposited in a bank account
3. A check is a written order for the bank to pay a person a specific amount of money
4. A check is negotiable; anyone who properly endorses the check is entitled to receive the money
5. Parties involved in a check:
   a. Drawer: the person writing the check
   b. Drawee: the bank
   c. Payee: the person who is to receive the money from the check

B. OPENING A CHECKING ACCOUNT

1. Requires approval from a bank official
2. Requires an initial deposit, in accordance with the bank's rules
3. Requires a signature card: the signature card contains the names and signatures of all persons who are authorized to access the checking account

C. DEPOSITS

1. Can be made by using:
   a. Paper money
      1) Arranged in order of denomination (smallest value bill on top)
      2) All bills should be arranged face up and top up
   b. Coins: a large quantity of coins should be wrapped in coin wrappers before deposit

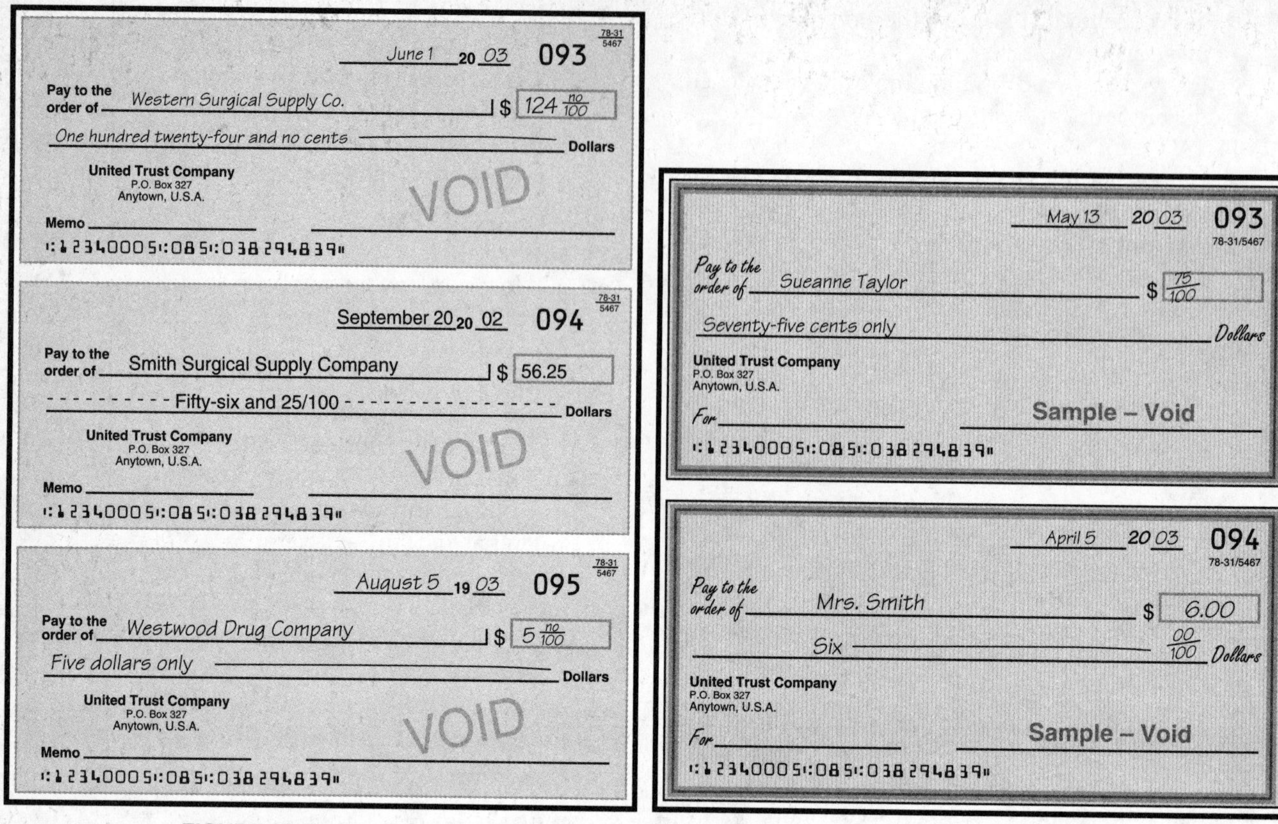

FIGURE 10-3. The first four examples illustrate the correct method of writing a check. The last example (bottom right) shows the incorrect method of writing a check, with incomplete name and space for altering (e.g., 6.00 might be made into 26.00 or more, and 00 could be made into 88). (Young AP, Kennedy DB: *Kinn's the medical assistant: an applied learning approach*, ed 9, Philadelphia, 2003, Saunders.)

c. Checks
1) Office personnel should verify each check for completeness
2) Each check must be endorsed (in writing or by stamp) directing how the check is to be applied
d. Deposit slip (see Figure 10-4): a preprinted form with account information; identifies all items being deposited
1) Enter the date of the deposit
2) Enter the total amount of coins and currency being deposited
3) Enter and note separately each check to be deposited
4) Record the total amount of the deposit
5) Withdraw cash by entering the amount to be withdrawn on the designated space on the deposit slip and subtracting this amount from the deposit total; if a withdrawal of cash is needed, the deposit slip must be signed

D. DISHONORED CHECKS
1. A check that the bank refuses to pay
2. Usually the result of insufficient funds in the account (*NSF*: not sufficient funds)

3. If a check is deposited and not accepted by the bank it is written on, the payee's bank will return the dishonored check back to the payee, will deduct the amount of that check from payee's account, and will normally assess the payee a fee for the work caused
a. Overdraft
1) Issuing a check without sufficient funds in the writer's account
2) Knowingly issuing a NSF check is illegal
b. Postdated check: issuing a check but putting a date in the future on the check; a bank may not honor a check until the date on the check

E. BANK STATEMENTS
1. Statement of account sent to each depositor once a month by the bank
2. Gives the account holder the following information:
a. Account balance at the beginning of the period
b. Amount of deposits made during the period
c. Amount of checks paid during the period
d. Other items paid or credited during the period
e. Account balance at the end of the period

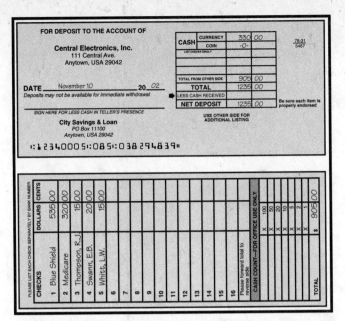

FIGURE 10-4. Front and back of a deposit slip. (Young AP, Kennedy DB: *Kinn's the medical assistant: an applied learning approach*, ed 9, Philadelphia, 2003, Saunders.)

3. Canceled checks may be enclosed with the statement
4. Statement needs to be reconciled (to ensure that the bank's balance agrees with the office's balance)
   a. Compare the deposited amounts recorded in the office files with the amounts recorded on the statement
   b. Compare the canceled check amounts with those on the statement and on the office check register
   c. Identify all debits and credits to the account between the bank's and the office's records
   d. Identify any errors found on the bank statement or on the office register
   e. Add and subtract all adjustments made to the bank statement and to the office register; both balances should be equal

11 Coding

I. Introduction To Coding

A. PURPOSE
1. Coding system translates descriptions of diseases, illnesses, injuries, and procedures into numeric codes
2. Helps insurance company quickly and accurately review what services the patient received and how they are related to the illness or injury
3. Facilitates the use of computers in insurance claim processing
4. Developed for:
   a. Tracking disease processes
   b. Classification of medical procedures
   c. Medical research
   d. Evaluation of hospital utilization

B. TYPES OF CODING SYSTEMS
1. ICD-9-CM
   a. *International Classification of Diseases*, ninth edition, Clinical Modification
   b. Used to code disease conditions or diagnosis
2. ICD-10-CM
   a. Will replace ICD-9-CM, volumes 1 and 2
   b. Changes will include organization overhaul, expansion of codes (50% more codes), new chapters (V- and E-codes in separate chapters), new categories and six-digit alphanumeric codes with greater specificity of site
3. CPT-4
   a. *Current Procedural Terminology*, fourth edition
   b. Used to code procedures and medical services provided by practitioner
4. HCPCS
   a. Health Care Financing Administration (HCFA) Common Procedural Coding System
   b. Used to report services performed to Medicare program
5. RVS
   a. Relative value scale
   b. Assigned unit value given to commonly performed medical procedures
   c. Based on time, knowledge, and skill required by the practitioner
   d. Point value is multiplied by a dollar factor to find a final fee amount
6. RBRVS
   a. Resource-based relative value scale
   b. Fee schedule for Medicare for services based on level of resources needed to provide the service
7. DRG
   a. Diagnosis-related groups
   b. Medicare-fixed fee structure for hospital billing of inpatient services
   c. Based on principal diagnosis

II. ICD-9-CM

A. GENERAL
1. Assigns numeric codes to illnesses, diseases, injuries, and health-related condition

B. ICD-9-CM SYSTEM
1. Volume I (Tabular List of Diseases): numeric arrangement of conditions
   a. 110 to 799: codes that refer to specific conditions by body systems
   b. 800 to 959, 990 to 999: codes that refer to injury
   c. 960 to 989: codes that refer to poisoning
   d. V-codes (V01 to V82): codes that refer to factors that influence health status (e.g., well-baby checks, annual physicals)
   e. E-codes: external causes of injury or poisonings
   f. M-codes: morphology of neoplasms
2. Volume II (Disease: Alphabetical List): three-part index for volume I
   a. Section I: alphabetical index of disease and injury
   b. Section II: table of adverse reactions to drugs and chemicals
   c. Section III: index of external causes (E-Codes)

3. Volume III (Tabular List and Alphabetical Index of Procedures)
   a. Used primarily in hospitals
   b. Procedures are arranged both alphabetically and numerically

C. ORGANIZATION OF VOLUMES
1. Volume I
   a. Codes 001 through 999 use a three-digit main number, with a specificity to cause identified with a fourth digit; a fifth digit may be required
   b. Chapter headings in bold uppercase letters
   c. Notes following the chapter headings give guidelines for coding within the chapter
   d. Major topic headings are in uppercase letters followed by inclusive codes in parentheses
   e. Exclusion statements tell what is *not* included in the specific code number
   f. Category headings further divide major topic headings
   g. Subcategory headings are indented and include a fourth-digit modifier
   h. Fifth-digit modifiers further subdivide the subcategory heading; generally flagged in some way (a section mark)
2. Volume II
   a. Alphabetical listing of conditions
   b. May be expressed as nouns, adjectives, or eponyms
   c. Main terms are highlighted in bold type followed by the code number
   d. Modifiers in parentheses may be present between the main term and the code number
   e. Subterms are indented, giving further subclassifications

D. CONVENTIONS
1. Volume I
   a. Colon (:): modifiers after the colon complete the statement before the colon
   b. Brace (}): term after the brace is a required modifier
   c. Section mark: identifies a code that needs a fifth-digit modifier
   d. Excludes: enclosed within a rectangle; conditions following this mark do not qualify for code assignment
   e. Includes: clarifies a description
2. Volume II
   a. Diagnoses are organized by main terms printed in boldface type
      1) Modifiers: specific factors that influence a diagnostic code
         a) Nonessential: main term followed by terms in parentheses; may be included with the main term
         b) Subterm: specific manifestations of a condition; these have a specific code number; indented below the main term

   c) Adjectives: appear as main terms with no code numbers; reference to *see condition*
   2) *See also:* directs researcher to another code number
   3) *See category:* directs the researcher to look into a synonym for the condition
   4) *See condition:* directs the researcher that the wrong word is being looked up
3. Volumes I and II
   a. Brackets ([ ]): enclosed terms are synonyms, explanatory phrases, or alternative words
   b. Parentheses (( )): enclosed terms may or may not affect a main term
   c. NEC (not elsewhere classified): used for ill-defined terms for which more precise information is not available
   d. NOS (not otherwise specified): general diagnosis term that may require more specific information
   e. Note: defines terms, or provides directions (fifth-digit modifier)
   f. *See:* directs researcher to look at another code

E. CODING STEPS
1. Locate the term in the alphabetical index of volume II
2. Read and act on the notes printed after the term
3. Consider modifiers of the term
4. Follow cross-references
5. Verify the code number in volume I and make modifications as instructed
6. Record the code assignment

F. TABLE GUIDELINES
1. Two coding tables in volume II:
   a. Hypertension table: three main column headings:
      1) Malignant: severe; vascular damage; diastolic blood pressure >130 mm Hg
      2) Benign: mild; in control
      3) Unspecified: no note of malignant or benign
   b. Neoplasm table
      1) Arranged by site
      2) Six classifications:
         a) Primary malignancy: original tumor site
         b) Secondary malignancy: tumor metastasized
         c) Carcinoma in situ: localized: noninvasive malignant tumor
         d) Benign: nonspreading, noninvasive tumor
         e) Uncertain behavior: impossible to predict behavior or morphology
         f) Unspecified: tumor with no indication of histology

III. CPT-4

A. GENERAL
1. Lists and codes procedures and services performed by practitioners

2. Each procedure is identified by a five-digit code
3. Simplifies reporting to insurance carriers
4. CPT book is divided into six sections; subsections include anatomic, procedural, conditions, and descriptors:
   a. Evaluation and Management (E&M): 99200 to 99499
   b. Anesthesia: 00100 to 01999
   c. Surgery: 10000 to 69999
   d. Radiology, Nuclear Medicine, and Diagnostic Ultrasound: 70000 to 79999
   e. Pathology and Lab: 80000 to 89999
   f. Medicine: 90701 to 99199

B. FORMAT AND CONVENTIONS

1. Main statement followed by semicolon; subordinate statement describes procedure or extent of services
2. Terms: indented below main statement giving additional statements
3. Guidelines: specific directions at the beginning of each section; necessary to code correctly
4. Modifiers: two-digit, terminal code; represents an alteration of the procedure or circumstances
5. Major headings are boldface
6. Notes: provide coding instructions
7. Descriptive qualifiers: descriptions surrounding a code provide more detailed information; sometimes in parentheses

C. CODING STEPS

1. Review the guidelines beginning each section
2. Turn to the index and locate the main term
3. Locate the subterm and follow the cross-references
4. Read the code descriptors of all code numbers
5. Record the proper code

D. E&M

1. Includes basic diagnostic and treatment services
2. E&M section divided into broad categories with two or more subdivisions
   a. New patient: patient who is new to the practice or who has not received any professional services by the practitioner for 3 or more years
   b. Established patient: patient who has received professional services from the practitioner within the last 3 years
   c. Concurrent care: rendering of similar services to the same patient by more than one practitioner on the same day
   d. Counseling: discussion with the patient and/or family regarding diagnosis, treatment, and patient education
3. The following *must* be determined within each category to select the correct E&M code:
   a. History
      1) Problem-focused: chief complaint and brief history of problem

2) Expanded problem-focused: chief complaint, brief history, and review of system affected by the problem
3) Detailed: chief complaint, expanded history of the problem, expanded review of system affected and pertinent past, family, and/or social history
   b. Examination
      1) Problem-focused: examination is limited to the affected body area or system
      2) Expanded problem-focused: examination is limited to the affected body area or system and other closely related systems
      3) Detailed: extended examination of the affected body area or system and other closely related systems
      4) Comprehensive: complete single-system specialty examination or a complete multisystem examination
   c. Complexity of medical decision-making (diagnosis and/or management)
      1) Straightforward: all three criteria are minimal
      2) Low complexity: low degree in each criterion
      3) Moderate complexity: moderate degree in each criterion
      4) High complexity: high degree of complexity in each criterion
4. Criteria to be considered at each complexity level:
   a. Number of diagnoses or management options available
   b. Amount and/or complexity of data
   c. Risk of complication, morbidity, and/or mortality

IV. HCPCS

A. GENERAL

1. HCFA: Health Care Financing Administration; government agency that regulates Medicaid and Medicare
2. Coding system that expands the CPT system
3. Provides a temporary list of new codes prior to inclusion in the CPT system
4. Three levels:
   a. Level I: existing CPT codes
   b. Level II: additional codes that provide greater precision in CPT categories; five-character alphanumeric system (A0000 to V5999); includes:
      1) Nonphysician services
      2) Codes not found within the existing CPT system
   c. Level III: codes used by private insurance companies contracted to process government claims (Medicare)

Health Insurance 12

I. General: Protection Against Financial Loss By Unplanned Events

A. TYPES OF HEALTH INSURANCE PROGRAMS
1. Commercial: policies created and sold by general companies
2. Health Maintenance Organization (HMO): organization that provides a comprehensive range of services for a prepaid fee
3. Preferred Provider Organization (PPO): agreement between employers and physician to provide services to employee subscribers at a discount

B. INSURANCE TERMS
1. Beneficiary: person designated to receive the benefits of the insurance policy
2. Carrier: insurance company; insurer
3. Co-payment: portion of the cost of service to be paid by the insured
4. Deductible: annual amount to be paid by the insured toward the cost of service before insurance policy benefits are paid
5. Exclusion: treatment or conditions not covered by the insurance policy
6. Explanation of benefits: document prepared by the carrier that identifies the services covered by the policy, the amount billed by the provider, and the amount paid by the carrier
7. Fee-for-service: provider bills for each service rendered
8. Group policy: policy purchased by an organization for the benefit of its members
9. Insured: policyholder; subscriber
10. Managed care: health care program that designates a primary care physician
11. Preexisting condition: medical conditions present and/or being treated at the time a health insurance application is made
12. Premium: the fees paid for the health insurance coverage
13. Provider: health professional who provides services
14. Rider: clauses to the health insurance policy designating coverage items in addition to those included within the standard contract

C. PLAN OPTIONS
1. Basic benefits include the following:
   a. Diagnostic studies
   b. Hospitalization
   c. Surgical treatments
   d. Obstetrical care
   e. Intensive care
   f. Chemotherapy
2. Major medical; services not normally covered by a basic plan may include the following:
   a. Outpatient visits
   b. Minor surgery
   c. Physical and occupational therapies
   d. Cost of medical equipment
   e. Mental health care
   f. Dental care
   g. Prescriptions
3. Companion plan: policy that pays in addition to health insurance policies carried; pays the fees not covered by conventional plans

D. METHODS OF PAYMENT
1. Physician fee profile: usual, customary, and reasonable charges
2. Assignment of benefits
   a. Gives the carrier instructions to send insurance payments directly to the provider
   b. Most commercial carriers will reimburse the patient unless instructed not to do so
   c. Assignment of benefits is accomplished by the patient (insured) signing the appropriate box on insurance claim form or completing a separate assignment of benefits form

d. Patient is responsible for paying the difference between the provider charge and the insurance benefits paid

e. If the provider accepts the assignment, the carrier then makes payment to the provider (in accordance with the policy language); if the claim is a government plan claim, the provider must then indicate on the claim form whether the assignment is accepted or rejected

f. If the provider rejects the assignment of benefits, then the provider may bill the patient the difference between the fee charged and the fee reimbursed

3. Medicaid and workers' compensation: provider must accept government reimbursement as payment in full if the provider agrees to treat Medicaid and/or workers' compensation patients

4. Deductibles and co-payments: patients are responsible to pay any deductible or co-payment according to the terms of the insurance policy

II. Sources Of Insurance

A. MEDICARE

1. Federal program administered by Health Care Financing Administration (HFCA)
2. Established in 1965 as Title 18 of the Social Security Act
3. Eligibility
   a. Age 65 or older
   b. Disabled under Medicare rules
4. Benefits
   a. Part A: covers inpatient care after applicable deductible is satisfied
   b. Part B: voluntary program; covers certain outpatient services
5. Medigap: commercial insurance policies available to cover the Medicare deductible, the co-insurance, and some specific treatments not covered by Medicare

B. MEDICAID

1. Federal program administered by each state
2. Established in 1965 as Title19 of the Social Security Act
3. Eligibility
   a. Determined by the state
   b. Available to persons with income levels below the federal poverty level
   c. Eligible patients receive an official identification card for their periods of eligibility
   d. Persons may be covered by both Medicare and Medicaid (Medi/Medi); Medicare is the primary carrier and is always billed first

C. TRICARE

1. Comprehensive health benefits program offering three types of plans for the dependents of men and women in the uniformed services
   a. TRICARE Standard: fee for service
   b. TRICARE Extra: PPO plan
   c. TRICARE Prime: HMO plan with a point-of-service option

D. WORKERS' COMPENSATION

1. State-administered program
2. Established to help pay the cost of medical care and lost wages associated with work-related injuries or illnesses
3. Patients are compensated in full for their related medical expenses and for a portion of their lost wages
4. Eligibility: patients must sustain an injury or illness while carrying out their job duties
5. Classification of cases
   a. Claim with no disability: filed for minor injuries or illnesses; patient returns to work in a few days
   b. Temporary disability: filed for injuries and illnesses requiring more than a few days of recuperation before returning to work
   c. Permanent disability: filed for injuries and illnesses resulting in diminished capacity of the patient; ranges from 10% to 100% disability
   d. Vocational rehabilitation: filed for permanently or temporarily disabled persons who require training or education to return to work

III. Insurance Claims

A. CMS-1500 CLAIM FORM (see Figure 12-1)

1. Universal health claim form developed by HCFA
2. Standardizes data required by most carriers so that claims can be processed
3. Before submitting a claim for payment, make sure patient information release forms are current
4. Type information onto the form using uppercase letters
5. Do not use periods, hyphens, commas, dollar signs, or slashes
6. Use two zeros (00) in the cents column for whole-dollar amounts
7. Dates should be filled in using six digits (mmddyy)
8. Boxes that should be checked are filled in with an X
9. Type corrections are made by permanent correction methods (correction fluid)
10. Completed forms should be maintained in provider files for 6 years

1500

HEALTH INSURANCE CLAIM FORM

APPROVED BY NATIONAL UNIFORM CLAIM COMMITTEE 08/05

PICA

| | | | | | | | | PICA |

1. MEDICARE (Medicare #) MEDICAID (Medicaid #) TRICARE CHAMPUS (Sponsor's SSN) CHAMPVA (Member ID#) GROUP HEALTH PLAN (SSN or ID) FECA BLK LUNG (SSN) OTHER (ID)

1a. INSURED'S I.D. NUMBER   (For Program in Item 1)

2. PATIENT'S NAME (Last Name, First Name, Middle Initial)

3. PATIENT'S BIRTH DATE   MM DD YY   SEX   M   F

4. INSURED'S NAME (Last Name, First Name, Middle Initial)

5. PATIENT'S ADDRESS (No., Street)

6. PATIENT RELATIONSHIP TO INSURED   Self   Spouse   Child   Other

7. INSURED'S ADDRESS (No., Street)

CITY   STATE

8. PATIENT STATUS   Single   Married   Other

CITY   STATE

ZIP CODE   TELEPHONE (Include Area Code) ( )

Employed   Full-Time Student   Part-Time Student

ZIP CODE   TELEPHONE (Include Area Code) ( )

9. OTHER INSURED'S NAME (Last Name, First Name, Middle Initial)

10. IS PATIENT'S CONDITION RELATED TO:

11. INSURED'S POLICY GROUP OR FECA NUMBER

a. OTHER INSURED'S POLICY OR GROUP NUMBER

a. EMPLOYMENT? (Current or Previous)   YES   NO

a. INSURED'S DATE OF BIRTH   MM DD YY   SEX   M   F

b. OTHER INSURED'S DATE OF BIRTH   MM DD YY   SEX   M   F

b. AUTO ACCIDENT?   PLACE (State)   YES   NO

b. EMPLOYER'S NAME OR SCHOOL NAME

c. EMPLOYER'S NAME OR SCHOOL NAME

c. OTHER ACCIDENT?   YES   NO

c. INSURANCE PLAN NAME OR PROGRAM NAME

d. INSURANCE PLAN NAME OR PROGRAM NAME

10d. RESERVED FOR LOCAL USE

d. IS THERE ANOTHER HEALTH BENEFIT PLAN?   YES   NO   *If yes*, return to and complete item 9 a-d.

READ BACK OF FORM BEFORE COMPLETING & SIGNING THIS FORM.

12. PATIENT'S OR AUTHORIZED PERSON'S SIGNATURE I authorize the release of any medical or other information necessary to process this claim. I also request payment of government benefits either to myself or to the party who accepts assignment below.

SIGNED _____ DATE _____

13. INSURED'S OR AUTHORIZED PERSON'S SIGNATURE I authorize payment of medical benefits to the undersigned physician or supplier for services described below.

SIGNED _____

14. DATE OF CURRENT: MM DD YY   ILLNESS (First symptom) OR INJURY (Accident) OR PREGNANCY(LMP)

15. IF PATIENT HAS HAD SAME OR SIMILAR ILLNESS. GIVE FIRST DATE MM DD YY

16. DATES PATIENT UNABLE TO WORK IN CURRENT OCCUPATION MM DD YY   FROM   TO MM DD YY

17. NAME OF REFERRING PROVIDER OR OTHER SOURCE   17a.   17b. NPI

18. HOSPITALIZATION DATES RELATED TO CURRENT SERVICES MM DD YY   FROM   TO MM DD YY

19. RESERVED FOR LOCAL USE

20. OUTSIDE LAB?   YES   NO $ CHARGES

21. DIAGNOSIS OR NATURE OF ILLNESS OR INJURY (Relate Items 1, 2, 3 or 4 to Item 24E by Line)

1. L____ . ____   3. L____ . ____

2. L____ . ____   4. L____ . ____

22. MEDICAID RESUBMISSION CODE   ORIGINAL REF. NO.

23. PRIOR AUTHORIZATION NUMBER

24. A. DATE(S) OF SERVICE						B. PLACE OF SERVICE	C. EMG	D. PROCEDURES, SERVICES, OR SUPPLIES (Explain Unusual Circumstances)		E. DIAGNOSIS POINTER	F. $ CHARGES	G. DAYS OR UNITS	H. EPSDT Family Plan	I. ID. QUAL.	J. RENDERING PROVIDER ID. #
From MM	DD	YY	To MM	DD	YY			CPT/HCPCS	MODIFIER						
1														NPI	
2														NPI	
3														NPI	
4														NPI	
5														NPI	
6														NPI	

25. FEDERAL TAX I.D. NUMBER   SSN   EIN

26. PATIENT'S ACCOUNT NO.

27. ACCEPT ASSIGNMENT? (For govt. claims, see back)   YES   NO

28. TOTAL CHARGE $

29. AMOUNT PAID $

30. BALANCE DUE $

31. SIGNATURE OF PHYSICIAN OR SUPPLIER INCLUDING DEGREES OR CREDENTIALS (I certify that the statements on the reverse apply to this bill and are made a part thereof.)

SIGNED _____ DATE _____

32. SERVICE FACILITY LOCATION INFORMATION

33. BILLING PROVIDER INFO & PH # ( )

a.   b.

a.   b.

NUCC Instruction Manual available at: www.nucc.org

OMB APPROVAL PENDING

CARRIER

PATIENT AND INSURED INFORMATION

PHYSICIAN OR SUPPLIER INFORMATION

FIGURE 12-1. CMS-1500 insurance claim form. (Courtesy U.S. Department of Health and Human Services, Centers for Medicare and Medicaid Services.)

B. MEDICARE

1. Requires the provider to report to the primary carrier on HCFA form
2. Filing deadline is December 31 of the year following service

C. MEDICAID

1. File this claim as soon as possible after service
2. Providers treating Medicaid patients must accept the assignment and accept Medicaid reimbursements as payment in full for the service
3. Patients cannot be billed for qualified services, regardless of the Medicaid amount reimbursed to the provider
4. Services not covered by Medicaid may be billed directly to the patient
5. Keep a copy of the patient's Medicaid identification card within his or her chart

D. WORKERS' COMPENSATION

1. Form completed in quadruplicate at patient's first visit to report the injury; copies are sent to the state workers' compensation board, compensation carrier, and employer; a copy is also inserted in the patient's chart
2. Filing deadlines may vary by state

3. Progress reports should be a narrative and should indicate any significant changes on the patient's current status
4. If an established patient seeks treatment for a work-related condition, create a separate chart and separate ledger card for the work-related condition
5. Provider must accept assignment and reimbursement as payment in full

E. REASONS CLAIMS CAN BE DELAYED OR REJECTED

1. Coding errors
2. Typographical errors
3. Missing dates
4. Incorrect identification or policy numbers
5. Diagnosis does not support treatment rendered
6. Patient names do not match the policyholder's names
7. Dates of treatments do not correspond with the dates on the documents
8. Missing attachments
9. Defacement of bar code area of the claim form
10. Submission of claim to the wrong carrier
11. Patient ineligible for benefits
12. Fee total calculated incorrectly

Office Management | 13

I. Introduction

A. GENERAL
1. Process of developing, implementing, and achieving organizational goals
2. Administration (nonhuman resources) and leadership (human resources) work together to achieve goals
3. Chain of command is the line of authority in clinics

B. PROCESS OF MANAGEMENT
1. Planning: development of goals
2. Organizing: assembling resources needed to achieve the goals
3. Coordinating: bringing various resources together to achieve the goals
4. Directing: supervising the use of resources to achieve the goals
5. Controlling: making necessary adjustments to achieve the goals

C. SUPERVISION
1. Begins with leadership
2. Leadership is the process of working with and through employees to achieve goals
3. Leadership requires two types of behavior:
   a. Task behavior: leader tells what, when, how, where, and who is to perform a specific task
   b. Relationship behavior: the way the leader communicates, listens, supports, and facilitates in assisting employees in performing a specific task
4. Leadership styles
   a. Telling: makes decisions and supervises employee performance
   b. Selling: makes and explains decisions to employees
   c. Participating: shares ideas and facilitates employee decision making
   d. Delegating: turns responsibility for making and implementing decisions over to the employees

D. HUMAN RESOURCES
1. Hiring process
   a. Recruiting: potential candidates are notified of an available position through advertisement
   b. Interviewing: face-to-face meeting and discussion with employee candidate
   c. Checking references: calling the references indicated by the employee candidate to verify the candidate's information
   d. Selection: choosing the best employee candidate based on the candidate's education, experience, references, and "*fit*"
   e. Offer: formally offering the position to the employee candidate, including wage and benefit information
   f. Negotiation: negotiating the specific terms of the employment offered
   g. Acceptance or rejection: employee candidate accepts the job offer and begins employment, or the candidate rejects the offer, and the employer again begins the process (or offers the position to the next-best candidate)
2. Job description should include:
   a. Job title
   b. Job summary
   c. Supervisor's title
   d. Job duties and employee responsibilities
   e. Job specifications
3. Orientation: transition from candidate to employee
4. Probation
   a. Time needed to determine whether the newly hired employee is a good "fit"
   b. Usually 60 to 90 days
5. Performance appraisal
   a. Objective employee performance assessment
   b. Should assess the employee's work, dependability, teamwork, appearance, and attitude
   c. Should be done regularly
   d. Result must be discussed with the employee

6. Discipline: all actions on employee performance should be recorded in the employee's personnel file
7. Professional development
   a. Encourage and subsidize professional development
   b. Encourage membership in professional organizations
   c. Promote the employee attendance at seminars, workshops, and conventions
   d. Enable the employee to obtain continuing education units (CEUs) or continuing medical education units (CMEs)

E. POLICY MANUAL
1. Information about the office for employees, which includes:
   a. Office or clinic mission statement
   b. Orientation information
   c. Dress code
   d. Job descriptions
   e. Holidays, leaves, vacations, and sick days
   f. Payroll and benefits
   g. Disciplinary actions

II. Meetings

A. GENERAL
1. Keep a calendar of all scheduled meetings (with date, time, place, and topic)
2. Meetings conducted in accordance with *Robert's Rules of Order*
3. Person chairing the meeting is responsible for all portions of the meeting process to ensure that objectives are met
4. Agenda should be typed and distributed to meeting members
5. Minutes are the record of the meeting; should include the date, time, place, and topic of the meeting; persons in attendance and those absent; issues discussed; and time of adjournment

III. Employer Travel

A. GENERAL
1. Travel arrangements may be made by the medical assistant, a travel agent, or both
2. Itinerary should be typed; must include departure and arrival times and locations, contact telephone numbers, destination ground transportation, hotel accommodations, and a schedule of events and activities involved in the travel function; a copy of the travel itinerary must be kept in the office; a copy of the itinerary is given to the traveler
3. If the travel function is a speaking arrangement, then confirm the time, place, and topic; also confirm the honorarium (payment)
4. Check with the airlines before leaving for the airport in case of flight delays
5. Confirm ground transportation at the destination location (courtesy car, taxi service, hotel shuttle, rental car)

6. Confirm hotel accommodations; copy the reservation confirmation number onto the travel itinerary

IV. Resource Management

A. FACILITY
1. Temperature: 68° to 74° F, with proper ventilation
2. Lighting: fluorescent lighting in all examination and working areas
3. Floor covering: carpeting in waiting room, office, and hallways; sheet vinyl flooring in all examination, bathroom, and laboratory areas
4. Walls: soft or pastel colors, paint or wallpaper
5. Storage: locked space for supplies, equipment, and patient charts; locked and secure cabinets for drugs
6. Noise control: examination rooms and physician offices should be arranged to keep sounds at a minimum
7. Patient rooms: arranged so that the patient cannot be seen by others when the door is opened
8. Offices: separate from the patient examination areas
9. Clinical areas: checked between patients to maintain cleanliness and to keep neat and well stocked with supplies
10. Laboratory area: well ventilated; ensure that contamination is well controlled
11. Bathrooms: clean and well stocked; patient bathrooms should be separate from staff facilities
12. Janitorial services: staff should keep all areas neat, clean, and repaired; staff should schedule janitorial services for the remainder of cleaning duties
13. Safety: continually monitor the office for hazards; smoke alarms and fire extinguishers should be strategically placed and checked often to ensure that they are properly functioning; fire exits should be clearly marked and kept free of obstacles
14. Security: an adequate number of security personnel should be readily available
15. Regulated waste disposal: schedule regular regulated waste removal and sharps biohazard waste removal

B. OFFICE EQUIPMENT
1. Keep warranties filed for future reference
2. Maintain a file for service agreements
3. Maintain a file with service technician telephone numbers
4. Keep inventories reports on file, with a physical inventory completed at least once a year; inventory should include:
   a. Name of item
   b. Model and serial number
   c. Date of purchase or lease (and price)
5. Inventory should be made of the following property:
   a. Laboratory equipment
   b. Clinical equipment
   c. Clinical instruments

d. Office equipment
e. Office furniture
f. Anything of value that is not consumed in the treatment of patients

C. SUPPLIES

1. Includes consumable items that are needed to operate the office, housekeeping supplies, and medical supplies
2. Ordered on an ongoing basis
3. One person within the office should be designated to order supplies and to maintain and inventory the supplies
4. Supply inventory (separate from office equipment inventory) should be kept up to date so that supplies never run out
5. Contents of supply deliveries should be checked in and verified against the purchase order and packing slip
6. Supplies must be stored in a neat and orderly fashion

14 Infection Control and Asepsis

I. Chain Of Infection (see Figure 14-1)

A. GENERAL
1. Growth of microorganisms in cycle
2. Break the cycle, break the process

B. RESERVOIR HOST
1. Start of the chain
2. May be an insect, animal, or human
3. Supplies nutrition to the microorganism
4. May not cause disease in the reservoir

C. MEANS OF EXIT
1. How the organism escapes the reservoir host
2. Exits include the mouth, nose, eyes, ears, intestines, urinary tract, reproductive tract, and open wounds

D. MEANS OF TRANSMISSION
1. Way organisms are spread
   a. Direct transmission: occurs from contact with an infected person or discharges of an infected person
   b. Indirect transmission: occurs from droplets in the air, vectors (insects) that harbor pathogens, contaminated food or drink, and fomites (contaminated objects)

E. MEANS OF ENTRY
1. How the organism gains entry into a new host
2. Entries include the mouth, nose, eyes, intestines, urinary tract, reproductive tract, and open wounds

F. SUSCEPTIBLE HOST
1. One that is capable of supporting the growth of a microorganism
2. Factors that affect susceptibility include:
   a. Location of entry
   b. Dose of organisms
   c. Physical condition of individual
3. If conditions are right, susceptible host becomes reservoir host; the chain or cycle begins again

G. INFLAMMATION
1. Trauma to the body alerts the protective mechanisms
2. The body responds
   a. Blood vessels at the site dilate; the number of white blood cells in the area increases, which causes redness
   b. White blood cells overpower and consume microorganisms (phagocytosis), which causes swelling
   c. Fluids in tissues increase and put pressure on nerves, which causes pain
   d. Blood supply to area increases and causes heat
3. The process creates four classic signs of inflammation: redness, swelling, pain, and heat

II. OSHA Standards

A. GENERAL
1. Occupational Safety and Health Administration (OSHA)
2. Sets standards and protocols for health and safety

B. BLOOD-BORNE PATHOGENS
1. Disease-causing microorganisms that may be present in the blood or bodily fluids
2. Concerned mainly with hepatitis B virus (HBV), hepatitis C virus (HCV), and human immunodeficiency virus (HIV)
3. Blood-borne pathogens are transmitted when infected blood comes into contact with nonintact skin or mucous membranes

C. STANDARD PRECAUTIONS
1. Concept of treating all blood and body fluids as if they are infected
2. Includes blood, body fluids, excretions, and secretions

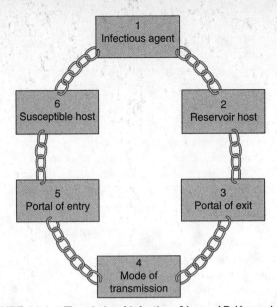

FIGURE 14-1. The chain of infection. (Young AP, Kennedy DB: *Kinn's the medical assistant: an applied learning approach*, ed 9, Philadelphia, 2003, Saunders.)

D. PREVENTION OF EXPOSURE

1. Immunization: all persons who come in contact with blood or body fluids should receive hepatitis B series
2. Engineering controls: mechanical devices designed to minimize exposure; include:
   a. Eyewash stations
   b. Sharps containers
   c. Biohazard waste containers and labels
   d. Hand-washing stations
3. Personal protection equipment: equipment that minimizes exposure beyond engineering controls; includes:
   a. Gloves
   b. Laboratory coats
   c. Eye and/or face shields

E. EXPOSURE CONTROL

1. Contaminated sharps placed in sharps container (puncture-resistant, leak-proof container) immediately after use
2. Do not bend, break, or recap used needles
3. Work surfaces and equipment should be cleaned and decontaminated with disinfectant after each use
4. Contaminated waste (except sharps) should be discarded in a clearly labeled biohazard waste container (*"red bag trash"*)
5. Employee exposure incidents should be reported as directed and properly followed up to ensure that they do not again occur

III. Hand Washing

A. GENERAL

1. Single most important defense against transmission of microorganisms

2. Proper hand washing depends on friction and running water
3. Hands should be washed:
   a. Between patients
   b. After handling specimens
   c. Before and after using the restroom
   d. After handling contaminated materials
   e. Before leaving the clinic at the end of the day
4. Hand-washing procedure
   a. Remove all jewelry except plain wedding band
   b. Using warm water, thoroughly wet the hands
   c. Apply soap; lather while keeping the fingers pointed downward
   d. Rub, using friction for 30 seconds; wash between the fingers
   e. Rinse; allow water to flow from the wrist to the fingertips
   f. Thoroughly dry the hands with paper towels, and turn off the faucet or faucets with the paper towels
   g. Apply lotion if desired

IV. Sanitization

A. GENERAL

1. Process of cleaning or removing materials from objects
2. Requires scrubbing objects with detergents and brushes
3. First step in the sterilization process
4. Methods include:
   a. Detergents: agents that remove bacteria, fats, oils, and protein substances (blood)
   b. Ultrasound: machine that uses sound waves through a liquid to cause a vibration
   c. Antiseptic: agent that sanitizes skin

V. Disinfection

A. GENERAL

1. Process of removing infectious material from objects
2. Processes include:
   a. Chemical
      1) Surface germicide
      2) Used on inanimate objects that are sensitive to heat
         a) Soap: mechanically removes bacteria but does not destroy them unless the soap is germicidal
         b) Alcohol: commonly used on skin
         c) Acids: solutions containing phenol
         d) Alkalis: bleach; used in the laboratory on flat surfaces
         e) Formalin: solution requires rinsing
   b. Ultraviolet radiation: ultraviolet light can have an effect on surfaces but does not penetrate surfaces
   c. Desiccation: drying; does not kill spores
   d. Boiling: kills most bacteria; does not kill some spores and viruses

VI. Sterilization

A. GENERAL
1. Complete destruction of microorganisms
2. Processes include:
   a. Chemical
      1) May be used for heat-sensitive materials
      2) Objects must be completely submerged for long periods
      3) Glutaraldehyde solutions commonly used
   b. Steam under pressure
      1) Autoclave
      2) Most common and effective sterilization method
   c. Gas: special chamber that uses a gas
   d. Oven: dry heat

VII. Use Of The Autoclave

A. PREPARING INSTRUMENTS AND SUPPLIES
1. Instruments are sanitized and dried before wrapping
2. Wrapping materials include:
   a. Muslin
   b. Disposable paper
   c. Peel-back pouches
3. Open any hinged instruments to allow steam to reach all surfaces
4. Items to be wrapped are placed in the center of the wrapping material, with corners of the wrap at the top, bottom, and sides; bring the bottom of the wrapper up over the instrument, folding back a small corner for a *handle*; bring in the sides, one at a time, also folding back the small corners; the top of the wrapper is brought around the object and secured with sterilizer tape

5. Label the tape with the identity of the contents, date, and operator's initials
6. Packs should be no larger than 12 × 12 × 20 inches
7. Sterilization indicator should be included in the pack to show that the proper time and temperature were achieved

B. LOADING THE AUTOCLAVE
1. Packs should be placed vertically, 1 to 3 inches apart, away from the sides of the chamber
2. Place hard goods underneath soft goods
3. Open glassware should be placed on its side

C. AUTOCLAVE PROCEDURE
1. Autoclave is a piece of equipment that provides steam under pressure
2. Autoclave is normally run at 250° F, 20 to 30 lb pressure, for 15 to 30 minutes
3. Moist heat in the form of steam circulates in a pattern throughout the autoclave chamber
4. Check the autoclave water level; add distilled water if necessary
5. Properly load the autoclave
6. Close the autoclave door securely; turn the unit on
7. Begin timing when the proper temperature and pressure are achieved
8. After the autoclave cycle is completed, vent the autoclave chamber
9. Open the autoclave door just slightly to allow the contents to dry
10. Remove the items and check the indicator on the sterilizer tape; wrapped items may be handled with clean hands
11. Store sterilized items in a clean, dust-proof area; the shelf life of sterilized items is approximately 28 days (resterilize the items after 28 days)

Vital Signs and Anthropometric Measurement 15

I. Vital Signs

A. GENERAL
1. Measurements that indicate the patient's general state of health and homeostasis
2. Can indicate a change in health and/or the presence or disappearance of a disease
3. Accuracy is essential
4. Includes temperature, pulse, respiration (TPR), and blood pressure (BP)

B. TEMPERATURE
1. Balance between heat lost and heat that the body produces
2. Heat is produced by metabolism
3. In illness, metabolism increases, increasing internal heat production and increasing the body temperature
4. Variation in patient's baseline temperature may be the first warning of an illness or change in condition
5. Body temperature is regulated by hypothalamus
6. Factors affecting body temperature
   a. Age: body heat decreases with age
   b. Environment: exposure, windchill, and temperature
   c. Activity: physical activity increases body temperature
   d. Diurnal variation: body temperature is lowest in the morning, highest in the evening
   e. Emotions: agitation increases body temperature; depression lowers body temperature
   f. Physiologic processes: body temperature increases with digestion, ovulation, and pregnancy
7. Normal ranges
   a. Oral: 97° to 99° F; 36° to 37.8° C
   b. Rectal: 1° higher than oral (most accurate measurement)
   c. Axillary: 1° lower than oral (least accurate measurement)
   d. Tympanic (aural): same as oral
8. Characteristics
   a. Fever: temperature >100° F; pyrexia; temperature ≥105° F can cause brain damage or death if untreated
   b. Febrile: having fever
   c. Afebrile: without fever
   d. Intermittent: fluctuation among normal, abnormal, and fever
   e. Remittent: elevated fluctuations that do not return to normal
   f. Lysis: gradual return to normal
   g. Crisis: sudden return to normal
9. Equipment: thermometer: device used to measure body temperature
   a. Electronic: consists of a battery-powered unit and a probe covered by a disposable plastic cover; temperature is displayed digitally; unit has blue (oral) and red (rectal) probes
   b. Tympanic (aural): handheld processor unit with a tympanic probe covered by a disposable cover: picks up infrared energy from the tympanic membrane: proper technique is important for correct results
10. Charting
    a. Record the patient's temperature within the patient chart
    b. Indicate (after the number) whether the patient's temperature was recorded by oral (O), rectal (R), axillary (A), or tympanic (T)
11. Procedure
    a. Oral: place the thermometer under the patient's tongue; instruct the patient to keep the lips closed around the thermometer and to breathe through the nose
    b. Axillary: wipe the axilla dry; place the thermometer under the patient's arm

c. Rectal: apply lubricating jelly to the thermometer; insert into the rectum approximately 1 inch

d. Tympanic (see Figure 15-1)
   1) For adult: gently pull the pinna up and back; insert the probe into the ear canal
   2) For child: gently pull the pinna down and back; insert the probe into the ear canal

C. PULSE

1. Palpable beat of arteries as they expand with the beat of the heart
2. Pulse in any artery will usually be the same as the heartbeat
3. Rate and characteristics can give information about the cardiovascular system
4. Factors affecting pulse
   a. Increased pulse rate: pain, fever, infection, and hyperthyroidism
   b. Decreased pulse rate: chronic pain, central nervous system disorders, and hypothyroidism
5. Characteristics
   a. Rate: number of beats per minute (bpm)
   b. Rhythm: time between beats
   c. Volume: force of beats

d. Condition of the arterial wall: springy, resilient, and elastic

6. Normal ranges
   a. Birth: 70 to 190 bpm
   b. 1 to 4 years: 80 to 120 bpm
   c. 6 to 12 years: 70 to 110 bpm
   d. 12 to 16 years: 75 to 90 bpm
   e. Adult: 60 to 80 bpm

7. Pulse sites (see Figure 15-2)
   a. Radial: most common; located on the thumb side of the wrist
   b. Carotid: located in the groove of the neck between the larynx and the sternocleidomastoid muscle; used in emergencies and during cardiopulmonary resuscitation (CPR)
   c. Brachial: located in the antecubital space; reference for BP
   d. Femoral: located in the groin
   e. Temporal: located over the temporal bone
   f. Popliteal: located at the back of the knee
   g. Dorsalis pedis: located on the top of the foot
   h. Apical: located just below the left nipple on the left side of the chest; taken with a stethoscope for 1 full minute; used for infants, young children, and cardiac patients

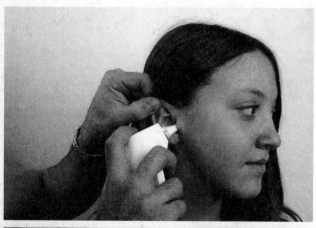
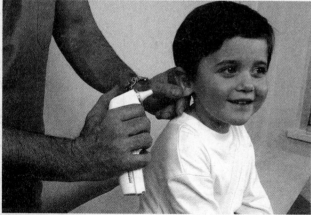

FIGURE 15-1. Positioning the ear for temperature taking. (Bonewit-West K: *Clinical procedures for medical assistants*, ed 6, St Louis, 2004, Saunders.)

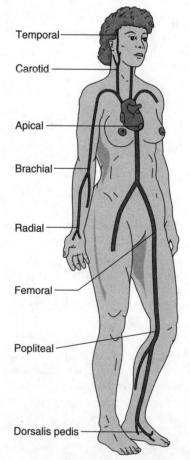

FIGURE 15-2. Pulse sites. (Young AP, Kennedy DB: *Kinn's the medical assistant: an applied learning approach*, ed 9, Philadelphia, 2003, Saunders.)

8. Procedure
   a. Radial pulse
      1) Have the patient in a sitting or lying position
      2) Gently press on the radial artery until the pulse is felt
      3) Count the beat for 30 seconds and multiply by 2; if the beat is irregular, then count for the full minute
      4) Chart the pulse; note the rate, rhythm, and strength
   b. Apical pulse
      1) Have the patient in a sitting or lying position
      2) Place the stethoscope below the patient's left nipple at the fifth intercostal space midclavicular line (apex of the heart)
      3) Count for 1 full minute
      4) Chart the pulse; note the rate, rhythm, and strength and indicate that the pulse was taken apically (A)

D. RESPIRATION

1. Involves the exchange of oxygen and carbon dioxide in lungs
2. Cycle consists of one inspiration and one expiration
3. Controlled by the medulla oblongata; the breathing rate is determined by the carbon dioxide level in the blood
4. Factors affecting respiration
   a. Disease
   b. Age
   c. Physical activity
   d. Emotional status
   e. Medications and drugs
   f. Body position
5. Characteristics
   a. Rate: number of respirations per minute
   b. Rhythm: breathing pattern
   c. Depth: amount of air being inhaled
6. Normal ranges (respirations per minute)
   a. Newborn: 30 to 40 breaths/min
   b. 1 to 6 years: 20 to 40 breaths/min
   c. 7 to 14 years: 15 to 25 breaths/min
   d. Adult: 16 to 20 breaths/min
7. Breathing patterns
   a. Eupnea: normal breathing
   b. Dyspnea: difficult, painful, or labored breathing
   c. Apnea: absence of breathing; temporary condition
   d. Orthopnea: difficulty breathing while lying down
   e. Hyperpnea: increased rate of breathing
   f. Tachypnea: excessively rapid breathing
   g. Rales: gurgling sounds caused by secretions
   h. Rhonchi: rattling sounds
   i. Cheyne-Stokes respirations: alternating periods of apnea and tachypnea; can indicate impending death

8. Procedure
   a. Respiration can be consciously controlled; the respiration rate should be counted without the patient's knowledge so that the patient is unaware of your respiration count; continue to act as if you are taking the pulse
   b. Watch the rise and fall of the patient's chest; count one inhalation and one exhalation as one respiration
   c. Count for 30 seconds and multiply by 2; if irregular, then count for a full minute
   d. Chart the respiration; note the rate, depth, and rhythm; note any irregularities

E. BLOOD PRESSURE

1. Measurement of the pressure of the blood against the walls of the arteries
2. Two readings
   a. Systolic pressure (systole): highest pressure; occurs when the heart contracts
   b. Diastolic pressure (diastole): lowest pressure; occurs when the heart relaxes
3. Systole + diastole = one cardiac cycle
4. Measured in millimeters of mercury (mm Hg)
5. Recorded as a fraction: systolic/diastolic
6. Factors affecting BP
   a. Age: BP increases with age
   b. Activity: BP increases with physical activity
   c. Gender
   d. Diurnal variation: BP is lower in the morning than it is at other times of the day
   e. Stress
   f. Disease state
   g. Medication
7. Normal ranges
   a. Newborn: 50/30 mm Hg
   b. 1 to 6 years: 95/65 mm Hg
   c. 6 to 12 years: 100/65 mm Hg
   d. 16 to adult: 118/75 mm Hg
   e. Adult: 120/80 mm Hg (average); normally ranges from 90/60 to <140/90 mm Hg
   f. Older adults: 140/90 mm Hg
8. Characteristics
   a. Hypertension (HTN): high BP
      1) BP >140/90 mm Hg
      2) Essential HTN: unknown cause
      3) Secondary HTN: associated with other disease processes
   b. Hypotension: low BP: < 90/60 mm Hg
   c. Orthostatic hypotension: temporary fall in BP that occurs when the patient rapidly changes from a lying or sitting position to a standing position
   d. Pulse pressure
      1) Difference between systolic and diastolic pressure
      2) Average is 40 mm Hg

9. Equipment
   a. Sphygmomanometer: consists of an inflatable cuff (various sizes for sizes of patient) with an inflation bulb (with control valve) and pressure gauge (mercury column or aneroid dial)
   b. Stethoscope; instrument used to listen to pulse
10. Procedure (see Figure 15-3)
   a. Objective
      1) Use of the inflatable cuff causes circulation in the artery to disappear
      2) As the cuff is slowly deflated, blood flow resumes, and cardiac cycle sounds are heard through the stethoscope
      3) Gauge readings are taken when the first sound is heard (systolic) and when the last sound is heard (diastolic)
   b. Palpate the brachial artery in the antecubital space
   c. Place the cuff snugly around the patient's arm approximately 1 to 2 inches above the arm fold, with the arrow on the cuff pointing to the brachial artery
   d. Place the stethoscope over the brachial artery
   e. Close the valve and inflate the cuff to approximately 200 mm Hg
   f. Slowly release the valve to deflate the cuff; the gauge needle should drop 2 mm Hg per second for proper release rate
   g. Note the gauge reading when the first beat is heard (systolic)
   h. Continue deflating the cuff until the last beat is heard (diastolic)
   i. Fully release the bulb valve, deflate the cuff, and remove it from the patient
   j. Record the result in the patient's chart; indicate which arm was used for reading (R or L); may also indicate the patient's position (sitting, standing, lying)
11. Korotkoff sounds: sounds heard during the measurement of BP
   a. Phase I: first sound heard as the cuff deflates; systolic reading
   b. Phase II: swishing sound; blood is flowing through the artery, and sounds may completely disappear and reappear later (auscultatory gap)
   c. Phase III: sharp, tapping sounds return and continue rhythmically
   d. Phase IV: soft tapping sound that becomes muffled and begins to grow fainter; may be recorded as the fading sound and recorded between the systolic and diastolic (e.g., 130/85/70 mm Hg)
   e. Phase V: sounds disappear; last sound heard; diastolic reading

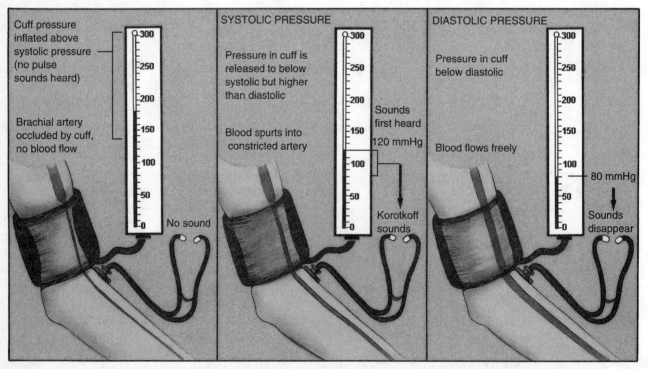

FIGURE 15-3. Measurement of blood pressure. (Applegate EJ: *The anatomy and physiology learning system*, ed 3, Philadelphia, 2006, Saunders.)

II. Anthropometric Measurement

A. GENERAL

1. Deals with the measurement of size, weight, and proportion of the human body
2. Often included with vital signs

B. WEIGHT

1. May be measured in pounds or kilograms
   a. Place a paper towel on the base of the scale if the patient removes his or her shoes; the patient should be weighed consistently with or without shoes, depending on office procedure
   b. Have the patient stand erect in the center of the base of the scale
   c. Move the large weight to the 50-lb notch nearest to, but under, the patient's weight
   d. Move the smaller weight to the right until the balance needle is in the middle of the frame
   e. Add the large and small weights together; record the result, in pounds, on the patient's chart to the nearest ¼ lb
   f. Return both weights to zero after the patient leaves the scale
   g. 1 kg = 2.2 lb; 1 lb = 0.45 kg

C. HEIGHT

1. May be measured in inches or centimeters
   a. Place a paper towel on the base of the scale if the patient removes his or her shoes (as previously described)
   b. Have the patient stand erect in the center of the base of the scale
   c. Lower the height bar until it rests on the top of the patient's head
   d. Note the height indicated on the height bar; record the result, in inches, or the patient's chart to the nearest ¼ inch
   e. Return the height bar to the lowest position
   f. 1 in = 2.54 cm; 1 cm = 0.39 in

D. BODY FAT

1. Measures percentage of body fat; percentage of body fat may be an indicator of cardiovascular disease, health, vitality, and appearance
2. Three methods:
   a. Body density measurement method
      1) Patient is submerged under water
      2) Most accurate and most difficult
   b. Electroimpedance method
      1) Electrodes are placed on the patient
      2) Computer determines body fat percentage on an impedance monitor
   c. Caliper method
      1) Measures the thickness of a fold of fat tissue
      2) Measurements are taken in three to four sites on the body; most common are
         a) Triceps
         b) Biceps
         c) Subscapular
         d) Suprailiac
      3) Indicates total percentage of body fat
      4) Normal range for men is 15% to 19%
      5) Normal range for women is 22% to 25%

16 *Patient Preparation*

I. General

A. THE MEDICAL ASSISTANT PREPARES THE PATIENT FOR EXAMINATION BY GOWNING, POSITIONING, AND DRAPING

II. Gowning

A. GENERAL
1. Patient must undress and put on a gown; makes performing the procedure easier for the healthcare provider
2. Principle of gowning: expose only the body part that needs to be examined or exposed

B. CONSIDERATIONS OF GOWNING
1. Patient's need for privacy and comfort
2. Type of examination or procedure to be performed
3. Patient's age and gender
4. Accessibility of the body part to be examined or exposed

C. TYPES OF GOWNS
1. Usually all patient clothing is removed under the gown
2. Gown will have an opening either in back or in front
   a. Full gown
      1) Knee length
      2) Opening extends the full length of the gown
      3) Closures of Velcro® or ties
      4) Can be paper or cloth material
   b. Partial gown
      1) Covers only the chest, back, and shoulders
      2) Opening extends the full length of the gown
      3) Can be paper or cloth material

III. Positioning And Draping

A. GENERAL
1. Patient is generally positioned on an examination table

2. Table should be long and wide enough to support any size patient
3. Table covered with a paper covering or cloth sheet; the covering is changed after each patient

B. POSITIONS (see Figure 16-1)
1. Erect
   a. Standing
   b. Patient is upright with arms at sides
   c. Used to examine musculoskeletal system and nervous system
2. Sitting (part A)
   a. Patient sits upright on the table with legs dangling over the edge of the table
   b. Used to examine the head, chest, heart, lungs, breasts, axilla, and upper extremities
   c. Draping: drape the sheet across the lap
3. Supine (part B)
   a. Dorsal recumbent
   b. Patient lies flat on the back with arms at the sides
   c. Used to examine the chest, abdominal area, heart, and extremities
   d. Draping: the drape sheet extends from under the arms
4. Dorsal recumbent (part C)
   a. Patient is supine with legs bent at the knees and feet flat on the table
   b. Used to examine the genital and rectal areas
   c. Draping: drape sheet is placed over that patient in a diamond-shaped fashion with side corners wrapped around each leg; upper and lower corners cover the chest, abdominal, and pubic areas
5. Lithotomy (part D)
   a. Patient is in dorsal recumbent position, except that the feet are placed in stirrups; knees are bent; buttocks are moved to the end of the table
   b. Used for vaginal examination, pelvic examination, and Papanicolaou (Pap) smear procedure
   c. Draping: same as for dorsal recumbent

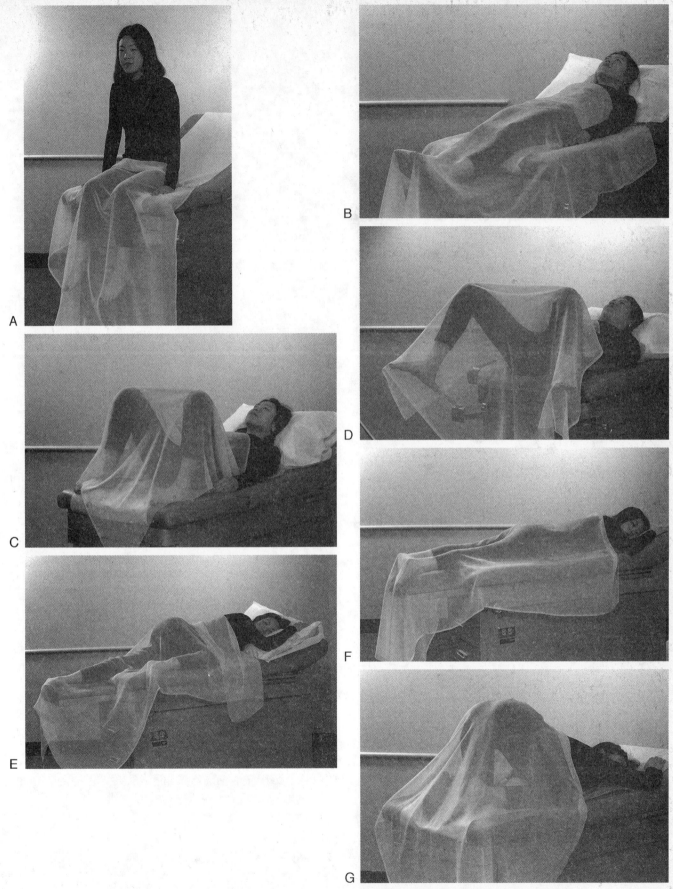

FIGURE 16-1. Positions for examination. (Young AP, Proctor DB: *Kinn's the medical assistant: an applied learning appraoch,* ed 9, Philadelphia, 2003, Saunders.)

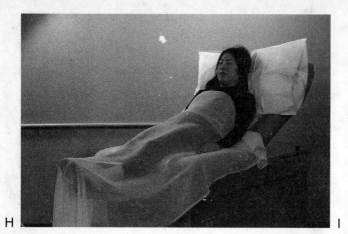
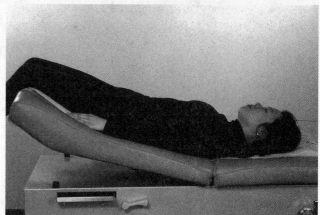

H   I

FIGURE 16-1, Cont'd

6. Sims' (part E)
   a. Lateral position
   b. Patient lies on the left side with the left arm behind the body and the right arm forward; both legs are flexed at the knees, but the right leg is sharply bent and positioned next to the left leg
   c. Used to examine the rectal area, perform enemas and douches, and insert suppositories
   d. Draping: drape sheet covers the patient from the shoulders to the toes; adjust to expose the necessary area
7. Prone (part F)
   a. Patient lies flat on the abdomen with the head turned to the side; arms are positioned above the head or at the sides of the body
   b. Used to examine the back, spine, and lower extremities
   c. Draping: drape sheet covers the patient from the waist to the knees; adjust to expose the necessary area
8. Knee-chest (part G)
   a. Genupectoral
   b. Patient assumes a kneeling position with the buttocks elevated, with head and chest on the table
   c. Used for proctologic examinations
   d. Draping: drape sheet covers the buttocks; adjust to expose the necessary area
9. Proctologic
   a. Knee-chest position facilitated by the use of a special table
   b. Used for a proctologic examination
   c. Draping: same as for knee-chest

10. Fowler's
    a. Patient sits on the examination table with the back supported at a 90-degree angle
    b. Used for examination and treatment of the head, neck, and chest; helpful for patients with breathing difficulties
    c. Draping: drape sheet covers the patient from the shoulders down; adjust to expose the necessary area
11. Semi-Fowler's (part H)
    a. Modification of Fowler's; back supported at a 45-degree angle
    b. Used for postsurgical examinations and for patients with head trauma or head pain
    c. Draping: same as for Fowler's
12. Trendelenburg (part I)
    a. Patient is supine with the foot of the table elevated 45 degrees (head lower than feet)
    b. Used for shock or abdominal surgery
    c. Draping: drape sheet covers the patient from underarms to below the knees; neck, head, and hands are left uncovered

C. GENERAL CONSIDERATIONS
1. Expose only the body part being examined or treated
2. Keep the patient as comfortable as possible
3. Provide a blanket for comfort and warmth
4. Modify the position to accommodate a weak or painful body part
5. Prevent the patient from falling from the table
6. Medical assistant should be present when a male physician examines a female patient

Assisting with Patient Examinations 17

I. Complete Physical Examinations

A. GENERAL
1. Normally performed on new patients to assess their health status and to establish the patient's base
2. Also performed on established patients for health maintenance
3. Medical assistant must be familiar with the process, principles, and methods to prepare the patient and to assist the provider

II. Diagnosis (see Figure 17-1)

A. SYMPTOMS
1. Conditions and feelings experienced by the patient

B. SIGNS
1. Observable characteristics by health care providers
2. May also be noticed by patient

C. DIFFERENTIAL DIAGNOSIS
1. Comparing certain diseases with others that have similar signs and symptoms
2. Process of ruling out (R/O)

D. IMPRESSION
1. Working diagnosis
2. Subject to change as the provider adds data from other diagnostic tools

E. DIAGNOSTIC TOOLS
1. Patient history
2. Physical examination
3. Vital signs
4. Laboratory and diagnostic tests
5. Patient's communications
6. Physician's perceptions

F. FINAL DIAGNOSIS
1. The provider's final conclusion

III. Methods of Examination

A. INSPECTION
1. Process of visual observation
2. Includes looking for abnormalities in size, shape, color, continuity, symmetry, and/or position

B. PALPATION
1. Process of touching and feeling
2. Can detect abnormalities of size, shape, texture, and tenderness

C. PERCUSSION
1. Process of tapping or striking the body
2. Done with fingers or small hammer
3. Aids in determination of size, position, or density of an organ or body cavity

D. MANIPULATION
1. Forceful passive movement of a joint to determine range of motion

E. AUSCULTATION
1. Process of listening to the body using a stethoscope

F. MENSURATION
1. Process of measurement

IV. Commonly Used Equipment (see Figure 17-2)

A. OPHTHALMOSCOPE
1. Instrument used to illuminate the internal eye for visual inspection
2. Runs off power source (battery or wall unit)

B. OTOSCOPE
1. Instrument used to illuminate the external and internal ear for visual examination
2. Runs off power source (battery or wall unit)

C. POCKET FLASHLIGHT OR HEADLIGHT
1. Instrument used to illuminate the mouth, throat, and nose for visual examination

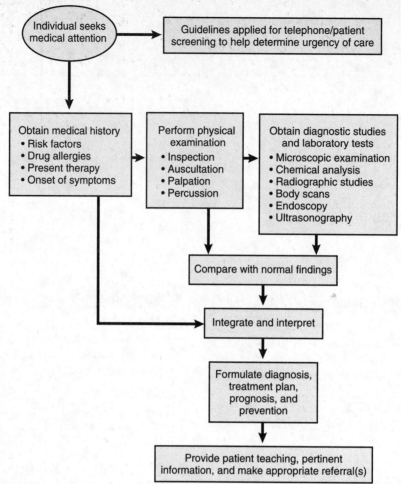

FIGURE 17-1. Essential steps in diagnosis. (Modified from Frazier MS, Drzymkowski JW: *Essentials of human diseases and conditions,* ed 3, Philadelphia, 2004, Saunders.)

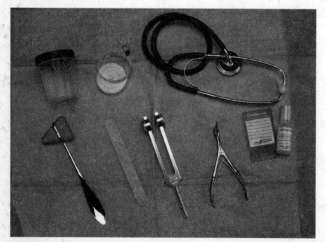

FIGURE 17-2. Physical examination instruments. (Young AP, Proctor DB: *Kinn's the medical assistant: an applied learning approach,* ed 9, Philadelphia, 2003, Saunders.)

D. TAPE MEASURE
1. Instrument used to measure body structures

E. TONGUE DEPRESSOR
1. Instrument used to control tongue movement while examining the mouth and throat
2. Disposable; nonsterile

F. STETHOSCOPE
1. Instrument used to listen to the sounds of the body

G. GLOVES AND LUBRICANT
1. Used for rectal and/or pelvic examinations

H. VAGINAL SPECULUM
1. Instrument inserted into the patient's vagina to allow visualization of the cervix and vagina

I. PERCUSSION HAMMER
1. Rubber-tipped hammer used to test patient's reflexes

J. TUNING FORK
1. Instrument used to test the patient's hearing; vibrates when struck to produce sound

K. MISCELLANEOUS
1. Cotton-tipped applicators
2. 2-inch × 2-inch gauze squares
3. Glass slides
4. Specimen and slide fixative
5. Tissues

V. Sequence of Events

A. PATIENT HEALTH HISTORY

B. VITAL SIGNS AND ANTHROPOMETRIC MEASUREMENTS

C. PHYSICAL EXAMINATION

D. SPECIMEN COLLECTION
1. Includes urine, blood, or other body fluids
2. Examination may be more comfortable if the patient's bladder is empty

E. DIAGNOSTIC TESTS
1. Includes electrocardiogram, x-ray, spirometry, and immunizations

F. PATIENT CONSULTATION OR DISCUSSION WITH PROVIDER

VI. Physical Examination Sequence

A. PRESENTING APPEARANCE (PATIENT'S GENERAL APPEARANCE)
1. General assessment of patient's state of health
2. Includes:
   a. Signs of distress
   b. Appearance of skin
   c. Posture, gait, and motor activity
   d. General grooming
   e. Presence of odors
   f. Speech patterns
   g. Body language and facial expressions

B. HEAD—PATIENT IN SITTING POSITION
1. Hair, scalp, and face
2. Eyes: ophthalmoscope used to visually examine the retina and vessels
3. Ears: otoscope used to examine the external ear and tympanic membrane
4. Nose and sinuses: otoscope or nasal speculum used to examine the nares and sinus cavities
5. Mouth and throat
   a. Lips, gums, teeth, and tongue
   b. Light source, tongue depressor (blade), and laryngeal mirror used to visually examine the throat
6. Neck: inspect and palpate the thyroid, trachea, and lymph nodes

C. THORAX—PATIENT IN A SITTING POSITION
1. Back
   a. Spine and muscles of the back are visually inspected
   b. Lungs are auscultated with a stethoscope
2. Chest
   a. Visually inspected for symmetry and expansion
   b. Inspirations auscultated
   c. Axillary nodes palpated
3. Heart
   a. Stethoscope used to listen to heart sounds
   b. Complete silence in the examination room is necessary to interpret the sounds
4. Breasts
   a. Examined for masses, tenderness, and discharge
   b. May also be examined with the patient in supine position

D. ABDOMEN—PATIENT IN THE SUPINE POSITION
1. Auscultated for the presence or absence of bowel sounds
2. Visually inspected for symmetry and contour
3. Manipulated and palpated for contours of the organs
4. Area needs to be relaxed for proper examination

E. GENITAL AND RECTAL—PATIENT IN THE SUPINE POSITION
1. Inguinal area: palpated for lymph nodes and hernias
2. Male genital and rectal: penis, scrotum, prostate, and anus palpated and inspected
3. Female genital and rectal—patient in the lithotomy position
   a. External genitalia, vagina, cervix, and anus inspected
   b. Pelvic examination
      1) Speculum inserted into the vagina to visualize the vaginal wall and cervix
      2) Bimanual examination done with a gloved hand inserted into the vagina and the other hand palpating the external abdomen to examine the uterus, ovaries, and fallopian tubes

F. LEGS—PATIENT IN THE STANDING POSITION
1. Inspected for pulse and varicosities

VII. Integumentary System (Dermatology)

A. DEFINITION
1. Deals with disorders of the skin, hair, glands, nails, and subcutaneous tissue
2. Specialized physician: dermatologist

B. GENERAL EXAMINATION
1. Skin, hair, and nails
2. Examined for:
   a. Color
   b. Consistency and texture
   c. Eruptions, lesions, growths

d. Tenderness

e. Irregularities

C. DIAGNOSTIC PROCEDURES

1. Fungal, bacterial, and viral cultures: tissue scrapings, purulent material, and exudate sent to the laboratory to identify pathogenic organisms

2. Potassium hydroxide (KOH) smears: skin scrapings immersed in 20% KOH; sample is examined for fungus

3. Biopsy

   a. Excisional: removal of the entire section of tissue for microscopic examination

   b. Incisional: removal of a portion of the tissue for microscopic examination

   c. Punch: use of an instrument (dermal punch) to remove only a small amount of tissue for microscopic examination

4. Allergy testing (see Figure 17-3)

   a. Patch test: a small piece of gauze with a small amount of allergen is placed on the skin; a positive reaction occurs if the skin becomes red or blistered after 48 hours

   b. Scratch test: a minute amount of allergen is placed, by scratch, in the skin; a positive reaction occurs if the scratch becomes red and swollen

   c. Intradermal: a small amount of allergen is injected intradermally; a positive reaction is determined by measuring the size of the wheals produced

5. Wood's light examination: examination to detect fluorescent characteristics of certain fungi; the skin is viewed in a darkened room under ultraviolet light that is filtered through Wood's glass

6. Antinuclear antibody titer (ANA): blood test used to screen for cutaneous lupus erythematosus and similar connective tissue diseases

7. Tuberculin (TB) skin testing: tests patient for tuberculosis antibodies

   a. Mantoux: intradermal injection using purified protein derivative (PPD)

   b. Tine: multipuncture method using a small plastic device

D. TREATMENT PROCEDURES

1. Cryosurgery: use of extreme cold (liquid nitrogen) to freeze and destroy unwanted tissue

2. Curettage: removal of the surface of the skin or a lesion by scraping with a sharp, spoon-shaped instrument (curette)

3. Dermabrasion: removal of scars or lesions by the use of mechanical or chemical abrasives

4. Electrodesiccation: destruction of growths, warts, or unwanted areas of tissue with electric current (diathermy)

5. Mohs' surgery: removal and microscopic examination of layers of malignant growth

E. MEDICATIONS

1. Antiacneics

   a. Used to treat acne

   b. Examples: Accutane, Retin-A, Cleocin, Persa-Gel

2. Antifungals

   a. Used to treat fungal infections

   b. Examples: Lotrimin, Monistat, Nizoral

3. Antihistamines

   a. Used to decrease allergic reactions

   b. Examples: Atarax, Benadryl

4. Antiinfectives

   a. Used to kill microorganisms

   b. Examples: Erythromycin, Keflex, Mycolog, Sumycin

5. Antivirals

   a. Used to inhibit viruses

   b. Example: Zovirax

6. Scabicides and pediculicides

   a. Used to kill scabies and lice

   b. Examples: Lindane, Kwell

7. Topical steroids

   a. Used externally to decrease inflammation

   b. Examples: Aristocort, Medrol, Topicort, Kenalog

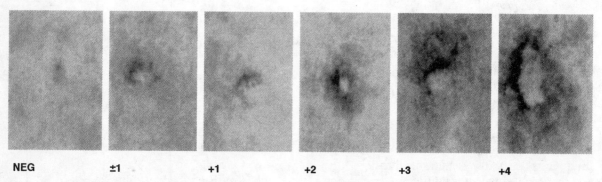

NEG   ±1   +1   +2   +3   +4

FIGURE 17-3. Skin-prick and intradermal skin test results. (Copyright and courtesy Hollister-Stier Spokane, Washington.)

VIII. Musculoskeletal System (Orthopedics)

A. DEFINITION
1. Deals with disorders of the musculoskeletal systems
2. Specialized physician: orthopedist, orthopod

B. GENERAL EXAMINATION
1. Observes for:
   a. Decreased range of motion (ROM)
   b. Tenderness and swelling
   c. Unequal or decreased strength
   d. Deformities or growths

C. DIAGNOSTIC PROCEDURES
1. Arthrocentesis: removal of joint fluid with a needle for analysis of fluid
2. Arthroscopy: examination of a joint with a viewing scope (arthroscope)
3. Electromyography: recording the strength of muscle contraction as a result of electrical stimulation
4. Muscle biopsy: removal of muscle tissue for examination
5. Bone scan: use of a machine to measure the uptake of a radioactive substance injected intravenously
6. Computerized axial tomography (CAT scan, CT scan): computer-assisted x-ray technique used to distinguish pathologic conditions such as tumors or fractures; a noninvasive method of viewing inside the body
7. Magnetic resonance imaging (MRI): production of detailed pictures of internal structures, using magnetism and computers; a noninvasive method of viewing inside the body
8. Skeletal x-ray: plain x-ray of the appropriate body part
9. Erythrocyte sedimentation rate (ESR; sed rate): blood test that can determine whether inflammation is present within the patient's body
10. Latex fixation: test for the presence of rheumatoid factor present in rheumatoid arthritis

D. TREATMENT PROCEDURES
1. Wrap or splint: cloth or elastic material or rigid material used to immobilize limbs or joints
2. Cast: application of material (plaster, resin, fiberglass) molded to the affected limb and allowed to harden; holds the affected limb or joint in a fixed position until healing is complete
3. Arthroscopic surgery: surgical procedures performed on joints using an arthroscope
4. Reduction: restoration of a fracture to normal position
   a. Closed reduction: manipulation without an incision
   b. Open reduction: incision is made at the fracture site
5. Physical therapy: use of exercise, heat, cold, and other physical means to reduce pain and swelling, to increase movement and circulation, and to promote healing

E. MEDICATIONS
1. Analgesics
   a. Used to reduce pain
   b. Examples: aspirin, Tylenol
2. Narcotic analgesics
   a. Used to reduce pain with narcotics
   b. Examples: Darvon, Lortab, Percodan
3. Antibiotics
   a. Used to kill microorganisms
   b. Examples: Cipro, Keflex
4. Nonsteroidal antiinflammatory drugs (NSAIDs)
   a. Used to reduce inflammation without the use of steroids
   b. Examples: Advil, Motrin, Naprosyn, Indocin, Clinoril
5. Muscle relaxants
   a. Used to relax skeletal muscles
   b. Examples: Flexeril, Valium

IX. Cardiovascular System (Cardiology)

A. DEFINITION
1. Deals with diseases and disorders of the heart and vessels
2. Specialized physician: cardiologist

B. GENERAL EXAMINATION
1. Listening to the heart with a stethoscope, noting heart sounds, rate, and rhythm

C. DIAGNOSTIC PROCEDURES
1. Cardiac catheterization
   a. Intensive study of the heart
   b. Uses catheters to perform angiocardiography and/or pressure-and-flow measurements
   c. Can determine the severity of heart disease and/or vessel blockage
   d. Medical assistant would schedule this procedure at the hospital
2. Echocardiogram: graphic recording of ultrasound waves from the heart
3. Electrocardiogram (ECG) (see details later): recording of the electrical activity of the heart
4. Holter monitor (see Figure 17-4)
   a. Portable ambulatory monitoring system
   b. Monitors ECG activity over a 24-hour period
   c. Designed so that the patient is able to maintain usual daily activities with minimal inconvenience while being monitored
   d. Device is connected to the patient by electrodes placed on the patient's chest and a special portable magnetic tape recorder that continually monitors the heart's activity
   e. Recorder is in a protective case that is either worn on a belt around the patient's waist or hung over the shoulder by a strap

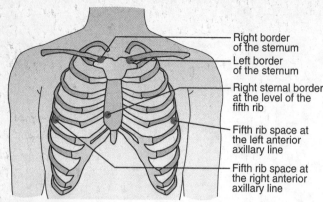

FIGURE 17-4. Holter monitor electrode positions. (Bonewit-West K: *Clinical procedures for medical assistants*, ed 6, Philadelphia, 2004, Saunders.)

f. Patient completes an activity diary; all activities and emotional states are recorded along with any symptoms experienced (chest pain, vertigo, palpitations)

g. Monitor is removed from patient after a 24-hour period, and the tape is evaluated and analyzed

h. Electrodes (floating electrodes) are placed as follows:
   1) Right border of the sternum (manubrium)
   2) Left border of the sternum (manubrium)
   3) Right sternal border at the level of the fifth rib
   4) Fifth rib space at the right anterior axillary line
   5) Fifth rib space at the left anterior axillary line

5. Treadmill: motorized machine that allows patient to walk in place; allows evaluation of the patient's heart function while exercising

6. Angiography: x-ray of blood vessels after an injection of radiopaque material

7. Arterial blood gases (ABGs): measures oxygen, carbon dioxide, and metabolic balance in an arterial blood sample

8. Cardiac enzymes
   a. Creatine phosphokinase (CPK): enzyme released into the blood when the heart or skeletal muscles are injured
   b. Aspartate aminotransferase (AST) (formerly serum glutamic-oxaloacetic transaminase [SGOT]): found in high concentration in heart muscle and in the liver
   c. Lactic dehydrogenase (LDH): enzyme found in heart muscle, skeletal muscles, kidneys, liver, and red blood cells

9. Prothrombin time (PT): tests coagulation of blood

D. TREATMENT PROCEDURES

1. Angioplasty: surgical repair of a blood vessel
2. Defibrillation (cardioversion): brief charges of electricity applied to the chest to stop cardiac arrhythmia
3. Coronary artery bypass: open-heart surgery for the purpose of bypassing an obstructed coronary artery
4. Endarterectomy: removal of the interior portion of an artery and occluding fatty deposits
5. Phlebotomy: opening into a vein; venipuncture
6. Vein stripping: removal of a diseased portion of a vein

E. MEDICATIONS

1. Diuretics
   a. Promote urination; decrease blood pressure
   b. Examples: Bumex, Dyazide, Lasix, Hydro-Diuril
2. Antihypertensives
   a. Decrease blood pressure
   b. Examples: Inderal, Lanoxin, Procardia, Tenormin, Minipress
3. Antilipemics
   a. Decrease cholesterol levels in blood
   b. Examples: Loped, Mevacor, Crestor, Lipitor
4. Antianginals
   a. Decrease chest pain
   b. Examples: Nitrostat, Transderm-Nitro

F. ECG (see Figure 17-5)

1. Cardiac electrical activity is generated, spreads through the heart, and creates an electrical wave
2. This electrical wave is measured as an ECG
   a. Electrical system of the heart
      1) Sinoatrial (SA) node (pacemaker)
      2) Atrioventricular (AV) node
      3) Bundle of His
      4) Right and left bundle branches
      5) Purkinje fibers
   b. Electrical states of the heart
      1) Polarization: cardiac muscle cells are resting
      2) Depolarization: cardiac muscle cells contract
      3) Repolarization: cardiac muscle cells transform from active to resting state for recharging

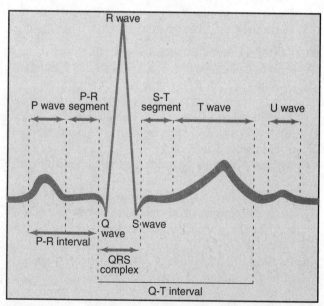

FIGURE 17-5. Cardiac cycle. (Bonewit-West K: *Clinical procedures for medical assistants*, ed 6, Philadelphia, 2004, Saunders.)

c. Normal ECG: all heartbeats appear as a pattern, consisting of:
  1) P-wave: impulse starting in the atria
  2) QRS complex: impulse going through ventricles
  3) T-wave: repolarization of ventricles
d. ECG leads (see Figure 17-6)
  1) Externally applied electrodes
  2) Relative to an axis (a direct line) between two poles
  3) Each lead makes up one positive pole, one negative pole, and one ground
  4) Leads give an electrical picture of the heart from different angles
  5) ECG uses 10 electrodes (four limb electrodes and six chest electrodes) to give 12 leads
    a) Bipolar (standard) limb leads (see Figure 17-7)
      • Six of the 12 leads
      • Electrodes are placed on the patient's extremities (upper arms and inside of calves)
      • Measures cardiac electrical activity between two extremities (negative and positive pole)
      • Right electrode is used for the ground
        (1) Lead I: measures activity from right arm to left arm (RA to LA)

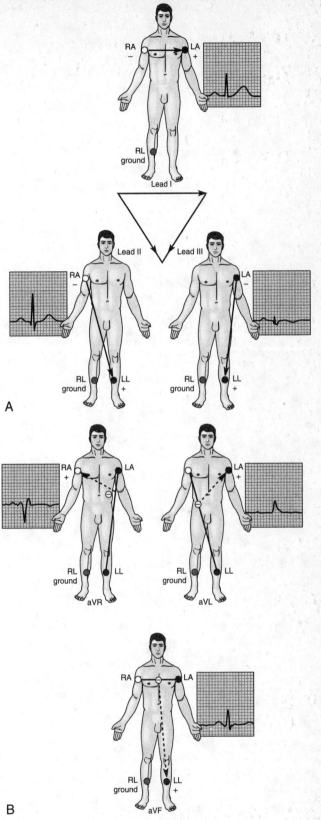

FIGURE 17-7.   Standard *(A)* and augmented *(B)* leads. (Hunt SA: *Saunders fundamentals of medical assisting,* Philadelphia, 2002, Saunders.)

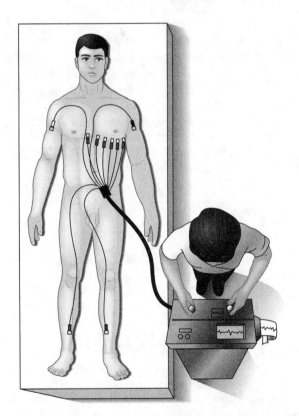

FIGURE 17-6.   ECG leads. *A,* Chest lead placement. *B,* Leg lead placement. *C,* Arm lead placement. (Hunt SA: *Saunders fundamentals of medical assisting,* Philadelphia, 2002, Saunders.)

(2) Lead II: measures activity from right arm to left leg (RA to LL)

(3) Lead III: measures activity from left arm to left leg (LA to LL)

b) Unipolar (augmented) limb leads (see Figure 17-7): measures cardiac electrical activity between the heart and one extremity
   - aVR: right side
   - aVL: left side
   - aVF: left foot

c) Precordial (chest) leads (see Figure 17-8)
   - Provide points of reference across the chest wall

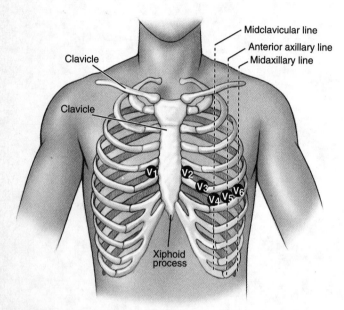

FIGURE 17-8. Chest leads. (Hunt SA: *Saunders fundamentals of medical assisting*, Philadelphia, 2002, Saunders.)

- Differentiate left- and right-sided heart events
   (1) Lead V1: electrode placed at the fourth intercostal space to the right of the sternum
   (2) Lead V2: electrode placed at the fourth intercostal space to the left of the sternum
   (3) Lead V3: electrode placed midway between leads V2 and V4
   (4) Lead V4: electrode placed left-midclavicular line in the fifth intercostal space
   (5) Lead V5: electrode placed at the level of V4 at axillary line
   (6) Lead V6: electrode placed at the level of V5 at the midaxillary line

d) Leads in relation to the anatomy of the heart
   - Right side of the heart: V1, aVR
   - Left side of the heart: V5, V6, I, aVL
   - Transition from right to left sides of the heart: V2, V3, V4
   - Inferior heart: II, III, aVF

e. ECG equipment
   1) Paper (see Figure 17-9)
      a) Records visible record of the heart's electrical activity
      b) Paper is heat-sensitive
      c) Heated stylus on the machine traces the heart activity onto the paper
      d) Composed of 1-mm squares: every fifth line is darkened, creating large blocks five squares wide and five squares high
      e) Cardiac voltage is measured on the vertical scale; time is measured on the horizontal scale
      f) Horizontally, each large block represents 0.2 second

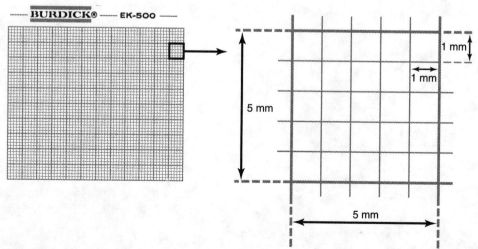

FIGURE 17-9. ECG paper. (Bonewit-West K: *Clinical procedures for medical assistants,* ed 6, Philadelphia, 2004, Saunders.)

g) Vertically, each large block represents 0.5 millivolt of electricity

h) Paper moves continuously through the machine at the rate of 1 inch per second on the standard machine setting

2) Controls

a) Main power switch: turns the machine on and off

b) RUN/STOP: activates (or stops) the amplifier so that the stylus can react to the heartbeat

c) Run-25: moves the paper 25 mm (1 inch) per second (standard speed)

d) Run-50: doubles the paper's speed to 50 mm (2 inches) per second

e) Sensitivity control: regulates the output of the amplifier

f) Standard (STD) button: manually checks the machine's calibration (stylus should deflect 10 mm, or two large squares)

g) Lead selector: changes leads

h) Marker button: allows manual identification of leads; uses codes of dots or dashes

3) Artifacts: abnormal ECG tracings not caused by heart activity

a) Somatic tremor: caused by the patient's muscle movement

b) Alternating current (AC) interference: caused by nearby operation of electrical equipment

c) Wandering baseline: caused by electrodes applied too loosely or too tightly

X. Blood (Hematology)

A. DEFINITION

1. Deals with blood disorders, bone marrow, and coagulation

2. Specialized physician: hematologist

B. GENERAL EXAMINATION

1. Obtain blood or bone marrow samples for testing

2. Palpation of spleen and liver

C. DIAGNOSTIC PROCEDURES

1. Bone marrow aspiration: insertion of a large needle into the sternum or iliac crest to remove bone marrow for testing

2. Blood cell counts (red blood cell [RBC] and white blood cell [WBC]): blood test to determine the number of RBCs and WBCs per cubic millimeter of blood

3. Differential: blood smear on glass slide; stain is applied to the smear; the smear is studied under a microscope to differentiate the types of WBCs

4. Hematocrit (HCT): measures the percentage of RBCs in volume of blood

5. Hemoglobin (Hgb): measures the grams of hemoglobin in volume of blood

6. Platelet count: estimates the number of platelets in volume of blood

7. Prothrombin time (PT): measures coagulation time of blood

D. MEDICATIONS

1. Anticoagulants
   a. Prevent blood from clotting
   b. Examples: Coumadin, Heparin

2. Stimulating factors
   a. Stimulate production of blood cells
   b. Examples: Neupogen, Leukine

3. Thrombolytic agents
   a. Dissolve clots
   b. Examples: Abbokinase, Streptase

4. Antianemics
   a. Treat anemias
   b. Examples: Epogen, Slow-Fe, vitamin B12

5. Antiplatelet agents
   a. Inhibit platelet aggregation; prolonged bleeding time
   b. Example: Plavix

XI. Respiratory System (Pulmonology)

A. DEFINITION

1. Deals with diseases and disorders of the lungs and respiratory system

2. Specialized physician: pulmonologist

B. GENERAL EXAMINATION

1. Inspection of the nose, face, and throat

2. Examination of the mucous membranes

3. Inspection and palpation of the sinuses, neck, and lymph nodes

4. Auscultation of the lungs

C. DIAGNOSTIC PROCEDURES

1. Bronchoscopy: visualization of the bronchi through a bronchoscope

2. Spirometry: measurement of the breathing capacity of the lungs

3. Lung biopsy: biopsy of tissue taken from the lungs

4. Pulmonary function test (PFT): evaluates how the patient breathes; determines lung volumes, pulmonary gas exchange, and flow rates

5. Thoracentesis: puncture of the chest wall with a needle to obtain fluid for testing

6. Tracheostomy: emergency or elective procedure that creates an opening through the neck into the trachea

7. Chest x-ray: full view of the lungs from the back (posteroanterior [PA]) and sides (lateral)

8. Sputum culture: collection of a sputum sample and testing it for microorganisms

9. Arterial blood gases (ABGs): measurement of hydrogen, carbon dioxide, pH, and oxygen pressure from an arterial blood sample

D. TREATMENT PROCEDURES

1. Endotracheal intubation: a procedure that establishes an airway by inserting a tube through the nose, pharynx, and larynx into the trachea
2. Thoracotomy: surgical insertion of a tube into the chest to drain fluid or air
3. Nebulizer: use of a machine to produce a fine mist of water and medication; the patient receives the medication by inhaling the mist

E. MEDICATIONS

1. Antibiotics
   a. Kill microorganisms
   b. Examples: Amoxil, Ampicillin, Biaxin, Ceclor, Keflex
2. Antihistamines
   a. Counteract the effects of histamine
   b. Examples: Benadryl, Phenergan, Seldane
3. Bronchodilators
   a. Dilate bronchial tubes
   b. Examples: Albuterol, Proventil, Ventolin, Aminophylline
4. Expectorants
   a. Produce productive cough
   b. Example: Humibid
5. Decongestants
   a. Decrease congestion in the nose and nasal passages
   b. Examples: Entex, Afrin, Sudafed

XII. Digestive System (Gastroenterology)

A. DEFINITION

1. Treats diseases and disorders of the digestive tract
2. Specialized physician: gastroenterologist

B. GENERAL EXAMINATION

1. Examination of the mouth
2. Palpation of the abdomen and intestines
3. Inspection of the rectum (can be accomplished with a scope)

C. DIAGNOSTIC PROCEDURES

1. Colonoscopy: visual examination of the colon using a lighted scope
2. Liver biopsy: removal of a tissue sample from the liver for microscopic examination
3. Proctoscopy (sigmoidoscopy): visual examination of the anus, the rectum, and part of the sigmoid colon
4. Barium enema (BE): infusion of barium into the rectum for visualization by x-ray
5. Cholecystogram: x-ray examination of the gallbladder
6. Upper gastrointestinal (GI) series: x-ray study of the esophagus, stomach, and duodenum; contrast medium is orally administered

7. Gastric analysis: aspiration of the stomach contents by a tube placed into the stomach, through the nose; contents analyzed
8. Occult blood (guaiac) test: test for hidden blood in the stool; Hemoccult
9. Ova and parasites (O&P): analysis of a stool sample for the presence of eggs and parasites
10. Liver function tests: tests performed to diagnose liver-related diseases or disorders

D. TREATMENT PROCEDURES

1. Appendectomy: removal of the appendix
2. Cholecystectomy: removal of the gallbladder
3. Colostomy: creation of an opening between the colon and the body surface
4. Hemorrhoid ligation: removal of hemorrhoids by using the rubber band technique (ligating)
5. Lithotripsy: crushing of stones
6. Hemorrhoidectomy: excision of hemorrhoids
7. Vagotomy: surgical transaction of the vagus nerve to decrease stomach acid secretion in patients with ulcers

E. MEDICATIONS

1. Antihelmintics
   a. Kill helminths (worms)
   b. Example: Vermox
2. Antibiotics
   a. Kill microorganisms
   b. Examples: Sumycin, Flagyl
3. Antispasmodics
   a. Decrease spasms of the GI tract
   b. Examples: Bentyl, Librax, Donnatal
4. Antidiarrheals
   a. Decrease or slow diarrhea
   b. Examples: Imodium, Lomotil, Pepto-Bismol
5. H_2 antagonists
   a. Decrease stomach acids
   b. Examples: Tagamet, Zantac, Axid, Pepcid
6. Laxatives
   a. Encourage bowel movements
   b. Examples: Colace, Dulcolax, Ex-Lax, Milk of Magnesia

XII. Urinary System (Urology)

A. DEFINITION

1. Treats diseases and disorders of the male and female urinary systems and the male reproductive system
2. Specialized physician: urologist

B. GENERAL EXAMINATION

1. Palpation of the kidneys and bladder
2. Inspection of the external genitalia
3. Palpation of the prostate gland through the rectum

C. DIAGNOSTIC PROCEDURES

1. Cystoscopy: visual examination of the bladder with a cystoscope

2. Retrograde pyelogram: x-ray of the kidney after introducing a contrast medium through the ureter
3. Intravenous pyelogram (IVP): study of the kidney using an intravenous contrast medium
4. Renal ultrasound: ultrasound of the kidneys
5. X-ray of the kidney, ureter, and bladder (KUB): x-ray done without injection of air or contrast medium; shows the size and location of the organs
6. Urinalysis (UA): analysis of urine to determine its physical, chemical, and microscopic properties
7. Blood urea nitrogen (BUN): measures the amount of urea in the blood; kidney function test
8. Semen analysis: measures the quantity and motility of sperm
9. Prostate specific antigen (PSA): blood test to check for the presence of prostate cancer

D. TREATMENT PROCEDURES
1. Dialysis: artificial means of removing waste products from the blood when the kidneys have failed
2. Lithotripsy: procedure to crush or break up stones in the urinary tract
3. Catheterization: introduction of a flexible tube through the urethra into the urinary bladder
4. Circumcision: removal of the foreskin of the penis
5. Prostatectomy: removal of the prostate
6. Transurethral resection of the prostate (TURP): prostatic tissue removed through an endoscope introduced through the urethra
7. Vasectomy: removal of a segment of the vas deferens; male sterilization technique

E. MEDICATIONS
1. Antibiotics
   a. Destroy microorganisms
   b. Examples: Bactrim, Furadantin, Gantrisin, Rocephin
2. Analgesics
   a. Reduce pain
   b. Example: Pyridium
3. Gonadotropins
   a. Stimulate gonads
   b. Example: Pergonal
4. For impotence
   a. Example: Viagra

XIV. Female Reproductive System (Obstetrics/Gynecology)

A. DEFINITION
1. Diagnosis and treatment of diseases and disorders of the female reproductive system and pregnancy
2. Specialized physician: obstetrician (pregnancy and childbirth) and/or gynecologist (female reproductive system)

B. GENERAL EXAMINATION
1. Inspection and palpation of the breasts
2. Inspection of the external genitalia, vagina, and cervix
3. Palpation of the uterus, ovaries, and fallopian tubes
4. Prenatal: includes initial general examination, as well as periodic examinations to monitor fetal growth and development

C. DIAGNOSTIC PROCEDURES
1. Amniocentesis
   a. Puncture of the amniotic sac with a needle to withdraw amniotic fluid for analysis
   b. Can detect genetic disorders
2. Cervical biopsy: removal of tissue to evaluate the presence of abnormalities
3. Colposcopy: examination of the cervix with a scope
4. Dilation and curettage (D&C): expansion of the cervix so that the uterine wall can be scraped
5. Fetal monitoring: recording of the fetal heart rate
6. Laparoscopy: examination of the abdomen by insertion of a laparoscope through the abdominal wall
7. Human chorionic gonadotropin (HCG)
   a. Hormone produced by the placenta during pregnancy
   b. Basis for pregnancy testing
   c. Testing performed on blood or urine
8. Chorionic villi sampling (CVS)
   a. Use of ultrasound to guide a needle into the uterine wall to obtain a sample of chorion
   b. Can detect chromosomal abnormalities
9. Endovaginal ultrasound: sound probe placed in the vagina for a closer, sharper look within the pelvis
10. Hysterosalpingography: x-ray of the uterus and fallopian tubes, using radiopaque material
11. Pelvimetry: measurement of the dimensions of the pelvis
12. Pap (Papanicolaou) smear (ThinPrep)
    a. Scrapings from the cervix used to detect tissue changes
    b. Screening test for cervical cancer

D. TREATMENT PROCEDURES
1. Abortion
   a. Premature termination of pregnancy
   b. May be spontaneous or therapeutic
2. Cauterization: use of heat to destroy abnormal tissue
3. Cesarean section (C-section): birth of an infant through a surgical incision into uterus
4. Conization: removal of a cone-shaped wedge of tissue from the cervix for examination
5. Cryosurgery: use of cold to destroy abnormal tissue
6. Hysterectomy: surgical removal of the uterus through the abdominal wall or vagina
7. Hysteroscopy: insertion of a scope into the uterus to view the endometrial cavity
8. Kegel exercises: simple exercises to strengthen the pubococcygeal muscles
9. Tubal ligation
   a. Tying off the fallopian tubes
   b. Female sterilization procedure

E. MEDICATIONS

1. Hormone replacement and hormones
   a. Examples: Premarin, Depo-Provera, Ogen
2. Ovulation stimulants
   a. Example: Clomid
3. Oral contraceptives
   a. Prevent pregnancy
   b. Examples: Triphasil, Ovral, Ortho-Novum, Ortho Tri-Cyclen
4. Supplements
   a. Vitamins and iron
   b. Examples: Ferro-Sequels, Natalins
5. Antifungals
   a. Treat fungal or yeast infections
   b. Examples: Monistat, Gyne-Lotrimin

XV. Endocrine System (Endocrinology)

A. DEFINITION

1. Diagnose and treats diseases and disorders of the endocrine system
2. Specialized physician: endocrinologist

B. GENERAL EXAMINATION

1. Complete physical examination

C. DIAGNOSTIC PROCEDURES

1. Radioactive iodine uptake: measures the uptake of a dose of radioactive iodine by the thyroid gland
2. Thyroid scan
   a. Administration of a radioactive compound to visualize the thyroid gland
   b. Used to detect tumors and nodules
3. CAT scans
   a. Can visualize the endocrine glands
   b. Can detect disease processes and masses
4. Ultrasonography: use of sound waves to obtain images
5. Blood tests
   a. Used to diagnose and manage endocrine disorders
   b. Blood tests for:
      1) Adrenocorticotropic hormone (ACTH): from the pituitary
      2) Aldosterone: from the adrenal cortex
      3) Thyroxin: from the thyroid
      4) Calcium: from the parathyroid
      5) Cortisol: from the adrenal cortex
      6) Electrolytes (sodium, potassium, and chloride): from the adrenal cortex
      7) Estradiol: from the ovaries
      8) Follicle-stimulating hormone (FSH): from the pituitary
      9) Growth hormone (GH): from the pituitary
      10) Glucose: from the pancreas
      11) Insulin: from the pancreas
      12) Luteinizing hormone (LH): from the pituitary
      13) Parathyroid hormone: from the parathyroid
      14) Triiodothyronine (T-3) and thyroxine (tetraiodothyronine [T-4]): from the thyroid
      15) Testosterone: from the testes

6. Basal metabolic rate (BMR)
   a. Not an often-ordered test
   b. Measures the energy exchange rate of the body in a state of rest
7. Glucose tolerance test (GTT)
   a. Blood is tested at specific intervals after the patient ingests a measured amount of glucose

D. TREATMENT PROCEDURES

1. Oophorectomy: surgical removal of the ovaries
2. Orchiectomy: surgical removal of the testes
3. Thyroidectomy: total or partial removal of thyroid gland

E. MEDICATIONS

1. Thyroid medications
   a. Replace thyroid hormones
   b. Examples: Synthroid, Euthroid
2. Corticosteroids
   a. Examples: Cortisone, Aristocort, Kenalog, Medrol, Decadron
3. GH
   a. Example: Humatrope
4. Antidiuretic hormones
   a. Example: Pitressin
5. Labor inducers
   a. Example: Pitocin
6. Oral antidiabetics
   a. Examples: Orinase, Glucotrol, Diabinese, Glucophage
7. Insulin
   a. Examples: Humulin, Novolin

XVI. Nervous System (Neurology)

A. DEFINITION

1. Diagnosis and treatment of diseases and disorders of the nervous system
2. Specialized physician: neurologist

B. GENERAL EXAMINATION

1. Mental status: includes assessment of intelligence; assessment of memory; orientation to person, place, and time; and general appearance
2. Evaluation of all cranial nerves
3. Motor nerves: includes coordination, strength, Romberg test, walking, and finger-to-nose exercise
4. Sensory nervous system
5. Reflexes

C. DIAGNOSTIC PROCEDURES

1. Electroencephalogram (EEG)
   a. Study of the electrical activity of the brain
   b. Uses electrodes attached to the scalp
2. Electromyogram (EMG): study of the contraction of a muscle as a result of electrical stimulation
3. Lumbar puncture: procedure for removal of cerebrospinal fluid (CSF) for analysis
4. Brain scan: procedure that uses radioactive chemicals and specialized machines to record the passage through, and absorption into, brain lesions

5. Myelography: x-ray of the spinal cord
6. Skull series: standard x-ray views of the skull
7. Cervical, thoracic, and lumbosacral spine: standard x-ray views of specific portions of the spine

D. TREATMENT PROCEDURES

1. Craniotomy: surgical opening into the cranium
2. Laminectomy: removal of laminae to decompress pinched spinal nerve roots
3. Halo traction: traction device for neck stability

E. MEDICATIONS

1. Anticonvulsants
   a. Decrease seizure activity
   b. Examples: Depakote, Dilantin, Tegretol
2. Antiemetics (antivertigo agents)
   a. Decrease vomiting, dizziness
   b. Examples: Antivert, Compazine, Dramamine
3. Anti-Parkinson's agents
   a. Decrease symptoms of Parkinson's disease
   b. Examples: Artane, Cogentin, Sinemet
4. Antidepressants
   a. Counteract depression
   b. Examples: Paxil, Prozac, Celexa

XVII. Sensory Systems (Eyes) (Ophthalmology)

A. DEFINITION

1. Diagnosis and treatment of diseases and disorders of the eye
2. Specialized physician: ophthalmologist

B. GENERAL EXAMINATION

1. Inspection and measurement of the external eye, eyelids, and accessory structures
2. Measurement of eye movements and pupillary distance

C. DIAGNOSTIC PROCEDURES

1. Keratometry (K-readings): measurement of the steepness of the cornea
2. Ophthalmoscopy: visual examination of the interior eye using an ophthalmoscope
3. Visual acuity
   a. Determines the amount of myopia, hyperopia, or astigmatism
   b. Uses the Snellen eye chart
4. Slit lamp examination: examines the cornea, conjunctiva, iris, lens, and vitreous humor using a slit light and biomicroscope
5. Tonometry
   a. Measures intraocular tension
   b. May indicate the presence of glaucoma
6. Ishihara color vision test: tests color vision

D. TREATMENT PROCEDURES

1. Blepharoplasty: surgical repair of the eyelids
2. Cataract extraction: removal of the lens of the eye
3. Enucleation: removal of the eye from the socket
4. Glaucoma operation: procedure that relieves increased intraocular pressure

E. MEDICATIONS

1. Antibiotic and steroid combinations
   a. Example: TobraDex
2. Antibiotics
   a. Examples: Tobrex, Bacitracin Opthalmic
3. Corticosteroids
   a. Examples: Decadron, Opticrom
4. Glaucoma treatment
   a. Examples: Timoptic, Propine, Betagan

XVIII. Ear, Nose, And Throat (ENT, Otorhinolaryngology)

A. DEFINITION

1. Diagnosis and treatment of diseases and disorders of the ear, nose, and throat
2. Specialized physician: otorhinolaryngologist

B. GENERAL EXAMINATION

1. Examination of the ear with an otoscope
2. Examination of the nasal structures, throat, and sinuses

C. DIAGNOSTIC PROCEDURES

1. Audiometry
   a. Use of an audiometer to deliver sound frequencies
   b. Determines the patient's hearing threshold
2. Laryngoscopy: visual examination of the larynx with a laryngoscope
3. Otoscopy: visual examination of the ear with an otoscope
4. Throat culture: inflamed areas of the throat are swabbed and analyzed for various pathogens
5. Nasal smear: removal of a specimen and analysis for pathogens
6. Skull, mastoid, sinus, and chest x-rays: standard views of specific body parts

D. TREATMENT PROCEDURES

1. Adenoidectomy: surgical excision of adenoids
2. Myringotomy: incision into the eardrum
3. Myringotomy with tubes: incision into the eardrum with placement of ventilation tubes
4. Rhinoplasty: reconstruction or plastic surgery of the nose
5. Tonsillectomy: surgical excision of tonsils
6. Ear irrigation: irrigation (washing) of external ear canal

E. MEDICATIONS

1. Antibiotics
   a. Examples: Amoxil, Ceclor, Erythromycin, Keflex
2. Otics
   a. Examples: Cerumenex, Cortisporin Otic

XIX. Pediatrics

A. DEFINITION

1. Diagnosis and treatment of diseases and disorders associated with childhood and health maintenance for infants, children, and adolescents
2. Specialized physician: pediatrician

B. GENERAL EXAMINATION

1. Similar to a complete physical examination for an adult
2. Examinations fall into two general categories:
   a. Well-child (well-baby) visit
      1) Evaluates the child's growth and development
      2) Physical examination is performed at this time
      3) Necessary immunizations are administered
   b. Sick-child (sick-baby) visit
      1) Child shows signs and symptoms of a disease process or injury
      2) Provider diagnoses and prescribes treatment

C. GROWTH CHART

1. Chart used to plot the physical growth pattern of a child
2. Includes height, weight, and head circumference
3. Identifies the percentile the child's growth falls into, as compared with the measurements listed on the standardized chart
4. Should be plotted at each well-baby visit
5. Separate charts
   a. Girls, 2 to 20 years (see Figure 17-10)
   b. Boys, birth to 36 months (see Figure 17-11)
   c. Girls, 2 to 18 years
   d. Boys, 2 to 18 years

D. IMMUNIZATIONS (see Figure 17-12)

1. Always refer to the Centers for Disease Control and Prevention (CDC) guidelines for current schedule
   a. Childhood diphtheria tetanus acellular pertussis vaccine (DtaP)
      1) Total of five doses required by law between 2 months and 6 years of age
      2) Administer: 0.5 mL intramuscularly (IM)
   b. Adolescent tetanus-diphtheria toxoids vaccine (Td): 11 and 12 years of age, Td booster
   c. Adult tetanus vaccine (Td)
      1) Given as a booster from age 7 through adult
      2) Adults are given one dose each 10 years for life
      3) For severe or dirty wounds, a booster is given if the last normal dose was more than 5 years ago
      4) For minor or clean wounds, a booster is given if the last normal dose was given 10 or more years ago
   d. *Haemophilus influenzae* type b (HiB)
      1) Four doses administered between 2 months and 18 months of age
      2) Administer: 0.5 mL IM
      3) Vaccine consists of killed virus grown in chicken embryo tissue
   e. Inactivated poliovirus (poliomyelitis) vaccine (IPV)
      1) Four doses administered between 2 months and 4 to 6 years of age

2) Administer: 0.5 mL IM
   f. Hepatitis B vaccine (HepB)
      1) Three doses administered between birth and 18 months of age
      2) Administer: 0.5 mL IM
   g. Mumps, measles, and rubella (MMR) vaccine
      1) Two doses administered between 12 months and 11 to 12 years of age
      2) Administer: 0.5 mL subcutaneously (SC)
      3) Vaccine consists of attenuated measles, mumps, and rubella virus
   h. Varicella vaccine (Var; chickenpox)
      1) Administered after 12 months of age
      2) Administer: 0.5 mL IM
   i. Pneumococcal vaccine (PCV)
      1) Three doses administered before age 12 months; last dose given after 12 months and before age 5
      2) Administer 0.5 mL IM
   j. Recommended immunization schedule (2006 CDC schedule)
      1) 2 months: HepB#1, DtaP#1, HIB#1, IPV#1, PCV#1
      2) 4 months: HepB#2, DtaP#2, HIB#2, IPV#2, PCV#2
      3) 6 months: HepB#3, DtaP#3, HIB#3, PCV#3
      4) 15 months: DtaP#4, HIB#4, MMR#1, IPV#3, PCV#, Var
      5) 18 months: Catch up
      6) 4 to 6 years: DtaP#5, IPV#4, MMR#2
      7) Over 12 years: HepB series if not vaccinated as an infant, Td every 10 years

XX. Geriatrics

A. DEFINITION

1. Treatment of the aged
2. Specialized physician: gerontologist and internist

B. AGING

1. Complex physiologic, psychological, and social process
2. Aging is not an illness; it is a normal life process
3. Changes occur in the patient's
   a. Appearance
   b. Abilities
   c. Vision
   d. Hearing
   e. Taste
   f. Smell

C. CARING FOR THE OLDER PATIENT

1. Speak slowly and distinctly if the person is hearing impaired
2. Use indirect lighting in examination rooms to decrease glare

2 to 20 years: Girls
Stature-for-age and Weight-for-age percentiles

NAME _____

RECORD # _____

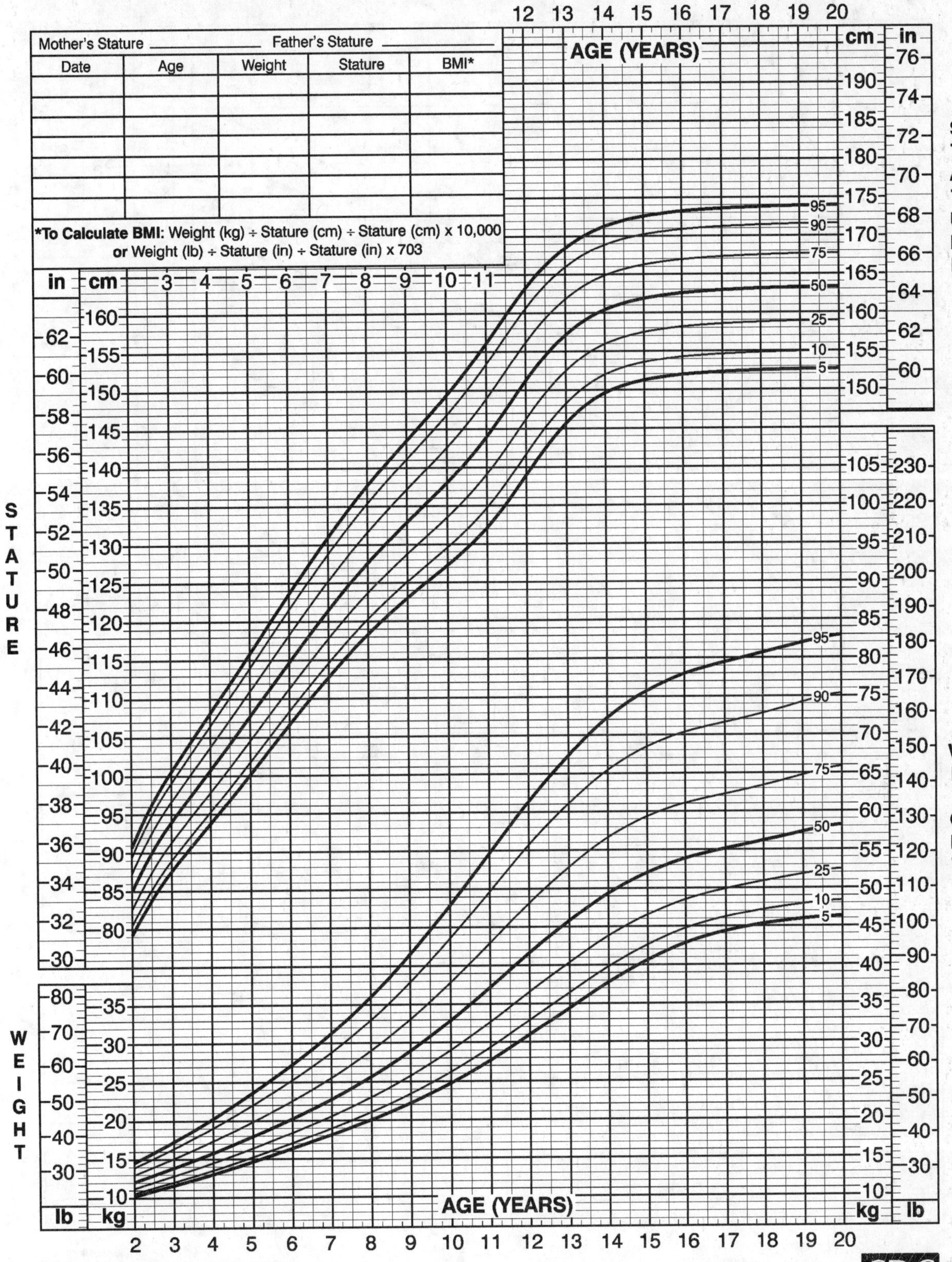

*To Calculate BMI: Weight (kg) ÷ Stature (cm) ÷ Stature (cm) x 10,000
or Weight (lb) ÷ Stature (in) ÷ Stature (in) x 703

Published May 30, 2000 (modified 11/21/00).
SOURCE: Developed by the National Center for Health Statistics in collaboration with
the National Center for Chronic Disease Prevention and Health Promotion (2000).
http://www.cdc.gov/growthcharts

CDC
SAFER·HEALTHIER·PEOPLE™

FIGURE 17-10. Growth rate graph: girls (2 to 20 years). (Developed by the National Center for Health Statistics in collaboration with the National Center for Chronic Disease Prevention and Health Promotion [2000]. Available at: http://www.cdc.gov/growthcharts. Published May 30, 2000.)

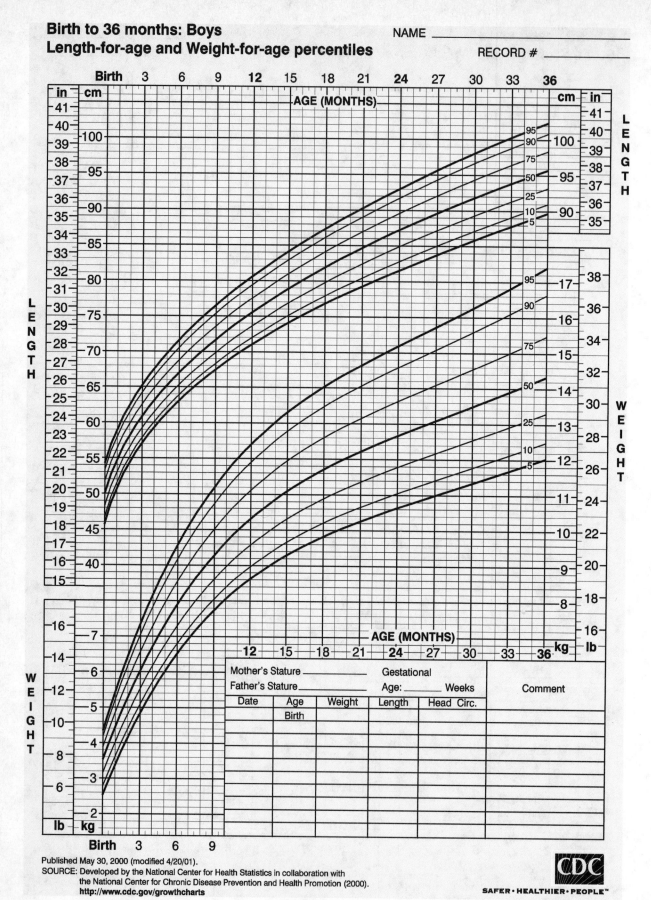

FIGURE 17-11. Growth rate graph: males (birth to 36 months). (Developed by the National Center for Health Statistics in collaboration with the National Center for Chronic Disease Prevention and Health Promotion [2000]. Available at: http://www.cdc.gov/growthcharts. Published May 30, 2000 [modified 4/20/01].)

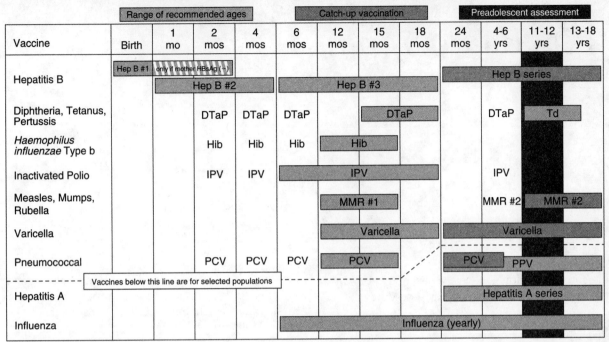

Recommended childhood immunization schedule*—United States, 2002

		Range of recommended ages			Catch-up vaccination				Preadolescent assessment			
Vaccine	Birth	1 mo	2 mos	4 mos	6 mos	12 mos	15 mos	18 mos	24 mos	4-6 yrs	11-12 yrs	13-18 yrs
Hepatitis B	Hep B #1 only if mother HBsAg (−)		Hep B #2			Hep B #3				Hep B series		
Diphtheria, Tetanus, Pertussis			DTaP	DTaP	DTaP		DTaP			DTaP	Td	
Haemophilus influenzae Type b			Hib	Hib	Hib	Hib						
Inactivated Polio			IPV	IPV		IPV				IPV		
Measles, Mumps, Rubella						MMR #1				MMR #2	MMR #2	
Varicella						Varicella				Varicella		
Pneumococcal			PCV	PCV	PCV	PCV			PCV	PPV		
Hepatitis A										Hepatitis A series		
Influenza					Influenza (yearly)							

Vaccines below this line are for selected populations

* Indicates the recommended ages for routine administration of currently licensed childhood vaccines, as of December 1, 2001, for children through age 18 years. Any dose not given at the recommended age should be given at any subsequent visit when indicated and feasible. ■ Indicates age groups that warrant special effort to administer those vaccines not given previously. Additional vaccines may be licensed and recommended during the year. Licensed combination vaccines may be used whenever any components of the combination are indicated and the vaccine's other components are not contraindicated. Providers should consult the manufacturers' package inserts for detailed recommendations.

Additional information about vaccines, vaccine supply, and contraindications for immunization is available at http://www.cdc.gov/nip or at the National Immunization hotline. 800-232-2522 (English), or 800-232-0233 (Spanish). Copies of the schedule can be obtained at http://www.cdc.gov/nip/recs/child-schedule.htm. Approved by the **Advisory Committee on Immunization Practices** (http://www.cdc.gov/nip/acip), the **American Academy of Pediatrics** (http://www.aap.org), and the **American Academy of Family Physicians** (http://www.aafp.org).

FIGURE 17-12. Immunization schedule. (From U.S. Department of Health and Human Services, Centers for Disease Control and Prevention.)

3. Do not carry on conversations with the patient where a large amount of background noise is present
4. Do not patronize the older patient
5. Touch the older patient as you would any other patient
6. Touch the older patient politely and affectionately, not in a controlling manner
7. Use eye contact when conversing with the older patient
8. Offer assistance to the older patient as needed
9. Treat the older patient as an individual
10. Reinforce treatment instructions by writing them down
11. Never approach a visually impaired person without making your presence known; identify yourself and others in the room

D. PROBLEMS ASSOCIATED WITH AGING

1. Inability to perform personal care, including bathing, dressing, eating, getting out of bed, and using the toilet
2. Inability to live independently, including preparing meals, shopping, managing money, using the telephone, and doing housework
3. Functioning such as walking, climbing stairs, lifting, and standing for periods of time

18 Radiography

(Depending on the location, a medical assistant may or may not be legally permitted to perform x-ray procedures.)

I. Introduction

A. GENERAL
1. High-energy, invisible, electromagnetic waves
2. Have the ability to penetrate body structures
3. Discovered by Wilhelm Konrad Roentgen in 1895
4. Some states may require a limited radiography license to take films

II. Functions

A. REVEALS THE PRESENCE OF FRACTURES AND/OR ABNORMALITIES OF BONES

B. REVEALS THE SIZE AND SHAPE OF ORGANS

C. REVEALS THE PRESENCE AND POSITION OF FOREIGN BODIES

D. DESTROYS PATHOLOGICAL CELLS

III. Equipment

A. TABLE
1. Supports the patient's body
2. Contains grids and Bucky mechanism for film placement

B. X-RAY TUBE
1. Glass vacuum tube that produces, focuses, and transmits the x-rays

C. COLLIMATOR
1. Apparatus below the tube that permits the radiographer to vary the size of the radiation field

D. CONTROL PANEL
1. Allows control of x-ray emissions
2. Regulates the machine
3. Should be located behind lead-lined wall so that the operator is protected from the rays
   a. Main switch: turns machine on and off
   b. Milliamperes (MA) setting: sets the amount of radiation that comes from the tube
   c. Time switch: number of seconds the patient is exposed to the x-rays
   d. Kilovolts peak (KVP) setting: penetrating power of the x-ray beam
   e. Bucky switch: turns on the Bucky mechanism
   f. Exposure switch: exposes the patient to the x-rays

E. GRID
1. Absorbs the scattered radiation
2. Prevents blurring of the film
3. Placed between the patient and the film to reduce secondary wave interference

F. POTTER-BUCKY DIAPHRAGM (BUCKY)
1. Framelike structure under the table
2. Holds the grid above the film
3. Used when thicker body parts are exposed to x-rays

G. CASSETTE
1. Device that holds the film

H. INTENSIFYING SCREEN
1. Special plates located within the cassette
2. Reduces the amount of exposure required, which reduces the time the patient is exposed to radiation

I. X-RAY FILM
1. Coated with special material that is sensitive to x-rays
2. Creates a visible record for viewing and archives
3. Film that receives x-ray appears black and gray; film that does not receive x-ray appears white; the more dense the object, the lighter the image is on the film
4. Use only under safety light in a darkroom to avoid exposure
5. Common sizes are 5 × 7, 8 × 10, 10 × 12, 11 × 14, and 14 × 17

J. VIEW BOX
1. Lighted box for viewing the developed x-ray film

K. CALIPER
1. Measures the thickness of body parts
2. Used to calculate the amount of x-ray exposure

IV. Safety

A. HAZARDS
1. Radiation has a cumulative effect on the body
2. Exposure damages body cells, especially gametes and the developing fetus
3. Eye exposure can cause cataracts
4. Exposure over a long period may cause cancer, sterility, or genetic defects
5. High exposure over a short period may cause radiation sickness (nausea, vomiting, diarrhea, and hair loss)

B. PRECAUTIONS
1. Keep appropriate equipment in good condition
2. Prevent exposure to gonads by using lead shields or lead aprons on both patients and operators
3. Always ask women of childbearing age whether any chance exists that they are pregnant; if so, the physician must approve the x-ray procedure
4. Wear a dosimeter (x-ray badge containing reactive material that is sensitive to radiation); must be checked periodically to measure the technician's exposure level
5. Wear the lead shield or lead apron

V. Patient Positioning
(see Figures 18-1, 18-2, 18-3, and 18-4)

A. THE BODY PART NEAREST THE FILM GIVES THE GREATEST DETAIL
1. Anteroposterior (AP): x-ray beam enters the anterior of the body surface and exits the posterior of the body surface before it hits the film
2. Posteroanterior (PA): x-ray beam enters the posterior of the body surface and exits the anterior of the body surface before it hits the film
3. Lateral: x-ray beam passes from one side to the other side before hitting the film; this x-ray order may be right lateral (from the right to the left side) or left lateral (from the left to the right)
4. Oblique: x-ray beam passes through the body part at an angle

VI. Procedure

A. SELECT THE FILM AND LOAD THE CASSETTE IN THE DARKROOM

B. IDENTIFY THE FILM
1. Each film is permanently identified
2. Include the patient's name and number and the date of the x-ray procedure

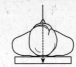
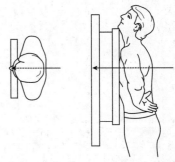

FIGURE 18-1. Anteroposterior view (Long BW et al: *Radiography essentials: for limited practice*, ed 2, St Louis, 2006, Saunders.)

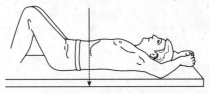

FIGURE 18-2. Posteroanterior view. (Long BW et al: *Radiography essentials: for limited practice*, ed 2, St Louis, 2006, Saunders.)

3. Indicate right (R) or left (L) body part to be examined using lead markers

C. POSITION THE PATIENT IN THE CENTER OF THE FILM

D. MEASURE THE BODY PART THROUGH THE THICKEST AREA

E. SHIELD THE PATIENT WITH THE LEAD SHIELD OR LEAD APRON

F. PLACE THE X-RAY FILM
1. Tabletop: most common use; the film cassette is placed on the table 40 inches from the tube
2. Bucky tray: the film cassette is placed in the tray under the table
3. Wall mount: the film is placed in the wall stand 72 inches from the tube

G. POSITION THE X-RAY TUBE DIRECTLY OVER THE BODY PART, CENTERING IT OVER THE FILM

H. ADJUST THE CONTROLS

I. POSITION YOURSELF BEHIND THE LEAD WALL

J. TAKE (EXPOSE) THE FILM

VII. Darkroom

A. LOCATION WHERE THE FILM IS HANDLED AND DEVELOPED

B. LIT BY A SAFETY LIGHT

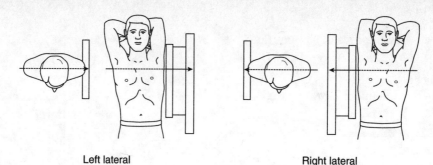

Left lateral   Right lateral

FIGURE 18-3. Lateral view. (Long BW et al: *Radiography essentials: for limited practice,* ed 2, St Louis, 2006, Saunders.)

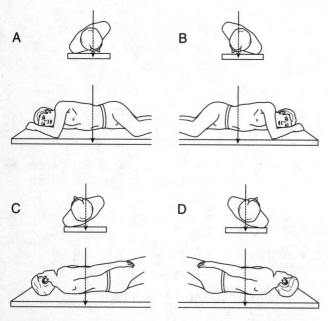

FIGURE 18-4. Oblique projections. **A,** right anterior oblique (RAO). **B,** left anterior oblique (LAO). **C,** Left posterior oblique (LPO). **D,** Right posterior oblique (RPO) (Long BW et al: *Radiography essentials: for limited practice,* ed 2, St Louis, 2006, Saunders.)

C. FILM DEVELOPER MAY BE MANUAL OR AUTOMATIC

D. DEVELOPMENT TECHNIQUE INCLUDES:
1. Developer
2. Water bath
3. Fixer

E. FILM SHOULD BE HANDLED BY THE EDGES ONLY AND BE ATTACHED TO A METAL HANGER (IF DEVELOPING MANUALLY)

F. AFTER THE FILM IS DEVELOPED AND DRIED, IT IS PLACED IN A STORAGE ENVELOPE OR FILE

G. USE A DEVELOPING TIMER

H. KEEP UNDEVELOPED FILM IN A LEAD-LINED VAULT

VIII. Special X-ray Studies

A. ANGIOGRAM
1. Contrast medium is injected intravenously
2. Can determine cardiovascular disease

B. ARTERIOGRAM
1. Similar to angiogram but specifically studies the arteries

C. BARIUM ENEMA (LOWER GASTROINTESTINAL [GI] SERIES)
1. Contrast medium is instilled by enema into the colon
2. Test is used to visualize the lower intestines

D. BARIUM MEAL (UPPER GI SERIES)
1. Contrast medium is orally administered
2. Test is used to visualize the esophagus, stomach, and duodenum

E. BRONCHOGRAM
1. Contrast medium is administered through the trachea and into the bronchial tree
2. Can detect cancer and other lung disorders

F. CHOLECYSTOGRAM
1. Tablet form of contrast medium is ingested by the patient the night before the procedure
2. The gallbladder is observed on film

G. HYSTEROSALPINGOGRAM
1. Contrast medium is injected into the fallopian tubes
2. Can detect the patency of the tubes

H. KIDNEY, URETER, BLADDER (KUB)
1. Basic flat x-ray of the abdominal area

I. INTRAVENOUS PYELOGRAM (IVP)
1. Contrast medium (dye) is injected intravenously, and the pathway of the contrast medium is observed as it is excreted through the kidneys; outline of the ureters and bladder can be visualized
2. Films are taken at intervals until the contrast medium is completely excreted

J. MAMMOGRAM
  1. X-ray of the breast; can detect cancer or abnormalities

K. COMPUTED AXIAL TOMOGRAPHY (CAT [OR CT] SCAN)
  1. Radiographic technique that produces a picture that represents a detailed cross section of tissue structures
  2. More sensitive than x-rays

L. MAGNETIC RESONANCE IMAGING (MRI)
  1. Uses a combination of radio waves and magnetic field to produce images of soft tissues

M. FLUOROSCOPY
  1. X-ray examination that permits visualization of internal body structures; contrast medium is used; motion of a body part can be observed

N. ULTRASOUND
  1. Not a radiologic procedure
  2. Permits visualization of internal structures by the use of high-frequency sound waves
  3. The sound waves echo off the body part and are displayed on a screen
  4. Useful for observation of obstetric and soft tissue (brain, eye, breast, reproductive) organs

19 *Therapeutic Modalities*

I. General

A. USE OF HEAT, COLD, MASSAGE, WATER, EXERCISE, AND/OR ELECTRICITY TO RESTORE NORMAL FUNCTION TO INJURED TISSUES; PHYSICAL THERAPY

B. OBJECTIVES INCLUDE:
1. Relief of the patient's pain
2. Increase or improve the patient's circulation
3. Increase or restore the patient's muscle function
4. Improve the patient's strength, range of motion, and joint mobility

C. PHYSICAL THERAPY PROGRAM MAY BE PRESCRIBED BY A PHYSICIAN AND IMPLEMENTED BY A PHYSICAL THERAPIST

II. Heat Application (Thermotherapy)

A. GENERAL
1. Relieves pain, inflammation, and congestion
2. Promotes muscle relaxation
3. Local effects
   a. Dilation of blood vessels, which results in increased blood supply and tissue metabolism
   b. Increases nutrients and oxygen to area and eliminates waste products

B. TYPES OF HEAT THERAPIES
1. Infrared therapy
   a. Administered by a heat lamp
   b. Lamp is placed 2 to 4 feet from the affected area for 15 to 20 minutes
2. Diathermy
   a. Electrical field that produces deep heat penetration
   b. Commonly used for muscular injuries and inflammation in joints
   c. Can be:
      1) Microwave: electromagnetic radiation
      2) Shortwave: high-frequency current
      3) Ultrasound: high-frequency sound waves
3. Ultrasound
   a. High-frequency sound waves used as deep-heating agent
   b. Used for strains, sprains, arthritis, edema, and dislocation
   c. Coupling agent (oil or gel) is used to increase conductivity
   d. Ordered by intensity of sound waves coupled with time
4. Paraffin wax
   a. Wax is melted and heated to approximately 125° F
   b. Affected part is immersed in the melted wax and lifted out
   c. Wax hardens and holds in the heat
   d. Used for arthritis, increase of circulation, and reduction of stiffness
5. Hot water bag
   a. Rubber bag filled approximately one-half full with hot water (115° to 125° F)
   b. Bag is applied to the affected body part for the prescribed period
   c. Place some sort of covering (towel, blanket) over the body part before positioning the hot water bag
6. Hot soaks
   a. Basin is filled with a warmed solution (105° to 110° F)
   b. Body part is immersed in the basin for the prescribed period
   c. As the solution cools, replace it with more warmed solution
7. Hot compress
   a. Immerse cloth or gauze squares in warm solution (105° to 110° F)
   b. Wring out excess fluid, and place the material over the affected body part
   c. Replace the hot compress every 2 to 3 minutes for the prescribed time

III. Cold Application (Cryotherapy)

A. GENERAL
1. Prevents edema by constricting vessels
2. Applied immediately after the trauma
3. Relieves pain by numbing
4. Local effects: vascular constriction, which leads to decreased blood supply to the area, decreased tissue metabolism, and decreased accumulation of wastes

B. TYPES OF COLD THERAPIES
1. Ice bag
   a. Ice bag is filled one-half to two-thirds full of ice
   b. Applied to the affected area for the prescribed time
   c. Place some sort of covering (towel, blanket) over the body part before positioning the ice bag
   d. Check for pallor, numbness, or cyanosis, and report any of these signs immediately
2. Cold compress
   a. Immerse cloth or gauze squares in a basin filled with cold water and ice
   b. Wring out excess fluid, and place the material over the affected body part
   c. Replace the cold compress every 2 to 3 minutes for the prescribed time

IV. Hydrotherapy

A. GENERAL
1. Use of external water applications for therapeutic purposes
2. Used for:
   a. Relaxation
   b. Increased circulation
   c. Improved mobility

B. MODALITIES
1. Whirlpool: moist heat with massage action
2. Contrast baths: patient moves affected part from hot, to cold, to hot baths
3. Underwater exercise: buoyant effect of water facilitates exercise

V. Ultraviolet (UV) Therapy

A. GENERAL
1. Produced by the sun and sunlamps
2. Capable of killing bacteria
3. Activates the formation of vitamin D in skin
4. Used to treat acne, psoriasis, wound applications, and pressure sores
5. Cover eyes when using UV therapy

VI. Exercise Therapy

A. GENERAL
1. Use of body motion to help the patient regain function
2. Dose must be constantly adjusted for the patient to benefit

3. Types include:
   a. Active: patient performs the exercise
   b. Passive: exercises are performed on the patient by someone else
   c. Aided: active exercise helped by a physical aid (such as a pool)
   d. Active resistance: counterpressure is applied
   e. Range of motion: active or passive joint mobility

VII. Massage

A. GENERAL
1. Manipulation of external body tissues to promote healing
2. Patient must be relaxed to receive benefit
3. Lubricating oil or cream should be used
4. Approaches
   a. Stroking: systematic movement of the hand across the patient's skin
   b. Compression: squeezing, kneading, or pressing the patient's soft tissues
   c. Percussion: thumping or striking the patient's skin with the hand
   d. Effleurage: stroking movement
   e. Friction: deep stroking or rubbing that involves the deeper tissues
   f. Pétrissage: kneading or rolling type of motion
   g. Tapotement: rapidly repeated light percussion or tapping

VII. Devices to Assist Patient Mobility

A. CRUTCHES
1. Wood or aluminum devices that serve as aids for walking
2. Patient's weight is transferred from the legs to the arms
3. Types
   a. Axillary crutches
      1) Crutch that extends from the patient's axillary region to the ground
      2) Used for temporary assistance
      3) Measured to fit for each individual patient
   b. Lofstrand crutches
      1) Cuff and handgrip that extend from the patient's forearm to the ground
      2) Used by patients who require permanent walking assistance
4. Crutch gaits
   a. Four-point gait
      1) Patient must be able to bear own weight on both legs
      2) Used for muscle weakness
      3) Right crutch moves forward, left foot moves to the level of the left crutch; left crutch moves forward, and right foot moves to the level of the right crutch

b. Three-point gait
  1) Used when the patient cannot bear his or her own weight on one leg
  2) Move both crutches and weak leg forward, then move the strong leg forward while balancing on both crutches
c. Two-point gait
  1) Similar to four-point gait
  2) Move the right crutch and left foot forward simultaneously, then move the left crutch and right foot forward simultaneously
d. Swing gait
  1) Used by patients with lower extremity paralysis
  2) Patient moves both crutches forward simultaneously then swings both legs through

B. CANES

1. Wood or aluminum pole with a handle or handgrip
2. Provides a balance point and/or support to the patient with leg weakness on one side
3. Used on the side of the strong leg
4. Measured so that the handle is level with the greater trochanter; the elbow should be flexed at 25 to 30 degrees
5. Types
   a. Standard cane: the least amount of support; used by patients who require slight assistance
   b. Tripod cane: three legs and a bent shaft; provides greater stability because of wider support base
   c. Quad cane: four legs and a bent shaft; provides the same support as a tripod
6. Gait
   a. Cane is held on the strong side; move the cane forward 12 inches, move the weak leg to the level of the cane, move the strong leg ahead of the weak leg and the cane
   b. Patient needs to stand erect and not lean on the cane to ensure good balance and support

C. WALKERS

1. Aluminum frame consisting of handgrips for both of the patient's hands and four squarely placed legs
2. Provides optimum balance for patients with balance problems
3. Gait: pick up the walker and move it forward 6 inches, move the right foot, then the left foot forward into the walker, then move the walker again

D. WHEELCHAIRS

1. Lock the wheels so the chair cannot move
2. Fold back the foot reats
3. Patient should back into the chair using the armrests
4. To leave the chair, lock the chair
5. Patient should place unaffected foot or feet flat on floor and lift her or his body, supporting him or herself on the armrests

Pharmacology 20

I. Definition

A. PHARMACOLOGY
1. Science that deals with the study of drugs and their actions, uses, properties, and origins

II. Drugs

A. GENERAL
1. Any substances that cause a change in body functions and/or structure

B. USES
1. Therapeutic
   a. Treats diseases
   b. Relieves symptoms
   c. Replaces a necessary body substance
2. Prophylactic: prevents disease
3. Diagnostic: helps diagnose diseases and disorders

C. SOURCES
1. Plant
   a. Naturally occurring substance from plants
   b. Parts used includes roots, leaves, and fruits
2. Animal
   a. Substances obtained from animals
   b. Includes glands, organs, and tissues
3. Mineral: naturally occurring substances obtained from the earth or soil
4. Synthetic
   a. Artificially prepared substances
   b. Prepared using chemicals and techniques in a laboratory

D. NAMES
1. Chemical name: drug's chemical formula that identifies its molecular structure
2. Generic name
   a. Official name of the drug
   b. Not capitalized
3. Trade name
   a. Brand name
   b. Name owned by the manufacturer and copyrighted (uses registered trademark [®])
   c. Always capitalized

E. DRUG REFERENCES
1. *Physicians' Desk Reference* (PDR)
   a. Common reference book
   b. Provides information on uses, precautions, indications, and doses for a variety of drugs
   c. Organized in color-coded sections
      1) Section 1 (white)
         a) Manufacturer's Index
         b) Lists manufacturers who have given product information for use in the book
      2) Section 2 (pink)
         a) Product Name Index
         b) Gives trade and generic names alphabetically
      3) Section 3 (blue)
         a) Product Category Index
         b) Drugs are listed according to their classification
      4) Section 4 (yellow)
         a) Generic and Chemical Name Index
         b) Lists drugs alphabetically according to the main ingredient
      5) Section 5 (noncolored pages)
         a) Product Identification
         b) Color photographs of the drugs on plain-color pages
      6) Section 6 (white)
         a) Product Information
         b) Detailed descriptions of the drugs
2. Product insert
   a. Folded sheet of paper within the drug container or box
   b. Contains information similar to the information on the drug contained in the PDR

3. United States Pharmacopoeia/National Formulary (USP/NF)
   a. Published every 5 years
   b. All drugs listed have met federal governmental standards
4. *Physicians' Desk Reference for Nonprescription Drugs and Dietary Supplements:* similar to PDR but for over-the-counter medications

F. DRUG FORMS

1. Syrup: drug is dissolved in water, mixed with sugar and flavoring
2. Solution: liquid preparation containing one or more solutes dissolved in a solvent
3. Suspension: drug that does not dissolve evenly in a liquid; must be shaken to mix before administration
4. Emulsion: mixture of water and oil; must be shaken to mix before administration
5. Tincture: drug is dissolved in alcohol
6. Elixir: drug is dissolved in a mixture of water, alcohol, and sugar
7. Lotion
   a. Topical preparation that is nongreasy
   b. Contains suspended particles of the drug mixed in an aqueous solution
8. Liniment
   a. Drug is mixed with soap, oil, or water
   b. Applied topically to produce a feeling of heat and warmth
9. Aerosol: drug is suspended in a liquid and administered in a spray or aerosol form
10. Capsule: powdered or liquid drug within a gelatin capsule
11. Gelcap: drug contained within gelatin-coated capsule
12. Spansule
    a. Granulated drug is enclosed within a capsule
    b. Designed to release the drug at various times after ingestion
13. Tablet
    a. Powdered medication is compressed into a disk shape
    b. May be scored for breaking into halves or quarters
    c. May be enteric-coated for dissolution in intestines instead of stomach
14. Caplet: capsule-shaped tablet
15. Geltab: gelatin-coated tablet
16. Suppository
    a. Drug is mixed with a base of fat or wax
    b. Shaped into a cone or cylinder
    c. Made to be inserted into the rectum, vagina, or urethra
    d. Suppository dissolves at body temperature
17. Ointment
    a. Semisolid preparation
    b. Drug is combined with oil or fat; topically applied

18. Lozenge (troche): medicine is mixed within a candylike base made to be dissolved within the mouth
19. Patch: transdermal administration of a medication
20. Time-release tablets, capsules, patches: medication dissolves or is administered over a period

G. TRANSACTIONS

1. Prescribe: an order for a medication by a practitioner
2. Administer: to give a medication that has been prescribed
3. Dispense: to prepare and give out to a patient
4. All practitioners who prescribe, administer, or dispense controlled substances *must* register with the Drug Enforcement Administration (DEA)
   a. Practitioner receives a DEA registration number that is valid for 3 years
   b. All controlled substances *must* be stored separately from other medications within the office; *must* be kept locked
   c. Separate records *must* be kept of all controlled substances
   d. Controlled substance inventory *must* be counted and recorded daily
   e. Discarded liquid controlled substances must be poured down the sink drains
   f. Discarded solid controlled substances must be crushed and flushed down the toilet

H. DRUG REGULATIONS AND CONTROLS

1. Controlled Substances Act of 1970
   a. Federal legislation designed to control dispensing of drugs that have a high potential for abuse
   b. Five schedules, based on medical usefulness and potential for abuse:
      1) Schedule I
         a) Drugs with a high potential for abuse and no acceptable medical use
         b) Examples: heroin and LSD (d-lysergic acid diethylamide)
      2) Schedule II
         a) Drugs with some accepted medical use but high potential for abuse
         b) Examples: morphine and cocaine
      3) Schedule III
         a) Drugs with moderate abuse potential; require prescription with refills limited to five within 6 months
         b) Example: Tylenol with codeine
      4) Schedule IV
         a) Drugs with low abuse potential; prescription is limited to five refills within 6 months
         b) Example: Valium, Darvon, and Librium
      5) Schedule V
         a) Low abuse potential; may include drug mixtures with a limited amount of narcotics
         b) Examples: cough medicines with codeine, Lomotil

2. Federal Food, Drug, and Cosmetic Act: allows U.S. Food and Drug Administration (FDA) to protect the public by requiring rigid standards for drug development
3. DEA: responsible for controlling narcotics abuse and illegal sales of drugs

I. PHARMACOKINETICS

1. Study of how drugs are used within the body
2. Process includes:
   a. Absorption
      1) How a drug enters the body
      2) Depends on how the drug is administered
   b. Distribution: how a drug is transported from the site of administration to the site or sites of action
   c. Action: changes that the drug causes when it reaches the site or sites of action
   d. Biotransformation
      1) How the drug is inactivated
      2) Usually occurs within the liver
   e. Elimination: route by which the drug is eliminated from the body

III. Prescriptions (see Figure 20-1)

A. GENERAL

1. An order written by the practitioner for the compounding, dispensing, and administration of a particular drug for a particular patient
2. A prescription is a legal document
3. Using common or accepted abbreviations is acceptable when writing a prescription; check with the agency for approved abbreviations

B. PARTS OF A PRESCRIPTION

1. Preprinted physician's name, address, telephone number, and DEA number

DEA#: 8543201   John Jones, M.D.   Tel: 544-8976
108 N. Main St.
City, State

Patient Ms. Jean Smith   DATE 10/7/02

ADDRESS 310 E. 10th St., Anytown, State

Rx: Zyrtec   10 mg tab

Disp: # 30

Sig: T hs

Refill 3 Times
Please label ☑   John Jones, M.D.

FIGURE 20-1. A sample prescription. (Young AP, Kennedy DB: *Kinn's the medical assistant: an applied learning approach*, ed 9, Philadelphia, 2003, Saunders.)

2. Date the prescription was written
3. Patient's name, address, telephone number, and age (if a child)
4. Superscription: symbol *Rx* means "take thou"
5. Inscription: name, form, and strength of drug prescribed
6. Subscription
   a. Practitioner's instructions to the pharmacist
   b. Includes the number of doses prescribed and special preparations
7. Signature
   a. *Sig* (label)
   b. Patient instructions for taking the drug
8. Refill information: number of refills allowed for the prescription, if any
9. Practitioner's handwritten signature

C. PRESCRIPTION PADS

1. Keep locked up except when being used
2. *Never* presign blank prescription forms
3. *Never* use blank prescription forms for scratch paper
4. *Never* leave blank pads in examination rooms

IV. Drug Classifications

A. ANTI-INFECTIVES

1. Antibiotic: destroys or inhibits the growth of microorganisms
2. Antifungal: kills or prevents the growth of fungi and yeast
3. Antiviral: prevents or treats viral infections
4. Antiparasitic: prevents or treats parasitic infections

B. DERMATOLOGIC AGENTS

1. Antiacneic: treats acne vulgaris
2. Antiseptic: kills or inhibits the growth of microorganisms
3. Anesthetic: causes loss of sensation and local numbing
4. Emollient: soothes skin and mucous membranes
5. Keratolytic: causes sloughing of hardened skin

C. MUSCULOSKELETAL AGENTS

1. Antiarthritic: treats arthritis
2. Antigout: treats gout (gouty arthritis)
3. Anti-inflammatory: decreases inflammation
4. Muscle relaxant: aids in the relaxation of skeletal muscles

D. CARDIOVASCULAR AGENTS

1. Angiotensin-converting enzyme (ACE) inhibitor: decreases blood pressure
2. Antianginal: reduces chest pain
3. Antiarrhythmic: regulates the heart rhythm and rate
4. Anticoagulant: prevents or delays blood clotting
5. Antihypertensive: decreases blood pressure
6. Calcium-channel blocker: decreases blood pressure
7. Cardiotonic: increases heart muscle strength

8. Hematenic: increases blood iron levels
9. Hemostatic: controls or stops bleeding
10. Vasoconstrictor: constricts blood vessels, raises blood pressure
11. Vasodilator: dilates blood vessels, lowers blood pressure

E. ENDOCRINE AGENTS

1. Contraceptive: prevents conception and pregnancy
2. Hypoglycemic: lowers blood glucose levels
3. Thyroid: replaces thyroid hormones
4. Hormone replacement therapy (HRT): replaces hormones lost through surgery, disease processes, aging, and so on

F. NERVOUS SYSTEM AGENTS

1. Central nervous system (CNS) stimulant: increases brain and body activity
2. CNS depressant: decreases brain and body activity
3. Analgesic: relieves pain
   a. Narcotic agents: highly addictive
   b. Non-narcotic agents
4. Antipyretic: reduces fever
5. Anticonvulsant: controls seizure activity
6. Antidepressant: relieves depression
7. Tranquilizer: reduces anxiety; calms the patient
8. Sedative: produces relaxation
9. Hypnotic: induces sleep

G. RESPIRATORY AGENTS

1. Antihistamine: relieves allergic symptoms; reduces secretions
2. Antitussive: suppresses cough
3. Bronchodilator: opens air passages (bronchi)
4. Decongestant: relieves congestion in respiratory tract
5. Expectorant: liquefies mucus; helps expel secretions

H. GASTROINTESTINAL (GI) AGENTS

1. Antacid: neutralizes stomach acid
2. Antiemetic: prevents nausea and vomiting
3. Antidiarrheal: controls or stops diarrhea
4. Cathartic, laxative: relieves constipation
5. Emetic: induces vomiting
6. Antispasmodic: prevents, controls, spasms of the GI tract
7. Antiulcer: treats gastric or duodenal ulcers

I. URINARY AGENTS

1. Diuretic: promotes or increases urination

J. CANCER AGENTS

1. Antineoplastic: Inhibits growth of malignant cells

V. 50 Most Prescribed Drugs of 2004

A. HYDROCODONE WITH APAP

1. *N*-acetyl-para-amino-phenol (acetaminophen)
2. Generic: same
3. Classification: analgesic
4. Indication: pain

B. LIPITOR

1. Generic: atorvastatin calcium
2. Classification: antilipemic
3. Indication: high cholesterol

C. ZESTRIL

1. Generic: lisinopril
2. Classification: antihypertensive
3. Indication: hypertension

D. TENORMIN

1. Generic: atenolol
2. Classification: antihypertensive
3. Indication: hypertension

E. SYNTHROID

1. Generic: levothyroxine sodium
2. Classification: hormone replacement
3. Indication: hypothyroidism

F. AMOXIL

1. Generic: amoxicillin
2. Classification: antiinfective
3. Indication: upper respiratory infection, urinary tract infection

G. HYDROCHLOROTHIAZIDE (HCTZ)

1. Generic: same
2. Classification: diuretic
3. Indication: edema, hypertension

H. ZITHROMAX Z-PAK

1. Generic: azithromycin
2. Classification: antiinfective
3. Indication: infections

I. LASIX

1. Generic: furosemide
2. Classification: diuretic
3. Indication: edema, hypertension

J. NORVASC

1. Generic: amlodipine
2. Classification: antianginal
3. Indication: angina

K. TOPROL-XL

1. Generic: metoprolol
2. Classification: antihypertensive
3. Indication: hypertension

L. XANAX

1. Generic: alprazolam
2. Classification: antianxiety
3. Indication: anxiety

M. ALBUTEROL

1. Generic: salbutamol
2. Classification: bronchodilator
3. Indication: asthma

N. ZOLOFT
1. Generic: sertraline
2. Classification: antidepressant
3. Indication: depression

O. ZOCOR
1. Generic: simvastatin
2. Classification: antilipemic
3. Indication: high cholesterol

P. GLUCOPHAGE
1. Generic: metformin
2. Classification: antidiabetic
3. Indication: diabetes

Q. IBUPROFEN
1. Generic: same
2. Classification: nonsteroidal antiinflammatory drug (NSAID)
3. Indication: inflammation, pain

R. DYAZIDE
1. Generic: triamterene w/HCTZ
2. Classification: antihypertensive
3. Indication: hypertension, edema

S. AMBIEN
1. Generic: imidazopyridine
2. Classification: hypnotic
3. Indication: insomnia

T. CEPHALEXIN
1. Generic: cephalexin monohydrate
2. Classification: antiinfective
3. Indication: infections

U. NEXIUM
1. Generic: esomeprazole magnesium
2. Classification: proton pump inhibitor
3. Indication: heartburn, gastroesophageal reflux disease (GERD)

V. PREVACID
1. Generic: lansoprazole
2. Classification: antiulcer
3. Indication: ulcers

W. LEXAPRO
1. Generic: escitalopram oxalate
2. Classification: selective serotonin-reuptake inhibitor (SSRI)
3. Indication: depression

X. PREDNISONE
1. Generic: prednisone
2. Classification: antiinflammatory
3. Indication: severe inflammation, immunosuppression

Y. ZYRTEC
1. Generic: cetirizine
2. Classification: antihistamine
3. Indication: seasonal allergies

Z. SINGULAIR
1. Generic: montelukast sodium
2. Classification: antiasthmatic
3. Indication: asthma

AA. CELEBREX
1. Generic: celecoxib
2. Classification: antiinflammatory
3. Indication: arthritis

BB. PROZAC
1. Generic: fluoxetine
2. Classification: antidepressant
3. Indication: depression

CC. FOSAMAX
1. Generic: alendronate sodium
2. Classification: bone growth regulator
3. Indication: osteoporosis

DD. LOPRESSOR
1. Generic: metoprolol tartrate
2. Classification: beta-adrenergic blocking agent
3. Indication: hypertension

EE. PREMARIN
1. Generic: estrogen
2. Classification: hormone replacement
3. Indication: hormone replacement

FF. LEVOXYL
1. Generic: levothyroxine sodium
2. Classification: hormone replacement
3. Indication: thyroid replacement

GG. ATIVAN
1. Generic: lorazepam
2. Classification: antianxiety
3. Indication: anxiety

HH. ALLEGRA
1. Generic: fexofenadine
2. Classification: antihistamine
3. Indication: allergy

II. PLAVIX
1. Generic: clopidogrel bisulfate
2. Classification: antiplatelet drug
3. Indication: myocardial infarction (MI), stroke, peripheral artery disease

JJ. EFFEXOR XR
1. Generic: venlafaxine hydrochloride
2. Classification: antidepressant
3. Indication: depression

KK. K-DUR
1. Generic: potassium chloride
2. Classification: electrolyte
3. Indication: electrolyte replacement

LL. PROTONIX
1. Generic: pantoprazole sodium

2. Classification: proton pump inhibitor
3. Indication: GERD, heartburn

MM. DARVON
1. Generic: propoxyphene-N
2. Classification: narcotic analgesic
3. Indication: pain

NN. ADVAIR DISCUS
1. Generic: fluticasone propionate/salmeterol
2. Classification: bronchodilator (inhalation powder)
3. Indication: asthma

OO. COUMADIN
1. Generic: warfarin sodium
2. Classification: anticoagulant
3. Indication: embolism, MI

PP. ACETAMINOPHEN WITH CODEINE
1. Generic: same
2. Classification: narcotic analgesic
3. Indication: pain

QQ. KLONOPIN
1. Generic: clonazepam
2. Classification: anticonvulsant
3. Indication: seizures

RR. NEURONTIN
1. Generic: gabapentin
2. Classification: anticonvulsant
3. Indication: seizures

SS. FLONASE
1. Generic: fluticasone
2. Classification: antihistamine
3. Indication: allergic rhinitis

TT. ELAVIL
1. Generic: amitriptyline hydrochloric acid (HCl)
2. Classification: antidepressant (tricyclic)
3. Indication: depression; anxiety; insomnia

UU. ZANTAC
1. Generic: ranitidine HCl
2. Classification: histamine H_2-receptor blocker
3. Indication: duodenal ulcers

VV. VIAGRA
1. Generic: sildenafil citrate
2. Classification: erectile dysfunction drug
3. Indication: erectile dysfunction

WW. NAPROSYN
1. Generic: naproxen
2. Classification: nonsteroidal antiinflammatory
3. Indication: pain

XX. AUGMENTIN
1. Generic: amoxicillin/clavulanate
2. Classification: antiinfective
3. Indication: respiratory and ear infections

VI. Calculation of Doses

A. METRIC SYSTEM
1. Based on multiples of 10
2. Used to weigh and measure
   a. Basic units of measure
      1) Gram (g): used to measure solids
      2) Liter (L): used to measure liquids (volume)
      3) Meter (m): used to measure length
   b. Basic metric prefixes
      1) Micro-: one millionth (0.000001)
      2) Milli-: one thousandth (0.001)
      3) Centi-: one hundredth (0.01)
      4) Deci-: one tenth (0.1)
      5) Unit (g, m, L): *one* (1.0)
      5) Deka-: ten (10.0)
      6) Hecto-: one hundred (100.0)
      7) Kilo-: one thousand (1000.0)
      8) Mega-: one million (1,000,000.0)
   c. Metric conversion
      1) Changing from larger unit to smaller unit
         a) Multiply by the number of smaller units that are in the larger unit
         b) Move the decimal point to the right the number of places equal to the number of zeros found in the smaller unit
      2) Changing from smaller unit to larger unit
         a) Divide by the number of smaller units that are in the larger unit
         b) Move the decimal point to the left the number of places equal to the number of zeros in the smaller unit

B. ADULT DOSE CALCULATION
1. Dose given is dose ordered divided by the available strength times the dose form:

$$\frac{\text{dose ordered}}{\text{available}} \times \text{form} = \text{dose given}$$

   a. Dose given: amount administered to the patient to fill the practitioner's order
   b. Dose ordered: amount of drug the practitioner orders to be given to the patient
   c. Available strength: concentration of medicine on hand
   d. Dose form: number of tablets (or capsules) or amount of liquid that contains the available strength
2. Example:
   Practitioner orders 500 mg amoxicillin; 250-mg/cap amoxicillin is available

$$\frac{500 \text{ mg}}{250 \text{ mg}} \times 1 = \text{two 250-mg caps administered}$$

C. PEDIATRIC DOSE CALCULATION
1. Young's rule

a. Used for children under 12, based on age

b. Formula: child's age divided by (child's age + 12) and multiplied by the average adult dose gives the amount administered to the child

2. Fried's rule

a. Used for infants and children under age 2, based on age in months

b. Formula: infant's age in months divided by 150 and multiplied by the average adult dose gives the amount administered to the child

3. Clark's rule

a. Used for children under 12, based on weight in pounds

b. Formula: (child's weight in pounds divided by 150) multiplied by the average adult dose gives the amount administered to the child

VII. Administration of Medications

A. ROUTES OF ADMINISTRATION

1. Buccal: medication is placed between cheek and gum and dissolves
2. Oral: medication is administered by mouth and swallowed
3. Sublingual: medication is placed under the tongue and dissolves
4. Inhalation: medication is delivered to lungs by means of a nebulizer (inhaler unit)
5. Topical: medication is externally applied to skin, eyes, ears, nose, or mucous membranes
6. Vaginal: medication is inserted into, or applied to, the vagina
7. Rectal: medication is inserted into the rectum and absorbed
8. Parenteral: medication is administered through a needle

B. SEVEN "RIGHTS" OF ADMINISTRATION

1. The right patient
2. The right drug
3. The right dose
4. The right route
5. The right time
6. The right technique
7. The right documentation

C. SAFETY

1. Three "befores": read the drug label three times when preparing the medication:
   a. Before removing the medication from storage
   b. Before preparing the medication for administration
   c. Before replacing the medication back in storage
2. Be familiar with the drug; use references
3. Prepare medication in a clean, quiet, well-lit area, away from distractions

4. Do not use a medication that does not appear normal (changes in color, odor, or appearance of sediment in the medication)
5. Check the expiration date; never administer a date-expired medication
6. Verify the patient's identity before administering (call by name; ask patient his or her name)
7. Always check for allergies
8. Correctly chart the procedure: include date, time, medication, dose, route, patient reactions, and medical assistant's initials

D. CONSIDERATIONS

1. Age: children and older adults require smaller doses than younger adults
2. Gender: women require smaller doses than men
3. Weight: smaller patients require smaller doses than larger persons
4. Tolerance: a patient who has taken this medication over a long period may require a larger dose for required results
5. Condition of the patient: physical and psychological conditions
6. Route: parenteral medications are absorbed more quickly than oral medications
7. Timing: medications are absorbed more quickly on an empty stomach

E. ALLERGIC REACTIONS

1. Mild reaction: rash, pruritus, and rhinitis
2. Severe reaction: (anaphylaxis): pruritus, edema, dyspnea, cyanosis, and shock; untreated, a severe reaction can lead to coma and/or death
3. Prevention
   a. Monitor the patient after administration of the drug
   b. Observe the patient for signs and symptoms
   c. Notify the practitioner immediately of any reaction
   d. Be prepared to provide emergency assistance

VIII. Parenteral Administration

A. EQUIPMENT

1. Syringe (see Figure 20-2)
   a. Parts include:
      1) Barrel: holds medication; calibrated for measuring (cc/mL and minims)
      2) Flange: rim at the end of the barrel; place to put the fingers while depressing the plunger and keeps the syringe from rolling off a flat surface
      3) Plunger: fits inside the barrel; brings the medication into and out of the barrel
      4) Tip: end of the barrel where the needle attaches
   b. Types include (see Figure 20-3):
      1) Regular hypodermic

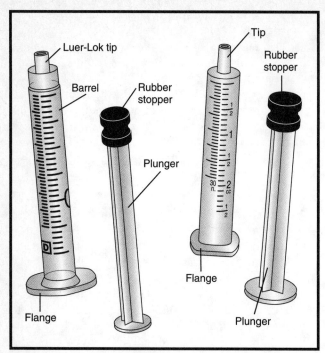

FIGURE 20-2. Parts of a syringe. (Young AP, Kennedy DB: *Kinn's the medical assistant: an applied learning approach,* ed 9, Philadelphia, 2003, Saunders.)

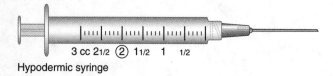

Hypodermic syringe

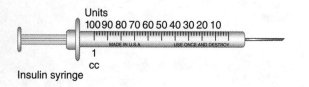

Insulin syringe

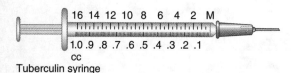

Tuberculin syringe

FIGURE 20-3. Various types of syringes used to administer injections. (Bonewit-West K: *Clinical procedures for medical assistants,* ed 6, St Louis, 2004, Saunders.)

      a) Most commonly calibrated in 2 cc, 3 cc, 5 cc, or 10 cc
      b) May be disposable (plastic) or nondisposable (glass)
      c) May come with needle attached or without needle
    2) Tuberculin (TB)
      a) Small syringe calibrated in 0.1 cc
      b) Holds up to a total volume of 1.0 cc
    3) Insulin

      a) Calibrated in units (U40, U80, U100)
      b) Used for insulin injections
      c) Syringe must correspond to the type of insulin prescribed
    4) Tubex, Carpuject
      a) Closed injection system
      b) Disposable medication cartridge-needle unit fits into a reusable plastic or metal holder
  2. Needle (see Figure 20-4)
    a. Parts include:
      1) Hub: the part of the needle that connects to the syringe
      2) Shaft: length of the needle; inserted into the body
      3) Point: sharpened end of the shaft
      4) Lumen: inside opening of the shaft
      5) Bevel: slant of the point
    b. Measured by:
      1) Gauge: size of the lumen
        a) The smaller the gauge, the larger the needle
        b) 13 G to 27 G
      2) Length
        a) Varies according to use
        b) ¼ inch to 6 inch

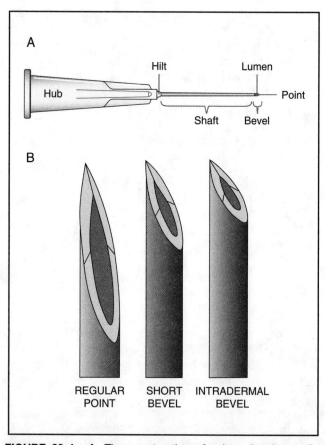

FIGURE 20-4. A, The construction of a hypodermic needle. **B,** Needle points. (A, Bonewit-West K: *Clinical procedures for medical assistants,* ed 6, St Louis, 2004, Saunders. B, Young AP, Kennedy DB: *Kinn's the medical assistant: an applied learning approach,* ed 9, Philadelphia, 2003, Saunders.)

B. ADMINISTRATION
1. Intradermal (ID)
   a. Needle and syringe size
      1) Syringes: TB (1 cc)
      2) Needle gauge: 26 G to 27 G
      3) Needle length: ⅜ inch to ½ inch
   b. Sites
      1) Anterior forearm
      2) Middle back
   c. Uses of route
      1) Allergy skin testing
      2) TB skin testing medication (Mantoux/purified protein derivative [PPD])
   d. Injection angle: 10 to 15 degrees (with bevel facing up)
   e. Goal of injection: formation of a wheal
   f. Amount given: 0.01 to 0.2 cc
2. Intramuscular (IM)
   a. Needle and syringe size
      1) Syringe: 1 cc to 2 cc (depending on the amount administered)
      2) Needle gauge: 22 G to 25 G (depending on the area of the body and the consistency of the medication)
      3) Needle length: 5/8 inch to 2 inches (depending on the size of the patient and the consistency of the medication)
   b. Sites
      1) Deltoid (not for infant or small child)
      2) Dorsogluteal (not for infant or small child)
      3) Vastus lateralis (used for infants and small children)
         a) Rectus femoris (medial to vastus lateralis; self-injection)

b) Ventrogluteal (side of hip ; all patients)
   c. Uses of route
      1) Adult and childhood immunizations (deltoid and vastus)
      2) Thick or oil-based medications (gluteal)
   d. Injection angle: 90 degrees
   e. Goal of injection: to deliver medication into muscle tissue
   f. Amount given
      1) less than 2 cc (deltoid and vastus)
      2) 2 to 5 cc (gluteal)
3. Subcutaneous (SC, SQ, subq)
   a. Needle and syringe size
      1) Syringe: insulin, TB, or 2 to 3 cc syringe
      2) Needle gauge: 25 G to 27 G
      3) Needle length: 3/8 inch to 5/8 inch
   b. Sites
      1) Upper arm (under deltoid, back of arm)
      2) Thigh
      3) Back
      4) Abdomen
      5) Any area where a fat surface exists
   c. Uses of route
      1) Insulin
      2) Allergy injections
      3) Mumps, measles, and rubella (MMR) immunization
      4) Epinephrine
   d. Injection angle: 45 degrees
   e. Goal of injection: delivery of medication into subcutaneous (fatty) tissue
   f. Amount given: less than 2 cc

21 | *Intravenous (IV) Therapy*

(Depending on location, a medical assistant may or may not be permitted to legally administer IV therapy.)

I. General

A. INTRODUCTION OF THERAPEUTIC FLUIDS DIRECTLY INTO THE VENOUS CIRCULATION

B. CAN BE USED FOR MAINTENANCE THERAPY, REPLACEMENT THERAPY, OR RESTORATION THERAPY

C. STRICT ASEPTIC TECHNIQUES MUST BE USED AT ALL TIMES

D. DANGER TO THE PATIENT CAN BE GREAT; MEDICAL ASSISTANT MUST BE ABLE TO EVALUATE ADVERSE REACTIONS AND FOLLOW PHYSICIAN'S ORDERS EXACTLY

II. Advantages and Uses of IV Therapy

A. ADVANTAGES
1. Entire amount of a medication is distributed in the bloodstream immediately after administration
2. No tissue barriers to cross
3. Route may be indicated for patients who cannot take oral or parenteral medications
4. Medications are not altered by gastrointestinal tract
5. Medications may be given to patients who are unconscious, vomiting, or uncooperative

B. USES
1. Maintenance therapy
   a. Provides necessary requirements for water, electrolytes, and nutrition
   b. Amount given depends on patient's age, height, weight, and amount of body fat
   c. Used for patients who have little or no intake of fluids by mouth; require supplements
2. Replacement therapy
   a. Replaces fluid and electrolyte deficits
   b. Indicated for vomiting and diarrhea, starvation, and hemorrhage
   c. Most common in ambulatory care settings
   d. Patient must be carefully monitored
3. Restorative therapy
   a. Daily restoration of fluids and electrolytes
   b. Fluids are physiologically the same as fluids being lost
   c. Several types of fluids are often given
   d. Done more often in in-patient settings

III. Dangers of IV Therapy

A. POSSIBLE INTRODUCTION OF MICROORGANISMS INTO THE BLOODSTREAM
1. Aseptic technique must be followed

B. INFECTION AT SITE
1. Site care and bandaging using medical and surgical asepsis must be used

C. HYPERTONIC AND HYPOTONIC SOLUTIONS MAY DESTROY RBCs
1. Can cause an embolus

D. FLUID OVERLOAD
1. Physician's order for amounts and rate must be carefully followed

E. INTRODUCTION OF MEDS INTO IV FLUIDS CANNOT BE REVERSED
1. Medications immediately travel throughout body once administered

IV. Types of IV Therapy

A. 0.9% SODIUM CHLORIDE
1. Normal saline
2. Isotonic
3. Maintains body fluid levels

B. GLUCOSE
1. Dextrose 5% in water (D_5W)

2. Saline (D_5NS)
3. Supply nutritional needs or part of daily caloric requirement

C. MULTIPLE ELECTROLYTE SOLUTION
1. Ringer's; lactated Ringer's
2. Contains sodium, calcium, chloride, and potassium
3. Usually does not supply calories

D. HYPOTONIC SOLUTION
1. Causes the flow of water into the cell
2. Hydrates cells leading to depletion in amount of fluid in circulation
3. Lowers blood pressure

E. HYPERTONIC SOLUTION
1. Causes the flow of water out of the cell
2. Increases blood volume
3. Used to replace electrolytes
4. Must be given slowly

F. ISOTONIC SOLUTION
1. Similar to body fluids
2. Can cause circulatory overload

G. ADDITIONS
1. Drugs
2. Supplements
3. Fat emulsions
4. Fluids

V. Equipment

A. USUALLY FOUND IN KITS CONTAINING ALL NECESSARY SUPPLIES

B. SET
1. Individually labeled with name, description, lot number, drops-per-milliliter rate for the chamber, usage description, and manufacturer

C. ADMINISTRATION SETS
1. Primary administration sets (see Figure 21-1)
   a. Puts medications directly into bloodstream
   b. Used for infusion in ambulatory care
   c. Gravity or infusion pumps
   d. Macrodrip (8 to 20 drops/mL) and microdrip (50 to 60 drops/mL)
2. Secondary infusion sets: used to add intermittent medications through secondary tubing
3. Blood administration sets: used to administer blood and blood products

D. TUBING
1. Varies in length
2. Has a sharp spike at the top for insertion into the fluid bag
3. May have injection port that acts as an access point for the addition of other fluids or secondary infusion sets

E. VENT
1. Located under spike
2. Allows air to displace the fluid

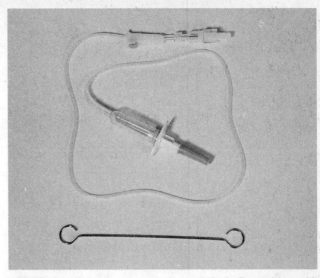

FIGURE 21-1. Intravenous equipment, including tubing, drip chamber, spike, flow-control clamp, and Luer-Lok connector. (Leahy JM, Kizilay PE: *Foundations of nursing practice: a nursing process approach,* Philadelphia, 1998, Saunders.)

F. DRIP CHAMBER
1. Under vent
2. Holds the fluids before infusion
3. Opening of drip chamber contains the drop orifice, which determines the size and shape of fluid drops

G. FLOW CONTROL CLAMP
1. Compresses the tubing to allow fluid to flow through tubing
2. Can be a roller or screw

H. FLUID CONTAINERS (see Figure 21-2)
1. Usually made of plastic
2. Bag collapses as fluid infuses

I. NEEDLES (see Figure 21-3)
1. Winged-tip (butterfly)
   a. Used for short-term therapy
   b. Gauge 17 to 25
   c. 0.5 to 1.0 inches
   d. Patient needs to remain inactive so the tip of the needle does not puncture the vein
2. Over-the-needle catheters
   a. Plastic sheath covers the distal point of the needle
   b. Needle is used to enter the vein and guide the catheter
   c. After entering the vein, the catheter is threaded off the needle and left in place
   d. Catheter comes in lengths of 0.5 to 2.0 inches
   e. Gauge 22 to 24

VI. Calculation of Flow Rates

A. PHYSICIAN ORDERS RATE OF FLOW OF FLUIDS

B. TO CALCULATE, THE MEDICAL ASSISTANT MUST KNOW:
1. Volume of fluid to be infused

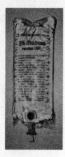
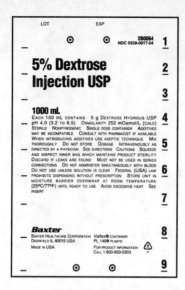
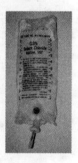
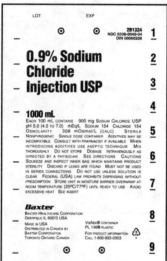

FIGURE 21-2. Examples of intravenous fluid bags and labels. (Brown M, Mulholland JM: *Drug calculations: process and problems for clinical practice*, ed 7, St Louis, 2004, Mosby.)

2. Length of time for the infusion
3. Manufacturer's drop rate (drops/mL)

C. TUBING MAY BE MACRODRIP OR MICRODRIP (MANUFACTURER PROVIDES THE DROPS/mL INFORMATION ON THE PACKAGE)

D. CALCULATION IS DONE IN TWO STEPS:

1. Calculate the total volume of fluid to be administered in an hour
   a. Total volume to be infused equals volume per hour
   b. Time in total hours
2. Calculate the drop-per-minute rate
   a. Volume to infuse per hour multiplied by the drops/mL (on tubing box) equals drop/min
   b. 60 min (1 hr)

E. SCREENING THE PATIENT BEFORE IV ADMINISTRATION

1. Provider performs a baseline screening

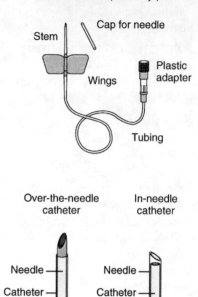

FIGURE 21-3. Equipment for starting short-term peripheral IV infusions: winged-infusion needle and over-the-needle catheter. (Leahy JM, Kizilay PE: *Foundations of nursing practice: a nursing process approach*, Philadelphia, 1998, Saunders.)

2. Patient's weight must be taken
3. Vital signs are taken and recorded

F. SCREENING THE PATIENT DURING IV INFUSION

1. Patient should be watched closely during infusion
2. Complications can be local or systemic
3. Can include:
   a. Infiltration
      1) Local complication
      2) Fluid enters the surrounding tissues
      3) Signs may include slowing or stoppage of flow, tissue induration, and swelling around the site
      4) Site should be changed; affected arm elevated and covered with warm compresses
   b. Phlebitis
      1) Not common in ambulatory care
      2) Can occur if fluids are given over successive days
      3) Patient may have redness, pain, swelling and warmth at the site; vein may feel similar to a cord
      4) If occurs, site should be moved; warm compresses are applied to the site
   c. Hematoma
      1) May be caused by nicking the vein during venipuncture
      2) Discoloration of the skin, swelling, and discomfort
   d. Local infection
      1) Site and catheter should be cultured
      2) Redness and purulent discharge may be present

3) Patient may have a fever and elevated white blood cell count
4) Infusion should be stopped; site covered with sterile dressings
e. Circulatory system overload
1) Too-rapid infusion of fluids
2) Monitor flow rate carefully
3) Notify physician immediately
4) Monitor vitals, check for shortness of breath, pitting edema, and increase in blood pressure
f. Sluggish infusion
1) Check tubing for kinking and obstruction
2) May need to reposition injection site
3) Obstructed line will need to be flushed
g. Venous spasm
1) Caused by the infusion of cold fluids
2) Sharp pain along the length of the vein
3) Fluids should be at room temperature before administration

G. PREPARING THE SITE AND INITIATING IV THERAPY: EQUIPMENT
1. Physician's order containing fluid to be used and length of the infusion
2. Proper fluids as ordered
3. Administration kit with correct drip chamber
4. IV pole
5. Gloves
6. Antiseptic skin preparation
7. Dressings and tape
8. Tourniquet
9. Sharps and biohazard containers
10. Sterile gauze sponges (2 inch × 2 inch)
11. Transparent dressing for the site

H. PROCEDURE
1. Identify the patient and explain the procedure
2. Wash hands; perform baseline vital signs
3. Place patient in comfortable position
4. Assemble supplies
5. Use *"seven rights"* and *"three befores"* to check medication order
6. Open sterile packages
7. Insert the spike into the fluid bag
8. Adjust the roller clamp on tubing (1 to 2 inches below drip chamber)
9. Allow fluids to fill chamber until one half full
10. Clamp the tubing when tubing is filled; replace protective cap on the end of tubing
11. Put on gloves
12. Inspect arm for an injection site
13. Apply tourniquet with adequate but not tight pressure
14. Cleanse site with soap and water, and follow with Betadine or alcohol in circular motion; allow site to dry
15. Insert the needle at a 20- to 30-degree angle; observe for flash of blood
16. Advance the needle or catheter approximately ¼ to ½ inch into the vein
17. Stabilize the needle and loosen the tourniquet
18. Connect the IV tubing to the hub of the needle
19. Secure the hub with tape or transparent dressing as per office policy
20. Open the roller and adjust the flow rate as ordered
21. Remove gloves, sanitize hands, and document procedure
a. Size of needle and catheter
b. Location of site
c. Type of fluid
d. Flow rate
e. Patient's reaction to procedure
f. Any adverse reactions

22 | *Clinical Lab*

I. Orientation to the Laboratory

A. LABORATORY DEPARTMENTS
1. Blood bank
   a. Analyzes blood and blood components for transfusions
   b. Examples: type and cross-match
2. Chemistry
   a. Analyzes blood and body fluids for presence and quantity of chemical substances
   b. Examples: glucose, cholesterol, and electrolytes
3. Cytology and histology
   a. Examines cells and tissues to diagnose diseases
   b. Examples: Papanicolaou (Pap) smear, biopsy
4. Hematology
   a. Performs tests on blood and blood components
   b. Examples: complete blood count (CBC), erythrocyte sedimentation rate (ESR, sed rate), and coagulation studies
5. Microbiology
   a. Identification and study of pathogenic microorganisms
   b. Includes bacteriology (bacteria), parasitology (parasites), and virology (viruses)
6. Serology
   a. Examination of blood to detect diseases through antigen-antibody reactions
   b. Examples: rubella titer and mononucleosis testing

B. LABORATORY PERSONNEL
1. Pathologist: physician in charge of the laboratory
2. Medical technologist: bachelor's degree–prepared laboratory technician
3. Medical laboratory technician: laboratory technician who has completed 1 to 2 years of training
4. Phlebotomist: obtains blood samples from patients

C. OCCUPATIONAL SAFETY AND HEALTH ADMINISTRATION (OSHA) STANDARDS
1. Hazard communication standard
   a. Employer must provide information and training to employees who are exposed to hazardous agents (chemicals, noise, radiation, infectious agents)
   b. Standards must be in writing and include:
      1) Training outline
      2) List of hazards and material safety data sheet (MSDS) forms
      3) Warning and labeling system
      4) Method of informing employees
   c. MSDS
      1) Must be kept for each hazardous substance on site
      2) Prepared by the manufacturer
      3) Describes chemical and physical properties, hazards, precautions, and first aid
      4) Signs posted in laboratory
   d. All hazardous agents must be labeled showing:
      1) Name of hazardous substance
      2) Specific product warnings
      3) Name and address of manufacturer
2. Blood-borne pathogen standard
   a. Disease-causing microorganisms transmitted through blood and body fluids
   b. OSHA requires employers to ensure the safety of employees and provide training about exposure
   c. Blood-borne pathogens transmitted when contaminated blood or body fluids come into contact with nonintact skin or mucous membranes of another person
   d. Prevention includes:
      1) Engineering controls: structural and mechanical devices that minimize exposure (sharps containers, eyewash stations)

2) Work practice controls: promotion of behaviors necessary to use the engineering controls properly

3) Personal protective equipment (PPE): equipment that decreases exposure (gloves, masks, laboratory aprons)

4) Standard precautions: concept that all bodily secretions should be treated as if they are contaminated

5) Body secretions include:
   a) Blood and body fluids containing blood
   b) Semen
   c) Cerebrospinal fluid
   d) Saliva
   e) Sputum
   f) Vaginal secretions
   g) Feces
   h) Urine
   i) Sweat and tears
   j) Vomitus
   k) Unidentifiable body fluids

D. LABORATORY SAFETY

1. Postevacuation routes
2. Postemergency telephone numbers (fire, police, poison control)
3. First-aid kit accessible and up to date
4. Safety equipment accessible and in working order, including:
   a. Eyewash station
   b. Shower
   c. Fire extinguisher
5. Laboratory coats or aprons worn at all times; remove before leaving the laboratory
6. Hair is pulled back; only minimal jewelry is allowed; fingernails are short
7. Dispose of sharps and broken glass immediately in a puncture-resistant container
8. Observe hazard identification labels
9. Work under the hood in a well-ventilated area when working with chemicals
10. *Never* pipette by mouth
11. Close all reagent containers when not in use
12. Label all reagent containers with name, expiration date, date of preparation, and preparer's initials
13. Pour acids into water when preparing solutions
14. Properly ground all electrical equipment
15. Wash hands after handling specimens and before leaving the laboratory
16. Do not eat, drink, smoke, apply makeup, or handle contact lenses in the laboratory
17. Do not store food in the laboratory refrigerator
18. Do not recap, break, or bend contaminated needles
19. Cap all tubes before centrifuging
20. Dispose of all contaminated nonsharps in labeled biohazard containers (red trash can or red trash bag)

E. CLINICAL LABORATORY IMPROVEMENT ACT OF 1988 (CLIA '88)

1. Federal legislation developed to regulate testing of specimens to diagnose, prevent, and treat diseases and disorders
2. Enforced by the Centers for Disease Control and Prevention (CDC) and Health Care Financing Administration (HCFA)
3. Laboratory must be in compliance with CLIA to receive Medicare and Medicaid reimbursement
4. Three main standards:
   a. Personnel standards
      1) Identify qualifications of persons directing or performing testing
      2) Qualifications depend on the complexity levels of the testing
   b. Testing standards: identify the tests that fall into one of three levels of complexity:
      1) Waived tests
         a) Not subject to personnel or quality assurance requirements
         b) Common in medical office (physician's office laboratory) [POL]
      2) Moderately complex tests
      3) Highly complex tests
   c. Quality assurance standards
      1) Identify quality assurance requirements for qualified laboratories
      2) Apply only to laboratories that perform moderately and highly complex testing
      3) Standards include:
         a) Written policies and standards
         b) Documented personnel training and proficiency testing
         c) Procedure manual
         d) Maintenance and documentation of the maintenance of instruments
         e) Quality control documentation

II. Collection of Specimens

A. URINE

1. Sterile liquid waste product
2. Should be analyzed within 30 minutes of collection but may be refrigerated for up to 8 hours
3. Specimen types include:
   a. First-morning specimen
      1) Specimen of choice
      2) Most concentrated
   b. Random specimen: specimen collected at any time of the day
   c. Midstream specimen
      1) Used for routine urinalysis
      2) Patient is instructed to retract foreskin or labia, void the first portion of the urine stream into the toilet, collect the midportion of the stream

into a sterile container, and void the remaining portion of the stream into the toilet
3) Properly label the container
d. Clean-catch specimen
1) Used for culture
2) Patient is instructed to thoroughly cleanse the glans penis or urethral meatus with an antiseptic solution, continue with the midstream specimen collection technique, and collect in a sterile container
e. 24-hour specimen
1) Used to measure volume
2) Used for quantitative analysis (amount) of chemicals
3) Specimen requires a preservative and refrigeration (specimen container usually provided by laboratory)
4) Patient is instructed to void first morning urine into the toilet; collect all urine into the same container for the next 24 hours, including the first morning specimen of the next day; bring the entire specimen in the container to the laboratory

B. BLOOD

1. Consists of liquid and cellular components
2. Sample can be separated into components by centrifuging or settling
a. Plasma
1) Liquid component of circulating blood; if whole blood is allowed to clot, the liquid portion is called serum; serum contains no clotting factors (formed clot)
2) Appears clear and light yellow
b. Buffy coat: consists of white blood cells and platelets
c. Red blood cells
3. Blood collection: Vacutainer Collection System
a. Vacuum tubes with color-coded stoppers
b. Tube used depends on the test to be performed on the sample
1) Yellow stopper
a) Used for serum collection
b) Contains no additive

c) Tube is sterile and used for bacteriologic testing
2) Red stopper
a) Used for serum collection
b) Contains no additives
c) Tube must sit for 15 minutes to allow a clot to form, then centrifuge
d) Used for samples for chemistry and serology
3) Tiger, speckled, SST (serum separator tube)
a) Red-and-black mottled stopper
b) Used to collect serum
c) Tube contains a silicon gel that creates a barrier between the serum and the clotted cells when centrifuged
d) Tube must sit for 15 minutes to allow a clot to form, then centrifuge
e) Used for the same purpose as red stopper
4) Lavender stopper
a) Used to collect plasma
b) Tube contains the anticoagulant EDTA (ethylenediaminetetraacetic acid)
c) Used for hematology
d) Tube must be gently mixed after collection
5) Blue stopper
a) Used to collect plasma
b) Contains anticoagulant sodium citrate
c) Used to perform coagulation testing
6) Green stopper
a) Used to collect plasma
b) Contains the anticoagulant sodium heparin
c) Used in chemistry for immediate (stat) testing
7) Gray stopper
a) Contains the anticoagulant sodium fluoride
b) Used in chemistry for glucose testing and alcohol testing
4. Order of collection: when multiple tubes are to be collected, collect in the following order (see Table 22-1):
a. Yellow stopper
b. Blue stopper
c. Red/SST stopper
d. Green stopper
e. Lavender stopper
f. Gray stopper

TABLE 22-1 Vaccum Tube Table

Colors of the Picture and the Plastic Vacutainer Tubes Placed in Order of Draw from Top to Bottom		Additives	Laboratory Uses
Blue sky	Blue topped	Citrate	Coagulation studies
Red rays and gold rays	Red topped "clot tube"	Clot activator in plastic tubes (Note: red glass tubes do not have clot activator)	Both yield serum commonly used for testing blood chemistry
	Gold topped "SST tube"	Clot activator and gel	
Green grass	Green topped	Heparin (with lithium or sodium)	Special tests such as electrolytes
Lavender flowers	Lavender topped	EDTA	Hematology tests
Gray rocks	Gray topped	Oxalate	For glucose testing

(From Garrels M, Oatis CS: *Laboratory testing for ambulatory settings: a guide for health care professionals*, St. Louis, 2006, Saunders.)

5. Venipuncture (phlebotomy) (see Figures 22-1 and 22-2)
   a. Puncture of vein to withdraw blood sample
   b. Usually performed on the median cubital vein in the antecubital area
      1) Apply tourniquet approximately 3 to 4 inches above site; palpate and observe for the vein; release the tourniquet (do not leave the tourniquet on for more than 60 seconds)
      2) Assemble all equipment
      3) Reapply the tourniquet
      4) Glove; cleanse the site with an alcohol wipe, and allow it to dry
      5) Anchor the vein; insert the needle at approximately 15 degrees, bevel up
      6) Fill the syringe by slowly pulling back on the plunger or by inserting the vacuum tube onto the needle in the holder
      7) As the blood fills, release the tourniquet
      8) After collection is complete, place a clean cotton ball or gauze over the site, and quickly withdraw the needle; instruct the patient to apply pressure to the site; apply a pressure dressing to the site
      9) Label the specimen; dispose of the needle into a sharps container
6. Butterfly-winged infusion set
   a. Used on small veins and for older adult and pediatric draws

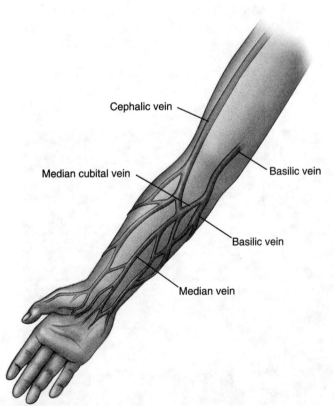

FIGURE 22-1. The veins of the forearm. (Hunt SA: *Saunders fundamentals of medical assisting,* St Louis, 2002, Saunders.)

Cephalic vein
Median cubital vein
Basilic vein
Basilic vein
Median vein

   b. Can be attached to a Vacutainer Collection System or syringe
7. Syringe method
   a. Used on fragile veins that might collapse under the pressure of the Vacutainer
   b. Same procedure as the Vacutainer except the phlebotomist pulls back on the plunger to draw the blood into the syringe
   c. Blood can be seen entering the tip of the syringe as soon as the needle enters the vein (flash)
   d. Blood must be transferred into vacuum tubes quickly so it does not clot
8. Capillary puncture (see Figure 22-3)
   a. Used to collect small amounts of blood
   b. Sites include:
      1) Middle or ring finger of the nondominant hand
      2) Earlobe
      3) Heel or big toe on an infant
   c. Procedure
      1) Cleanse the site with alcohol, and allow it to dry
      2) Quickly puncture the skin with a lancet; wipe away the first drop of blood
      3) Collect a sample in the appropriate container

C. CEREBROSPINAL FLUID (CSF)
1. Fluid that surrounds the brain and spinal cord
2. Normal CSF is clear and colorless
3. Collected by lumbar puncture procedure between L3, L4, or L5
4. Fluid may be cultured for bacteria, analyzed for chemical components (glucose and protein), or tested for the presence of blood cells

D. SEROUS FLUIDS
1. Includes pericardial, plural, and peritoneal fluids
2. Normal fluids appear clear and light yellow
3. May be tested for chemical components, cultured and smeared for bacteria, or tested for cell counts

E. SYNOVIAL FLUID
1. Fluid that lines and lubricates joints
2. Normal fluid appears yellow and viscous
3. Collected through joint puncture
4. May be cultured, analyzed for cells and crystals, and tested for glucose and protein

F. FECES
1. Collected in a clean container
2. Avoid contamination from water or urine
3. Tests include:
   a. Occult blood (stool guaiac test)
      1) Detects hidden blood
      2) Helps diagnosis of cancer or bleeding
      3) Hemoccult; ColoScreen
   b. Ova and parasites (O&P): detects eggs and parasites in the intestinal tract
   c. Culture: detects microorganisms

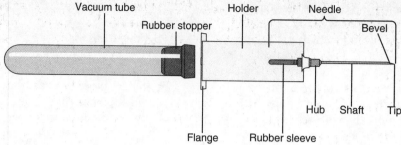

FIGURE 22-2.   Vacuum tube system. (Hunt SA: *Saunders fundamentals of medical assisting*, St Louis, 2002, Saunders.)

G. SPUTUM
1. Secretions of trachea and bronchi
2. Avoid contamination with saliva and nasal secretions
3. Patient is instructed to cough deeply into the container for the culture

H. OTHER SECRETIONS
1. Collected with sterile swabs for cultures, includes:
   a. Wound secretions
   b. Throat secretions
   c. Genital secretions

III. Microscope

A. GENERAL
1. Precision magnifying instrument used to view objects too small to be seen with the naked eye
2. Total magnification equals objective lens magnification times ocular lens magnification

B. PARTS OF THE MICROSCOPE (see Figure 22-4)
1. Base: portion that supports the microscope
2. Arm: supports lenses and focus knobs
3. Stage: platform that holds the objects being observed; contains clips for holding the objects on the stage

4. Light source: light bulb in base that illuminates the objects; knob controls the intensity of the light
5. Condenser: lens over the light source that directs and focuses the light on the object
6. Iris diaphragm: shutter mechanism on the bottom of condenser; regulates the amount of light passing through the object
7. Ocular: one or two eyepieces; contains a lens that magnifies the image
8. Objectives: lenses mounted on a revolving nosepiece; microscope usually contains three lenses on the nosepiece
   a. Low power: usually 10×; used for initial focusing
   b. High-dry power: usually 40×; used for cellular specimens, wet preparations, and urine sediment
   c. Oil immersion: usually 100×; requires the use of immersion oil to prevent refraction; used to study cell detail and bacteria
9. Coarse adjustment: large focusing knob; moves the stage up or down for rough focus
10. Fine adjustment: small focusing knob; allows for precise focusing

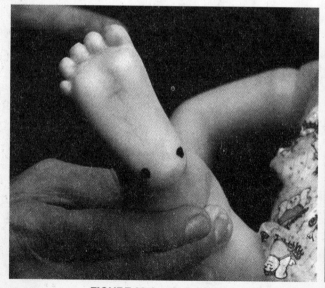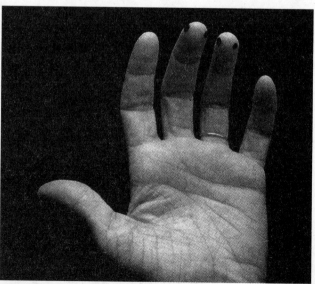

FIGURE 22-3.   Skin puncture sites for microcapillary blood collection. (Young AP, Kennedy DB: *Kinn's the medical assistant: an applied learning approach*, ed 9, St Louis, 2003, Saunders.)

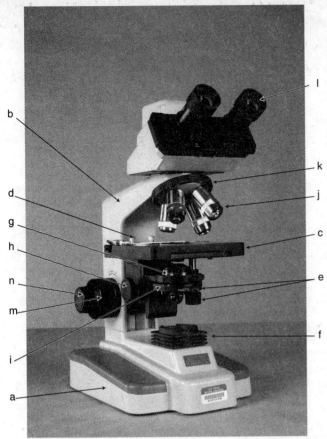

FIGURE 22-4. Microscope. *A*, Base; *B*, arm; *C*, stage; *D*, slide holder; *E*, mechanical slide controls; *F*, light source; *G*, condenser; *H*, condenser adjustment; *I*, diaphragm lever; *J*, low power objective; *K*, nosepiece; *L*, ocular lens; *M*, coarse focus objective; *N*, fine focus adjustment (Garrels M, Oatis CS: *Laboratory testing for ambulatory settings: a guide for health care professionals*, St Louis, 2006, Saunders.)

C. CARE
1. Transport with one hand under the base, the other on the arm
2. Wipe immersion oil off the objective immediately after use
3. Store with 10× objective over the stage; bring the stage to the lowest level and cover
4. Lenses should be cleaned only with lens paper to decrease the possibility of scratches

IV. Urinalysis

A. GENERAL
1. Physical, chemical, and microscopic examination of urine
2. Provides information about the conditions of the kidneys and urinary tract
3. Can help in the diagnosis of metabolic and systemic disorders

B. PHYSICAL EXAMINATION
1. Color
   a. Normal: yellow; color is due to urochrome pigment
   b. Pale (straw): dilute urine
   c. Dark yellow (amber): concentrated urine; may be seen in person with fever or dehydration
   d. Yellow-brown or green/brown: presence of bilirubin; will foam when shaken
   e. Bright orange: seen in patients taking Pyridium; will interfere with reagent strips
   f. Red: clear red may indicate hemoglobin; cloudy red indicates the presence of red blood cells (hematuria)
   g. Dark brown or black: presence of melanin
   h. Pink, green, or blue: results from foods, dyes, chemicals, or vitamins
2. Clarity
   a. Normal: clear but becomes cloudy on standing
   b. Hazy: solid particles make urine appear hazy; print is not distorted when viewed through the sample
   c. Cloudy: solid particles make print difficult to see through the sample
   d. Turbid: solid particles make print impossible to see through the sample
   e. Normal cloudiness may be caused by:
      1) Mucus
      2) Certain crystals
      3) Epithelial cells
      4) Sperm cells
   f. Abnormal cloudiness may be caused by:
      1) Certain crystals
      2) White and red blood cells (WBCs and RBCs)
      3) Pus
      4) Epithelial cells
      5) Casts
      6) Fats
3. Specific gravity (SG)
   a. Measures the amount of dissolved solids in urine
   b. Compares weight to an equal amount of distilled water
      1) Normal SG is 1.005 to 1.035: SG inverses with volume
         a) Low volume has high specific gravity (concentrated urine)
         b) High volume has low specific gravity (diluted urine)
      2) Methods of measuring SG
         a) Reagent strip
         b) Urinometer
         c) Refractometer
4. Odor: may be noted if abnormal
   a. Normal: faintly aromatic; not unpleasant
   b. Ketones: sweet or fruity odor
   c. Ammonia: caused by bacterial growth that breaks down urea
   d. Strong food ingestion may cause odor

C. CHEMICAL EXAMINATION
1. Chemical components are measured by use of a reagent strip
2. Presence of a chemical causes a color change on the reagent pad on the strip

3. Tests are qualitative
4. Specimen should be well mixed before testing
5. Completely immerse the strip into the sample
6. Remove the strip and keep it in a horizontal position (avoids cross-contamination of pads)
7. Compare the color of the reagent pad with the color on the bottle or chart at the time specified
8. Testing includes:
   a. pH: measures acidity and alkalinity of urine; normal is 5 to 7
   b. Protein: significant for renal disease; normal is *negative*
   c. Blood: significant for kidney disease or hemorrhage in the urinary tract; normal is *negative*
   d. Nitrite: significant for urinary tract infection (UTI) (some bacteria convert nitrate to nitrite); normal is *negative*
   e. Leukocytes: significant for UTI; normal is *negative*
   f. Glucose: significant for diabetes mellitus; normal is *negative*
   g. Ketones: end product of metabolism; significant for diabetes mellitus and starvation; normal is *negative*
   h. Bilirubin: by-product of RBC destruction; significant for liver disease or bile duct obstruction; normal is *negative*
   i. Urobilinogen: result of breakdown of bilirubin in the intestine; significant for anemias and malaria; normal is *small amount*
9. Automated (Clinitek) method
   a. Analyzer that automatically reads the reagent strips
   b. Based on principle of photometry
   c. Timing and color interpretation are consistent

D. MICROSCOPIC EXAMINATION

1. Consists of examining, counting, and categorizing the solid material
2. Standardized method (Kova Urine Sediment system) is used
3. Sample is centrifuged, supernatant (liquid portion) is poured off, and sediment is stained
4. Medical assistant may prepare the slide; practitioner interprets the results
   a. Examined under low power (10×)
   b. Examined under high power (40×) for cells and bacteria
   c. Examination includes:
      1) RBCs: normal is zero to two per high-powered field (HPF); cells appear small, round, and clear
      2) WBCs: normal is zero to five per HPF; cells appear two to three times the size of RBCs and round with a grainy appearance
      3) Epithelial cells
         a) Squamous epithelial cells: normal: not significant unless a large quantity per HPF; appear approximately the same size as WBCs
         b) Renal epithelial cells: normal is zero per HPF; presence indicates renal tubule destruction; appear round and grainy, approximately twice the size of WBCs
      4) Bacteria: normal are a few per HPF; more indicates UTI; appear as tiny grains
      5) Yeast: normal are a few per HPF; more indicates yeast infection (*Candida albicans*); they appear as round, clear bodies; some have buds (hyphae); may be confused with RBCs
      6) Mucous threads: wavy, threadlike structures
      7) Spermatozoa: appear as small oval bodies, with tail; normal in men, contamination in women
      8) Casts: structures formed in nephron tubules; material solidifies in tubules and may contain cells, fat, and bacteria; normal is zero to two per LPF; appear as cylindrical bodies, longer than wide: types include:
         a) Hyaline: colorless and semitransparent
         b) Fatty cast: contains fat globules
         c) RBC cast: orange-yellow in color
         d) WBC cast: contains WBCs
         e) Granular cast: sandlike granules
         f) Waxy cast: yellowish, wide cast with irregular edges
      9) Crystals
         a) Normal crystals found in acidic urine
            • Uric acid: appears lemon shaped
            • Calcium oxalate: square shape with an X
         b) Normal crystals found in alkaline urine
            • Triple phosphate: coffin-lid-shaped
            • Calcium phosphate: flat plates
         c) Abnormal crystals found in acidic urine
            • Cystine: hexagonal plates
            • Tyrosine: fine needles
            • Leucine: yellow spheres
            • Sulfonamides: large needles in rosettes
            • Cholesterol: large, flat, hexagonal plates with notched corners

V. Serology and Immunology

A. GENERAL

1. Tests done on serum to evaluate antigen-antibody reaction
2. Helps detect disease or amount of antibodies present (titer)
3. Some tests available in kit and/or *rapid* forms
4. Test reactions include:
   a. Precipitation: antigen-antibody complex visibly settles out of solution
   b. Agglutination: type of precipitation method that creates visible clumping

B. INFECTIOUS MONONUCLEOSIS

1. Disease caused by Epstein-Barr virus
2. Body produces heterophil antibodies in response

3. Tests (Monospot, QuickVue+) are designed to detect heterophile antibody

C. STREPTOCOCCUS

1. Group A beta hemolytic *Streptococcus* causes strep throat, rheumatic fever, and impetigo
2. Tests detect antibody antistreptolysin-O (ASO)

D. RHEUMATOID FACTOR

1. Group of proteins (autoantibodies)
2. Causes rheumatoid arthritis
3. Test detects antibodies against factor

E. HUMAN CHORIONIC GONADOTROPIN (HCG)

1. Hormone produced by the placenta
2. Test for hormone in blood and urine
3. Basis of pregnancy testing

F. BLOOD GROUPS

1. Blood cells are mixed with antisera; agglutination indicates the presence of antigens on RBCs
2. Can detect ABO group (A, B, AB, or O)
3. Can detect Rh (Rh+, or Rh–)

G. SYPHILIS

1. Antibody test for *Treponema pallidum*
2. Tests include:
   a. Rapid plasma reagin (RPR)
   b. Venereal disease research laboratory (VDRL)

H. SYSTEMIC LUPUS ERYTHEMATOSUS

1. Testing to detect antinuclear antibodies (ANA)

I. *HELICOBACTER PYLORI*

1. Spiral-shaped bacteria believed to be the cause of the majority of peptic ulcers
2. QuickVue *Helicobacter pylori* gII Test is performed from a finger stick

VI. Chemistry

A. LIPIDS

1. Before lipid testing, the patient should fast for 12 to 14 hours; the patient should consume no alcohol for 24 hours before the test; the patient should reduce fat intake for 2 weeks before the test
2. These tests can assess the risk of coronary and vascular disease
3. Lipid profile is made up of the following tests:
   a. Cholesterol
      1) Fatty compound
      2) Necessary for production of sex hormones and bile
      3) Helps in formation of cell membranes
      4) Normal range: <200 mg/dL
   b. High-density lipoproteins (HDLs)
      1) "*Good*" cholesterol
      2) Removes excess cholesterol from cells and carries it back to the liver for excretions
      3) Normal range: >50 mg/dL
   c. Low-density lipoproteins (LDLs)
      1) "*Bad*" cholesterol
      2) Picks up fat from liver and carries it in the blood
      3) Normal range: <100 mg/dL
   d. Triglycerides
      1) Form fat in the bloodstream
      2) Transported in blood by LDLs
      3) Make up most of the fat in the body
      4) Normal range: 30 to 150 mg/dL

B. GLUCOSE

1. Simple sugar from the breakdown of carbohydrates
2. Provides energy for cells and tissues
3. Excess is stored as glycogen in the liver
4. Blood levels regulated by hormones produced by pancreas
   a. Glucagon: converts glycogen to glucose (increased blood levels)
   b. Insulin: transports glucose into cells (decreased blood levels)
5. Tests include:
   a. Fasting blood glucose (FBG)
      1) Testing done on blood sample of patient after fasting for 8 to 12 hours (water permitted)
      2) Test is commonly used in the diagnosis or evaluation of diabetes mellitus
      3) Normal range: 65 to 110 mg/dL
   b. Postprandial glucose (2-hour postprandial blood sugar [PPBS])
      1) Measures the amount of glucose in the patient's blood after a meal is ingested
      2) Blood level should return to the premeal range within 2 hours
      3) Normal range: 65 to 110 mg/dL
   c. Glucose tolerance test (GTT)
      1) Assists in the diagnosis of diabetes mellitus
      2) Patient's blood glucose levels are evaluated at fasting, then 30, 60, 120, and 180 minutes after ingestion of a standard oral glucose solution
      3) Urine samples are evaluated at the same time
      4) Patient is to fast 12 hours before the test
      5) Fasting blood sugar is drawn
      6) Patient drinks 75 g of glucose solution
      7) Collect blood samples and urine samples 30, 60, 120, and 180 minutes (or any combination of these times) after the patient takes the glucose solution
      8) Patient may drink water during the test, but *no* coffee, tea, or tobacco
      9) Normal glucose ranges:
         a) Fasting: 65 to 110 mg/dL
         b) 30 min: 200 mg/dL
         c) 1 hour: 200 mg/dL
         d) 2 hours: 140 mg/dL
         e) 3 hours: 65 to 115 mg/dL

C. ELECTROLYTES

1. Charged particles of the body

2. Includes:
   a. Cation: positively charged ions
   b. Anion: negatively charged ions
3. Found in extracellular fluids
4. Body strives for neutrality (balance of anions and cations); if balance is not achieved, can be dangerous or fatal for the patient
5. Lungs and kidneys control the electrolyte balance
6. Functions of electrolytes
   a. Maintain water balance in the body
   b. Maintain pH of the body
   c. Help with blood coagulation
   d. Control neuromuscular excitability
7. Sodium (Na^+)
   a. Major extracellular cation
   b. Helps maintain osmotic pressure
   c. Low sodium level: hyponatremia
   d. High sodium level: hypernatremia
   e. Normal range: 135 to 146 mEq/L
8. Potassium (K^+)
   a. Major intracellular cation
   b. Influences muscle activity of heart
   c. Works with sodium for acid-base balance
   d. Low K^+ level: hypokalemia
   e. High K^+ level: hyperkalemia
   f. Normal range: 3.5 to 5.3 mEq/L
9. Chloride (Cl^-)
   a. Major extracellular anion
   b. Counterbalances sodium for neutrality in body fluids
   c. Helps maintain osmotic pressure (water distribution between cells), plasma, and interstitial fluid
   d. Helps maintain acid-base balance
   e. Normal range: 98 to 108 mEq/L
10. Bicarbonate ($HCO3^-$)
    a. Major anion
    b. Measured by blood carbon dioxide levels
    c. Works with Cl^-
    d. Normal range: 21 to 31 mEq/L

D. BILIRUBIN

1. Yellow pigment in bile
2. Comes from heme portion of hemoglobin (heme released when RBCs break down)
3. Two types
   a. Unconjugated (indirect): transported by albumin to the liver
   b. Conjugated (direct): becomes water soluble in the liver and enters the bile; transported to the small intestine, where it is converted into urobilinogen
4. Increased levels may indicate:
   a. Destruction of RBCs
   b. Impaired liver function
   c. Obstruction of flow of bile
5. Exposure to ultraviolet lights results in oxidation of bilirubin

6. Normal range: 0.1 to 1.2 mg/dL

E. PROTEINS

1. Make up muscles, enzymes, hormones, hemoglobin, and other important functional and structural substances in the body
2. Albumin
   a. Principal plasma protein
   b. Found in liver
   c. Functions
      1) Maintenance of osmotic pressure
      2) Transportation of drugs, hormones, and enzymes
   d. Can be a measure of nutritional status
   e. Normal range: 3.5 to 5.0 g/dL
3. Globulin
   a. Building block of antibodies, lipids, and clotting factors
   b. Transport mechanism
   c. Can be measure of nutritional status
   d. Normal range: 1.7 to 3.5 g/dL
4. Albumin to globulin (A/G) ratio
   a. Normal range: 1.1 to 2.5
5. Total protein
   a. Albumin plus globulin
   b. Component of osmotic pressure (keeps fluids within vascular system)
   c. Normal range: 6.0 to 8.5 g/dL

F. NITROGENOUS COMPOUNDS

1. Forms of nitrogen in the body
2. Waste product of metabolism
3. Blood urea nitrogen (BUN)
   a. Main indicator of kidney function
   b. Urea is main nonprotein nitrogen in blood
   c. Urea is formed in the liver and is the waste product of the breakdown of protein
   d. Normal range: 8 to 26 mg/dL
4. Creatinine
   a. End product of creatine metabolism in muscles
   b. Constantly being formed; the amount has a direct relationship to muscle mass
   c. Filtered by the kidneys and excreted in urine
   d. Reliable screening test for renal function
   e. Normal range: 0.7 to 1.4 mg/dL
5. Uric acid
   a. By-product of protein metabolism
   b. Blood levels from food metabolism (high-protein diet) and muscle tissue breakdown
   c. Normal range: men: 3.6 to 8.0 mg/dL; women: 2.5 to 6.8 mg/dL

G. ENZYMES

1. Substances that speed up chemical reactions but remain unchanged themselves
2. Values expressed in International Units (IU)
3. Always end with the suffix -*ase*
4. Can originate in cells, specific organs, or tissues
5. Release may be caused by damage or disease of tissues

6. Alanine aminotransferase (ALT)
   a. Formerly serum glutamic-oxaloacetic transaminase (SGOT)
   b. Found in highly metabolic tissues (heart muscle, liver, skeletal muscles)
   c. Levels increase post–myocardial infarction (MI) (indication of MI)
   d. Normal range: men: 0 to 37 U/L; women: 0 to 31 U/L
7. Creatine phosphokinase (CPK, CK)
   a. Enzyme found in mitochondria of cells
   b. High concentration in the heart, skeletal muscles, and brain
   c. Useful in diagnosis of MI and muscle disease
   d. Normal range: 25 to 130 IU/L
8. Alkaline phosphatase (ALP)
   a. High concentration in bone and liver
   b. Bone growth or liver disease can cause levels to rise
   c. Normal range: child: 117 to 390 U/L; adult: 39 to 117 U/L
9. Acid phosphatase
   a. Largest source is the prostate gland
   b. Elevated in prostate cancer
   c. Normal value: 0 to 0.8 IU/L

H. MINERALS
1. Inorganic chemical elements needed in small amounts but essential for life
2. May be part of hormones or enzymes or work with vitamins
3. Calcium (Ca)
   a. Found in bone tissue
   b. Required for:
      1) Bone development
      2) Cardiac function
      3) Blood clotting
      4) Transmission of nerve impulses
      5) Muscle contractions
   c. Normal range: 8.5 to 11.5 mg/dL
4. Phosphorus (P)
   a. Required for metabolism of protein, calcium, and glucose
   b. Combines with calcium
   c. Normal range: 2.5 to 4.5 mg/dL
5. Magnesium (Mg)
   a. Found in bone
   b. Binds with adenosine triphosphate (ATP) molecule for energy
   c. Required for:
      1) Muscle action
      2) Nerve impulse transmission
      3) Calcium regulation
      4) Enzyme activity
   d. Normal range: 1.2 to 2.0 mEq/L

I. THYROID
1. Triiodothyronine (T3)
   a. Evaluates thyroid function (hyperthyroidism, hypothyroidism)
   b. Monitors thyroid replacement and suppressive therapy
   c. Normal range: 70 to 205 ng/dL
2. Thyroxine (tetraiodothyronine) (T4)
   a. Initial test done for assessing thyroid function
   b. Used to diagnose thyroid function
   c. Used to monitor replacement and suppressive therapy
   d. Normal range: women: 5 to 12 µg/dL; men: 4 to 12 µg/dL

VII. Hematology

A. GENERAL
1. Study of blood and blood components

B. BLOOD COMPONENTS
1. Part of the circulatory system
2. Functions as transport mechanism for nutrients, waste, and defense agents to tissues and cells
3. Specimens collected by venipuncture (anticoagulated specimens) or capillary puncture
4. Plasma
   a. Liquid portion of circulating, unclotted blood
   b. 55% of total blood volume made up of:
      1) 90% water
      2) 10% solutes (proteins, hormones, vitamins, carbohydrates, enzymes, lipids, and salts)
5. Formed elements
   a. Blood cells
   b. 45% of total blood volume made up of:
      1) Erythrocytes (RBCs)
      2) Leukocytes (WBCs)
      3) Thrombocytes (platelets)

C. ERYTHROCYTES
1. Mature cells are anuclear biconcave discs
2. Contain hemoglobin (Hgb)
   a. Heme (iron-containing portion) plus globin (protein-containing portion)
   b. Transports oxygen
3. Color
   a. Normally appear pinkish-red (depends on Hgb concentration)
   b. Anisochromia: variations in color (depends on Hgb concentration)
4. Size
   a. Normally 6 to 8 micrometers
   b. Anisocytosis: variation in size
5. Shape
   a. Normally appear round
   b. Poikilocytosis: variation in shape
6. Diseases and disorders
   a. Anemia: caused by:
      1) Blood loss
      2) Increase in plasma volume (overhydration, pregnancy)

3) Iron deficiency caused by Hgb decrease
  b. Polycythemia: increase in RBC numbers
7. Laboratory testing
  a. Hgb (hemoglobin) test
    1) Measures the total amount of Hgb in the blood
    2) Rapid indirect measurement of RBC count
    3) Evaluates anemic patients
    4) Routine portion of CBC
    5) Blood sample is diluted with Drabkin solution; lyses RBCs and releases Hgb into the solution; chemicals in the reagent react with released Hgb and forms the pigment cyanmethemoglobin, which can be measured by photometer
    6) Normal Hgb ranges:
      a) Newborn: 17 to 21 g/dL
      b) Infant: 10 to 15 g/dL
      c) Child: 11 to 16 g/dL
      d) Male adult: 15 to 18 g/dL
      e) Female adult: 12 to 16 g/dL
  b. Hematocrit (HCT, microhematocrit, crit)
    1) Direct measurement of percentage of RBCs in total blood volume
    2) Indirect measurement of RBC number and volume
    3) Rapid measurement of RBC count
    4) Routine portion of CBC
    5) Height of RBC column is measured after the blood sample is centrifuged; compared with the height of the column of whole blood (height of the column of whole blood is 100%)
    6) After centrifuging, blood separates into three layers:
      a) Plasma (top) layer
      b) Buffy coat: thin middle layer made up of WBCs and platelets
      c) RBCs (bottom) layer
    7) Hgb value multiplied by 3 gives the HCT value (±3)
    8) Procedure
      a) Two tubes needed (for comparison; to balance centrifuge; if one breaks)
      b) Fill two capillary tubes three-quarters full with blood from capillary puncture or lavender-stoppered tube from venipuncture
      c) Wipe the ends to remove blood from the outside of the tubes and seal with clay (Critoseal)
      d) Place in a HCT centrifuge with the sealed ends facing outward; spin for 5 minutes
      e) Read tubes by comparing them to the printed reading device
      f) To be valid, the tubes should read within 2% of each other; report the average reading; repeat the test if not within 2%
    9) Normal HCT ranges:

      a) Newborn: 44% to 64%
      b) Infant: 30% to 40%
      c) Child: 35% to 41%
      d) Female adult: 37% to 47%
      e) Male adult: 42% to 52%
  c. RBC count
    1) Counts the number of circulating RBCs in 1 mm³ of peripheral venous blood
    2) Routine portion of CBC
    3) Closely related to Hgb and HCT values
    4) Normal RBC ranges (in million/mm³):
      a) Newborn: 4.8 to 7.1
      b) Infant: 3.5 to 5.5
      c) Child: 4.5 to 4.8
      d) Female adult: 4.0 to 5.5
      e) Male adult: 4.5 to 6.0
  d. Indices
    1) Provide information about RBC size, weight, and Hgb concentration
    2) Part of automated CBC
    3) Results of RBC count, HCT, and Hgb necessary to calculate indices
      a) Mean corpuscular volume (MCV)
        • Measure of average size per volume of an RBC
        • Used to classify anemias
        • HCT (%) × 10 MCV = RBC (in million/mm³)
        • Normal ranges:
          (1) Newborn: 96 to 108
          (2) Child and adult: 82 to 98
      b) Mean corpuscular hemoglobin (MCH)
        • Measures amount per weight of Hgb within an RBC
        • Hgb (g/dL) × 10 MCH = RBC (in million/mm³)
        • Normal ranges:
          (1) Newborn: 32 to 34 pg
          (2) Child and adult: 26 to 34 pg
      c) Mean corpuscular hemoglobin concentration (MCHC)
        • Measure of average concentration per percentage of Hgb in a single RBC
        • Hgb (g/dL) × 100 HCT = g/dL or (%)
        • Normal ranges:
          (1) Newborn: 31 to 33 g/dL
          (2) Child and adult: 31 to 37 g/dL
  e. Reticulocyte count
    1) Reticulocytes are immature RBCs
    2) Indication of ability of bone marrow to respond to anemia and make RBCs
    3) Used to classify and monitor anemia therapy
    4) Count is percentage of total number of RBCs
    5) Normal ranges:
      a) Newborn: 0.5% to 2% of total RBCs
      b) Infant: 0.5% to 3.1% of total RBCs
      c) Child and adult: 0.5% to 2% of total RBCs
  f. ESR (sed rate; erythrocyte sedimentation rate)

1) Nonspecific test used to detect illnesses associated with acute and chronic infection, inflammation, and neoplasms
2) Measures the rate at which RBCs settle in plasma over a specified time period (1 hour)
3) Methods include:
   a) Wintrobe
   b) Westergren
   c) Landau-Adams
4) All methods are based on the same principle, although they vary in the amount of blood needed, the tube size, and calibration
5) Procedure
   a) Fill the tube according to manufacturer's directions
   b) Place the tube perfectly upright in the rack; let the tube sit for 1 hour without being disturbed
   c) After 1 hour, note how many millimeters cells fall (settle)
6) Normal ranges:
   a) Newborn: 0 to 2 mm/hr
   b) Child: 0 to 10 mm/hr
   c) Female adult: 0 to 30 mm/hr
   d) Male adult: 0 to 20 mm/hr

D. LEUKOCYTES

1. Mature cells vary in morphology depending on type
2. Neutrophil (segmented neutrophil [seg], poly, polymorphonuclear [PMN]): most numerous of granulocytes
   a. Size: 10 to 15 micrometers
   b. Nucleus: contains two to five lobes with constrictions (as sausage links); stains deep reddish-purple
   c. Cytoplasm: abundant; stains light to medium pink, with many small granules
   d. Distribution: 35% to 70% of circulating WBCs
   e. Increased number: shift to the right
3. Bands (stabs): immature form of segmented neutrophil
   a. Size: 10 to 15 micrometers
   b. Nucleus: peanut-, band-, or rod-shaped; no lobes or constrictions
   c. Cytoplasm: same as segmented neutrophil
   d. Distribution: 1% to 5% of circulating WBCs
   e. Increased number: shift to the left
4. Eosinophil (eos): granulocyte
   a. Size: 11 to 16 micrometers
   b. Nucleus: not significant; stains dark pinkish-red
   c. Cytoplasm: stains pink; contains large, reddish-orange granules
   d. Distribution: 1% to 5% of circulating WBCs; increase seen in allergic reactions, parasite infestation, and inflammation
5. Basophil (baso): granulocyte
   a. Size: 10 to 15 micrometers
   b. Nucleus: indistinct; usually occluded by granules
   c. Cytoplasm: small amount; stains purplish-blue; contains large, dark-purple-to-black granules; granules contain histamine and heparin
   d. Distribution: 0% to 1% of circulating WBCs; increase seen in allergic reactions, radiation exposure, and after splenectomy
6. Monocytes (mono): agranulocyte
   a. Size: 15 to 20 micrometers
   b. Nucleus: large, foamy, and round; stains reddish-purple to medium purple
   c. Cytoplasm: large amount; may appear foamy; stains sky-blue to blue-gray
   d. Distribution: 3% to 5% of circulating WBCs
7. Lymphocyte (lymph): agranulocyte
   a. Smallest in size of all WBCs
   b. Size: 6 to 10 micrometers
   c. Nucleus: round; fills most of the cell; stains dark purple
   d. Cytoplasm: small amount; encircles the nucleus; stains sky-blue to medium blue
   e. Distribution: 30% to 40% of circulating WBCs; infants and children normally have more than adults; increase seen in acute and chronic infections
8. Laboratory testing
   a. WBC count
      1) Measurement of total number of WBCs
      2) Routine part of CBC
      3) Helps evaluate and diagnose infection, allergy, neoplasm, or immunosuppression
      4) Normal ranges
         a) Newborn: 9000 to 30,000/mm^3
         b) Child: 5000 to 13,000/mm^3
         c) Adult: 5000 to 10,000/mm^3
   b. Differential (diff)
      1) Measurement of different WBCs in a smear
      2) Smear is stained with polychromatic stain (Wright's)
      3) Preparation of smear
         a) Small drop of blood is placed approximately 1/2 inch from the end of the slide
         b) Spreader slide is held at a 35- to 40-degree angle and moved back into the drop of blood slide; blood should be completely spread across the edge of the spreader's edge; push the spreader smoothly from the blood across the slide
         c) Allow to air dry; a smooth feather edge should be seen
         d) Stain the smear following the manufacturer's directions and completely air dry
      4) Normal ranges adult:
         a) Segs: 50 to 65
         b) Bands: 0 to 7
         c) Lymphs: 25 to 40
         d) Monos: 3 to 9
         e) EOS: 1 to 3
         f) BASO: 0 to 1

E. THROMBOCYTES

1. Platelet count test
    a. Actual count of the number of platelets in a cubic millimeter of blood
    b. Used to monitor the course of disease and therapy for thrombocytopenia and bone marrow failure
    c. Small round or oval bodies; no nucleus
    d. Stain dark blue on a different smear
    e. Normal ranges
        1) Newborn: 140,000 to 300,000/mm³
        2) Infant: 200,000 to 473,000/mm³
        3) Child/adult: 150,000 to 400,000/mm³
2. Bleeding time
    a. Measures platelet function by noting the length of time required for bleeding to stop
    b. Two methods:
        1) Ivy method: small incision in the patient's arm
        2) Duke method: small incision in the patient's earlobe (not commonly performed)
        3) Normal range: 1 to 9 minutes for bleeding to stop
3. Prothrombin time (PT, pro-time)
    a. Used to evaluate clotting mechanism
    b. Used to monitor Coumadin therapy
    c. Normal range: 11 to 12.5 seconds
4. Partial thromboplastin time (PTT)
    a. Used to evaluate the pathway to clot formation
    b. Used to monitor heparin therapy
    c. Normal range: 60 to 70 seconds

VIII. Microbiology

A. GENERAL

1. Study of microorganisms
2. Includes:
    a. Bacteria
    b. Fungi
    c. Viruses
    d. Rickettsiae
    e. Mycobacteria
    f. Parasites
3. Main objective is to identify the organism so that the practitioner can properly treat

B. CLASSIFICATION OF ORGANISMS

1. Scientific study of classification process is taxonomy
2. Simple, orderly method
3. Places organisms into categories according to similar morphologic and biochemical properties
    a. Species: basic unit; based on reproduction (members of the same species can mate successfully)
    b. Genus: share biological likenesses
    c. Family: similar genera
    d. Order: related families
    e. Class: related orders
    f. Phylum: classes with common characteristics
4. Organisms in laboratory setting have two separate names:

a. Genus: name is capitalized; often abbreviated, using the first initial
b. Species: name in lowercase
5. Both names are underlined or italicized when written

C. BACTERIA (BACTERIOLOGY)

1. Characteristics: help with identification of organisms in the laboratory (see Figure 22-5)
    a. Shape
        1) Cocci: round (singular: coccus)
        2) Bacilli: rod shaped (singular: bacillus)
        3) Vibrio: comma shaped
        4) Spirilla: spiral shaped (singular: spirillum)
    b. Arrangement
        1) Diplo: arranged in pairs
        2) Strepto: arranged in chains
        3) Staphylo: arranged in grapelike clusters
        4) Tetra: four cocci together in capsule
    c. Staining properties
        1) Gram stain
            a) Gram-positive: stain blue or dark purple
            b) Gram-negative: stain pink or red
        2) Acid-fast stain: type of stain used on bacteria that are difficult to stain with other stains

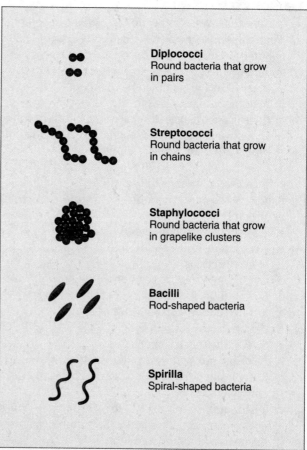

Diplococci
Round bacteria that grow in pairs

Streptococci
Round bacteria that grow in chains

Staphylococci
Round bacteria that grow in grapelike clusters

Bacilli
Rod-shaped bacteria

Spirilla
Spiral-shaped bacteria

FIGURE 22-5. Classification of bacteria by shape. (From Bonewit-West K: *Clinical procedures for medical assistants*, ed 6, Philadelphia, 2004, Saunders.)

d. Oxygen requirements
   1) Aerobic: requires oxygen to survive
   2) Anaerobic: requires no oxygen to survive
   3) Facultative: can survive in either environment
e. Colony growth
   1) Size
   2) Color
   3) Shape
   4) Elevation
   5) Texture
   6) Margins
   7) Hemolysis (present or absent)
f. Chemical reactions: bacteria respond differently to chemical reagents
3. Common pathogenic bacteria
   a. Gram-positive cocci
      1) *Staphylococcus* (appears in clusters, dark purple)
         a) *S. aureus:* skin infections, impetigo
         b) *S. epidermis:* normal flora of the skin
         c) *S. saprophyticus:* UTI
      2) *Streptococcus* (appears in chains, dark purple)
         a) *S. pyogenes:* URI, rheumatic fever
         b) *S. pneumoniae:* otitis media, pneumonia, meningitis
         c) *S. viridans:* gum disease, endocarditis
   b. Gram-negative cocci: *Neisseria* (appears as diplococci, pink)
      1) *N. gonorrhoeae:* gonorrhea
      2) *N. meningitidis:* meningitis
   c. Gram-negative bacilli
      1) *Escherichia coli:* normal flora of the colon; UTI
      2) *Salmonella*
         a) *S. typhi:* constipation
         b) *S. enteritidis:* gastroenteritis
      3) *Shigella dysenteriae:* severe dysentery
      4) *Klebsiella pneumoniae*
         a) Normal flora of the colon and respiratory tract
         b) UTI, wound infections, pneumonia
      5) *Proteus vulgaris:* normal flora of the gastrointestinal tract; UTI, wound infections
      6) *Pseudomonas aeruginosa:* UTI, wound and burn infection
      7) *Haemophilus influenzae:* severe meningitis, otitis media (HiB vaccination)
   d. Gram-negative vibrio and spirochetes
      1) *Treponema pallidum* (spirochete): syphilis
      2) *Borrelia burgdorferi* (spirochete): Lyme disease
      3) *Vibrio cholerae* (vibrio): cholera
   e. Gram-positive bacilli
      1) *Corynebacterium diphtheriae:* diphtheria
      2) *Mycobacterium tuberculosis:* tuberculosis
      3) *Mycobacterium leprae:* leprosy
4. Rickettsia
   a. Extremely small, gram-negative bacteria
   b. Parasites; require living cells to live
   c. Transmitted by the bite of fleas, ticks, lice, and mites

d. *Rickettsia rickettsii:* Rocky Mountain spotted fever
5. *Chlamydia*
   a. Gram-negative cocci
   b. Parasites; depend on host for food and energy source
      1) *C. psittaci:* parrot fever
      2) *C. trachomatis:* conjunctivitis; pelvic inflammatory disease (PID)
6. *Mycoplasma*
   a. Simplest form of bacteria
   b. Normal flora of the respiratory system and genitalia

D. CULTURE MEDIA

1. Contains known amount of substances for optimal growth and diagnostic properties of bacteria
2. May contain:
   a. Sugar
   b. Vitamins and minerals
   c. Proteins
   d. Dyes for diagnostics
3. Forms
   a. Semisolid and solid
      1) Usually made of agar (from seaweed)
      2) Allows for general growth
      3) Allows for identification of colony size, color, and shape
   b. Liquid
      1) Broth
      2) Allows for general growth
      3) Allows for study of gas production or patient changes
4. Bacterial growth requirements
   a. Nutrients: differ among species
   b. Temperature: usually thrive at normal body temperature (98.6° F, 37° C)
   c. Oxygen: differs among species (aerobic or anaerobic)
   d. pH: human pathogens thrive at 7 (neutral); blood, milk, and seawater are neutral
   e. Sterile: medium must be sterile and uncontaminated for use
   f. Moisture: most bacteria require some level of moisture
5. Classification of media
   a. Differential: contains substances (dyes) that give organisms easily identifiable characteristics
   b. Selective: inhibits growth of some species
   c. Supportive: allows most organisms to grow equally
6. Common media
   a. Blood agar
      1) Used for primary plating
      2) Contains sheep's blood
      3) Demonstrates hemolysis (staphylococcal and streptococcal cultures)
   b. Chocolate agar
      1) Contains denatured blood

2) Used for organisms that require a rich food source and moisture

c. Mueller-Hinton: selective for *Neisseria;* used for sensitivity testing

d. Thayer-Martin (TM): selective for *N. gonorrhoeae* and *N. meningitidis*

E. PROCEDURE FOR STREAKING CULTURE PLATES (PLATING) (see Figure 22-6)

1. Used to culture bacteria and isolate colonies for identification
2. Collect a specimen with a sterile swab; may use a sterile inoculating loop if already plated
3. Primary streak: streak a swab (or loop) over one fourth of the plate using a back-and-forth motion; do not gorge or break the agar
4. Secondary streak
   a. Sterilize (or flame) the loop, and let it cool
   b. Turn the plate counterclockwise 45 degrees
   c. Touch the primary streak with the loop, and draw a new streak to cover one fourth of the plate (carry the material from the primary streak into a secondary streak)
5. Tertiary streak
   a. Sterilize (or flame) the loop, and let it cool
   b. Repeat the secondary procedure for this streak
6. Quaternary streak
   a. Repeat the process as previously described
   b. Carry the last streak into the center part of the plate that had not been streaked
7. Sterilize (or flame) the loop
8. Incubate the plate
   a. Place into the incubator face down

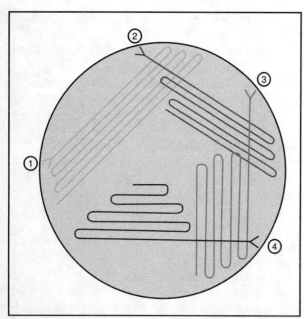

FIGURE 22-6. Quadrant streaking. (From Garrels M, Oatis CS: *Laboratory testing for ambulatory settings: a guide for health care professionals,* St Louis, 2006, Saunders.)

b. Identify the plate (name, date, source) on the plate, not the lid

F. COLLECTION OF MOST COMMON SPECIMENS

1. Throat culture
   a. Use a sterile swab and swab the back of throat in a *rainbow* or *figure-8* pattern
   b. Collect any material in the area
   c. Transport or send the specimen to the laboratory using a transport medium or streak immediately
2. Urine culture
   a. Collect a clean-catch specimen in a sterile container
   b. Use a sterile loop to streak the plate
3. Genitourinary culture
   a. Collect a specimen using a sterile swab
   b. Roll the swab over the plate in a Z or W pattern
   c. Streak across the Z or W, using a sterile loop
4. Blood culture
   a. Collect a specimen in a yellow-stoppered tube
   b. Cleanse the skin with Betadine before venipuncture
   c. Inject approximately 10 mL of the specimen into two separate blood culture bottles
5. Wound culture
   a. Collect a specimen with a sterile swab
   b. Streak the plate using the Z or W method
6. Fecal culture
   a. Collect a specimen in a clean container
   b. Streak the plate with a sterile loop

G. CULTURE AND SENSITIVITY (C&S)

1. Determines an organism's susceptibility to selected antibiotics
2. Streak the plate with culture; cover the entire plate, rotating 45 degrees between each streak
3. Apply antibody disks using a dispenser or sterile forceps; make sure the disk is in contact with the medium
4. Incubate; check after 24 hours
5. Measure the zones of inhibition around each disk; compare with the chart provided by the manufacturer
6. Report the results

H. MYCOLOGY

1. Study of fungus
2. Medical mycology fungal forms
   a. Molds
      1) Multicellular organisms made up of hyphae
      2) Produce powdery, fuzzy, or fluffy colonies on media
   b. Yeasts
      1) Single-cell organisms
      2) Multiply by budding
      3) Produce moist, creamy colonies on media
3. Common pathogenic fungi
   a. *Trichophyton:* causes various forms of tinea infections
   b. *Microsporum:* transmitted by animals and humans; causes ringworm

c. *Candida albicans:* yeast; normal flora of bowel and skin; causes thrush and vaginal yeast infections

d. *Aspergillus fumigatus:* affects respiratory tract and ears

e. *Penicillium notatum:* used to make penicillin; causes pulmonary infections, UTI

f. *Phycomycetes mucor:* causes opportunistic infections in poorly managed patients with diabetes

4. Identification methods
   a. Potassium hydroxide (KOH) preparation
      1) Place the specimen on a slide
      2) Mix KOH with the specimen and allow to sit for 15 to 20 minutes
      3) Observe under low power
   b. India ink
      1) Helps identify capsules
      2) Mix bodily fluid with ink on the slide
      3) Observe under low power
      4) Cells will appear to have halo around them

I. VIROLOGY

1. Study of viruses
2. Intracellular parasites that require a host to carry out their functions
3. Do not have cellular structure (nucleic acid and protein layer)
4. Reproductive by replication
5. Common viruses
   a. Adenovirus: conjunctivitis
   b. Arbovirus: yellow fever, encephalitis (carried by insects)
   c. Coxsackie: herpangina
   d. Echovirus: meningitis, encephalitis
   e. Hepatitis B virus (HBV): hepatitis B
   f. Herpes virus: herpes simplex, varicella (chickenpox), varicella zoster (shingles), Epstein-Barr
   g. Human immunodeficiency virus (HIV): acquired immunodeficiency syndrome (AIDS)
   h. Myxovirus: influenza
   i. Paramyxovirus: mumps, rubeola (measles)
   j. Papillomavirus: verruca (warts)
   k. Poliomyelitis: polio
   l. Rhabdovirus: rabies
   m. Rhinovirus: common cold

J. PARASITOLOGY

1. Study of parasites
2. Organisms that live in or on a host and derive nourishment from the host
3. Can be one-celled (protozoa) or many-celled (helminths) parasites
4. Relationships
   a. Commensalism: neither organism harmed; one benefits
   b. Mutualism: both organisms benefit
   c. Parasitism: one organism benefits at the expense of the other

d. Symbiosis: dependant relationship between two dissimilar organisms

5. Infection: invasion of microscopic parasites causing disease
6. Infestation: external or internal invasion of animal-like parasites
7. Classifications
   a. Protozoa: unicellular organisms
      1) Transmission
         a) Ingestion of cysts in fecally contaminated water or food
         b) Become adults after infection; they multiply in the intestine and are passed in feces
      2) Amoeba
         a) Move by means of pseudopods (*false foot*)
         b) *Entamoeba histolytica:* amebic dysentery
      3) Flagellates
         a) Move by flagella
         b) *Trichomonas vaginalis:* vaginal flagellate; vaginitis
      4) Ciliates
         a) Move by cilia
         b) *Balantidium coli:* largest protozoan; causes dysentery
      5) Sporozoans
         a) Have sexual and asexual reproductive cycles
         b) *Plasmodium:* malaria
         c) *Pneumocystis carinii:* pneumonia in patients with AIDS
   b. Helminths: parasitic worms
      1) Nematodes: roundworms
         a) *Ascaris lumbricoides:* intestinal roundworms
         b) *Enterobius vermicularis:* pinworms
         c) *Necator americanus:* hookworms
         d) *Trichuris trichiura:* whipworms
         e) *Strongyloides stercoralis:* threadworms
      2) Cestodes: tapeworms
         a) *Diphyllobothrium latum:* broad tapeworms
         b) *Taenia saginata:* beef tapeworms
         c) *Taenia solium:* pork tapeworm
      3) Trematodes (flukes): *Schistosoma:* blood fluke
   c. Arthropods: organisms with exoskeletons and jointed appendages; can serve as vector or as intermediate host
      1) Insects: *Pediculosis species:* head and body lice
      2) Fleas
      3) Mosquitoes: *Anopheles* species: malaria
      4) Arachnids: *Sarcoptes scabiei:* scabies (itch mite)
8. Diagnostic procedures
   a. O&P: examination of feces for parasites and/or eggs
      1) Collect a sample in a clean, dry container; do not allow the specimen to touch water or urine
      2) Scoop out an amount of specimen and place in prepared specimen containers as directed by the manufacturer

b. Cellophane-tape test
   1) Pinworm diagnosis
   2) Female adult lays eggs in area around anus
      a) Affix tape onto the end of a slide and drape over the slide so that the adhesive side faces outward

b) Gently touch the anal area with the adhesive side of the tape
c) Undrape the tape and stick it to the slide
d) Send the slide with tape on it to the laboratory

Minor Surgery 23

I. General

A. SURGICAL PROCEDURE PERFORMED WITHIN THE MEDICAL OFFICE

B. DOES NOT REQUIRE GENERAL ANESTHESIA

II. Surgical Instruments

A. GENERAL
1. Have clearly identifiable parts for visual identification
2. Classified according to use

B. CUTTING AND DISSECTING INSTRUMENTS
1. Scissors (see Figure 23-1)
   a. Used to cut tissue and sutures
   b. Blades touch at the tip; can be curved or straight
   c. Blade combinations include:
      1) Sharp/sharp (S/S)
      2) Blunt/blunt (B/B)
      3) Sharp/blunt (S/B)
   d. Bandage scissors
      1) Blunt probe tip for easy insertion under bandage
      2) Used to remove bandages and dressings
   e. Operating scissors
      1) Metzenbaum scissors: dissects tissues
      2) Mayo scissors: cuts and dissects fascia and muscle
      3) Iris scissors: general use
   f. Gauze shears: used to cut gauze, tubing, and adhesive
   g. Stitch (or suture) scissors (Littauer)
      1) One blade has a hook to slide under sutures
      2) Used to remove sutures
2. Scalpel (see Figure 23-2)
   a. Surgical knife used to make incision
   b. May be reusable or disposable
   c. Parts include:
      1) Handle
         a) Holds the blade
         b) Many sizes and shapes (#3 is standard)
      2) Scalpel blade
         a) Disposable
         b) Fits onto handle
         c) Different sizes and shapes (#15 is standard)

C. GRASPING AND CLAMPING INSTRUMENTS (see Figures 23-3, 23-4, 23-5, 23-6, and 23-7, pp. 211-213)
Used to retract, clamp, hold, or manipulate tissue, other instruments, or sterilized materials
1. Hemostat forceps (hemostats)
   a. Jaws may or may not be serrated
   b. Used to clamp small vessels or hold tissue
      1) Kelly hemostats
      2) Mosquito hemostats
2. Needle holders (needle pushers)
   a. Jaws shorter and look stronger than hemostats
   b. Used to grasp suture needles
3. Splinter forceps
   a. Fine tip for foreign body retrieval or removal
   b. Various designs and construction
4. Thumb forceps (dressing forceps)
   a. Serrated jaws with teeth
   b. Used to insert packing into a wound or to remove objects from cavities
5. Allis tissue forceps
   a. Blunt teeth
   b. Used to grasp tissue, muscle, or skin surrounding a wound
6. Adson thumb forceps (tissue forceps)
   a. Teeth for grasping tissue
   b. Used to grasp tissue and in suturing
7. Bayonet forceps
   a. Smooth-tipped
   b. Used to insert or remove objects from nose and ear
8. Towel clamps (forceps)
   a. Very sharp hooks
   b. Various lengths
   c. Used to hold drapes in place during surgery

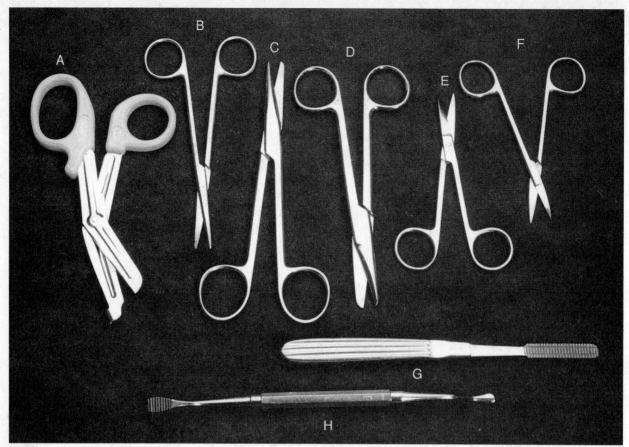

FIGURE 23-1. Operating scissors. **A,** Bandage scissors. **B,** Metzenbaum (Metz) scissors. **C,** Curved Mayo scissors. **D,** Straight Mayo scissors. **E,** Straight ins scissors. **F,** Curved ins scissors. **G,** Bone rasp, single ended. **H,** Bone rasp, double ended. (Young AP, Kennedy DB: *Kinn's the medical assistant: an applied learning approach,* ed 9, Philadelphia, 2003, Saunders.)

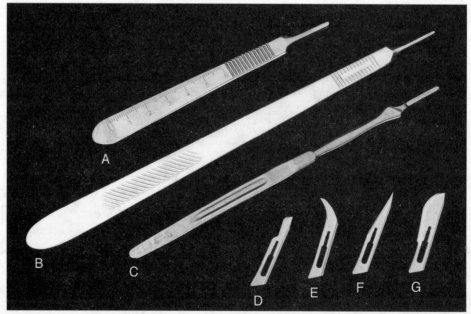

FIGURE 23-2. Scalpels. **A,** No. 3 scalpel blade. **B,** No. 3 long scalpel handle. **C,** No. 7 scalpel handle. **D,** No. 15 blade. **E,** No. 12 blade. **F,** No. 11 blade. **G,** No. 10 blade. (Young AP, Kennedy DB: *Kinn's the medical assistant: an applied learning approach,* ed 9, Philadelphia, 2003, Saunders.)

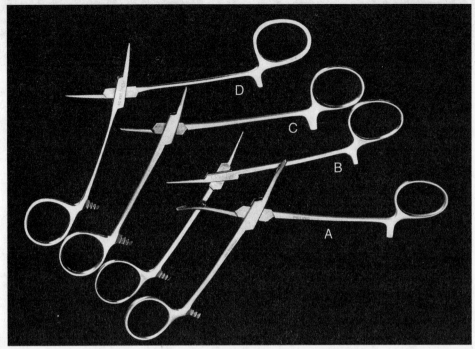

FIGURE 23-3. **A**, Kelly hemostat forceps. **B**, Mosquito hemostat forceps. **C**, Needle holder. **D**, Smooth-tip needle holder. (Young AP, Kennedy DB: *Kinn's the medical assistant: an applied learning approach*, ed 9, Philadelphia, 2003, Saunders.)

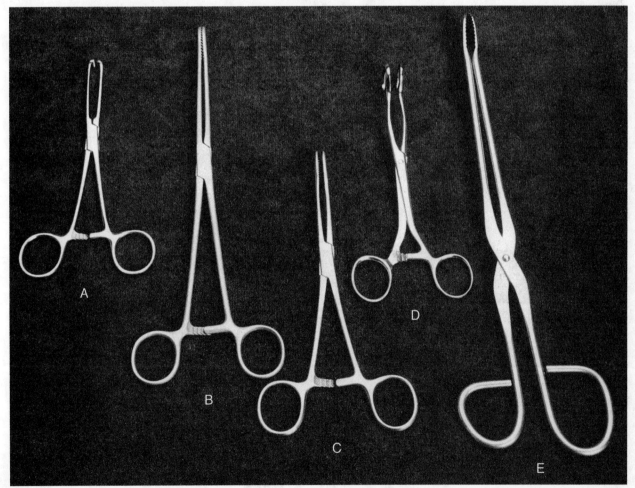

FIGURE 23-4. **A**, Allis forceps. **B**, Foerster sponge forceps. **C**, Straight transfer forceps. **D**, Short transfer forceps. **E**, Long transfer forceps. (Young AP, Kennedy DB: *Kinn's the medical assistant: an applied learning approach*, ed 9, Philadelphia, 2003, Saunders.)

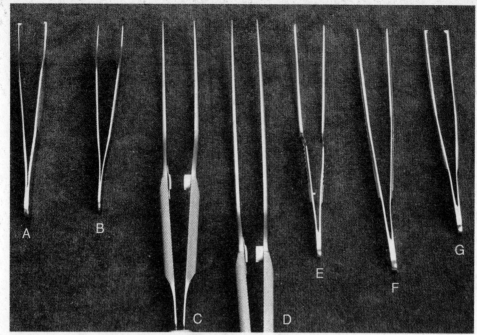

FIGURE 23-5. **A**, Toothed Adson forceps. **B**, Smooth Adson forceps. **C**, Medium long bayonet forceps. **D**, Long bayonet forceps. **E**, Short bayonet forceps. **F**, Plain-tip tissue forceps. **G**, Toothed tissue forceps. (Young AP, Kennedy DB: *Kinn's the medical assistant: an applied learning approach,* ed 9, Philadelphia, 2003, Saunders.)

9. Transfer forceps
   a. Many sizes and lengths
   b. Sterile forceps used to arrange objects on sterile field

D. RETRACTING INSTRUMENTS (see Figure 23-8)
Holds tissue away from surgical incision
   1. Rake retractor: as pronged end
   2. Senn retractor

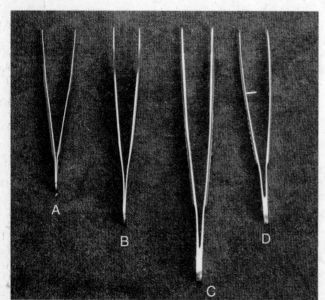

FIGURE 23-6. **A**, Splinter forceps. **B**, Smooth Adson forceps. **C**, Long plain-tip forceps. **D**, Short plain-tip tissue forceps. (Young AP, Kennedy DB: *Kinn's the medical assistant: an applied learning approach,* ed 9, Philadelphia, 2003, Saunders.)

   a. Pronged end may be sharp or dull
   b. Flat end is blunt retractor
   3. Skin hook: sharp point is used to retract small incisions or to secure skin edge for suturing
   4. Ribbon retractor (Crile malleable retractor): used to hold back tissues and organs in large wounds

E. PROBING AND DILATING INSTRUMENTS
(see Figures 23-9 and 23-10)
   1. Used for surgery and examinations
   2. Probes search a cavity or wound
   3. Dilators used to stretch a cavity or opening
      a. Specula
         1) Most common dilator used
         2) Valves spread apart and dilate the opening
         3) Includes vaginal, nasal, rectal, and ear specula
      b. Trocars and obturators
         1) Consist of sharply pointed instrument (trocar) contained within an outer tube
         2) Used to withdraw fluids from cavities or for draining and irrigating with a catheter
      c. Probes
         1) Different lengths (from 4 inches to 12 inches)
         2) Used to enter body cavities
      d. Sound: long, slender probe

F. SPECIALTY INSTRUMENTS
   1. Fall into the four main categories
   2. Specific for particular examinations in a specialty
      a. Gynecology (see Figure 23-11, p. 213)
         1) Sponge forceps: used the way dressing forceps are used
         2) Uterine dressing forceps

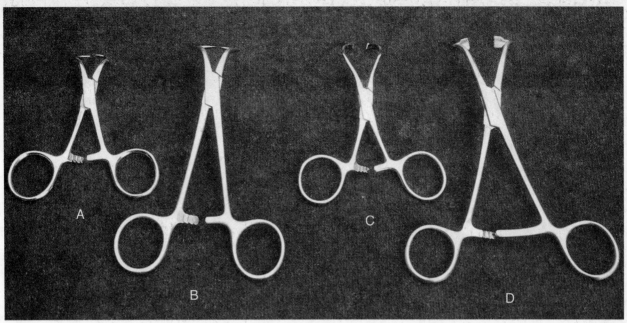

FIGURE 23-7. **A**, Small sharp towel forceps. **B**, Large sharp towel forceps. **C**, Small atraumatic towel forceps. **D**, Large atraumatic towel forceps. (Young AP, Kennedy DB: *Kinn's the medical assistant: an applied learning approach,* ed 9, Philadelphia, 2003, Saunders.)

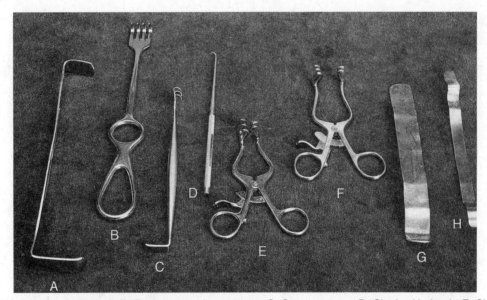

FIGURE 23-8. **A**, Army-Navy retractor. **B**, Four-prong rake retractor. **C**, Senn retractor. **D**, Single skin hook. **E**, Sharp 3/2 Weitlaner retractor. **F**, Dull 3/2 Weitlaner retractor. **G**, Wide Crile (ribbon) retractor. **H**, Narrow Crile (ribbon) retractor. (Young AP, Kennedy DB: *Kinn's the medical assistant: an applied learning approach,* ed 9, Philadelphia, 2003, Saunders.)

a) Can reach the cervix and vagina
b) Used to swab the area or to apply medications
3) Curettes (endocervical and uterine Sims)
   a) Hollow and spoon shaped
   b) Used to remove polyps, secretions, and tissue
4) Schroeder tenaculum forceps
   a) Sharp, pointed tips
   b) Used to hold tissue or cervix while obtaining specimen

5) Hegar uterine dilators: used to dilate the cervix for dilation and curettage (D&C)
b. Ophthalmology and otolaryngology (see Figure 23-12)
  1) Krause nasal snare
   a) Wire loop on tip
   b) Used to remove polyps
  2) Alligator ear forceps: used to remove foreign bodies

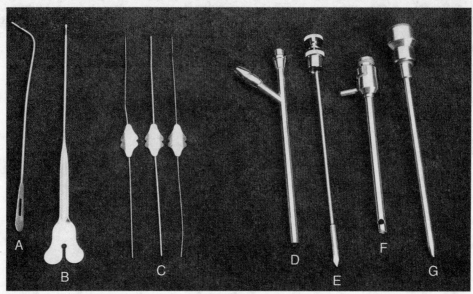

FIGURE 23-9. **A,** Probe. **B,** Grooved director. **C,** Lacrimal duct probes. **D,** Double-ended cannula. **E,** Sharp trocar. **F,** Cannula. **G,** Blunt-tip obturator. (Young AP, Kennedy DB: *Kinn's the medical assistant: an applied learning approach,* ed 9, Philadelphia, 2003, Saunders.)

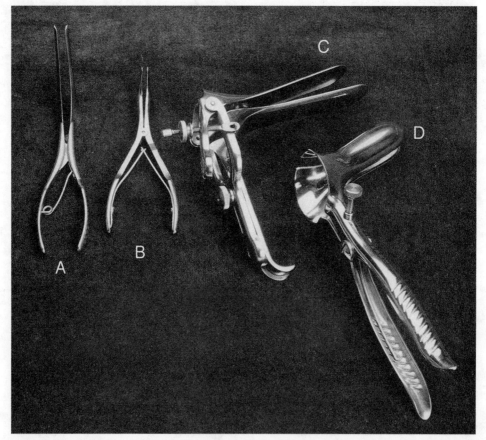

FIGURE 23-10. **A,** Long nasal speculum. **B,** Short nasal speculum. **C,** Graves vaginal speculum. **D,** Anal speculum, self-retaining. (Young AP, Kennedy DB: *Kinn's the medical assistant: an applied learning approach,* ed 9, Philadelphia, 2003, Saunders.)

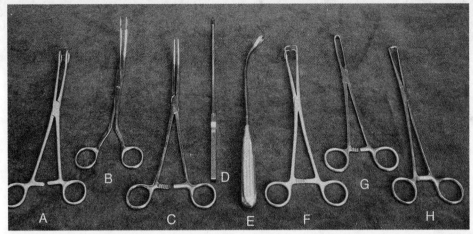

FIGURE 23-11.   **A,** Foerster sponge forceps. **B,** Placenta forceps. **C,** Bozeman uterine dressing forceps. **D,** Endocervical curette. **E,** Sims uterine curette. **F,** Schroeder uterine vulsellum forceps. **G,** Long Allis forceps. **H,** Schroeder uterine tenaculum forceps. (Young AP, Kennedy DB: *Kinn's the medical assistant: an applied learning approach,* ed 9, Philadelphia, 2003, Saunders.)

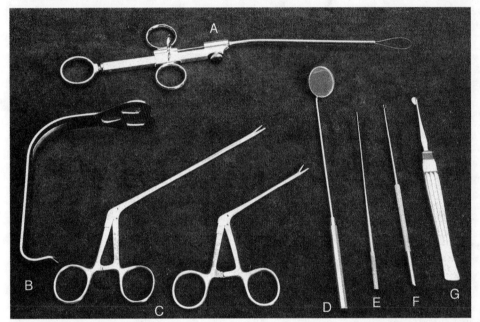

FIGURE 23-12.   **A,** Krause nasal snare. **B,** Metal tongue depressor. **C,** Long and short alligator forceps. **D,** Laryngeal mirror. **E,** Ivan metal applicator. **F,** Buck ear curette. **G,** Sharp ear dissector. (Young AP, Kennedy DB: *Kinn's the medical assistant: an applied learning approach,* ed 9, Philadelphia, 2003, Saunders.)

3) Laryngeal mirror
   a) Various sizes
   b) Used to examine larynx and postnasal area
4) Buck ear curette
   a) Sharp or blunt scraper end
   b) Used to remove foreign matter from ear canals
c. Biopsy
   1) Cervical biopsy forceps: used to obtain specimens
   2) Punch biopsy: used to remove tissue specimens

3) Biopsy needle: works on the same principle as an obturator
4) Abscess needle
   a) Used to withdraw fluids or pus from cyst or abscess
   b) Usually disposable
d. Genitourinary: Foley catheter
   1) Manufactured in sizes 8 to 32 (French)
   2) Used as an indwelling catheter
e. Endoscopes
   1) Hollow, cylindrical instruments
   2) Used to visualize the interior of a cavity or opening

a) Sigmoidoscope: used to visualize the sigmoid colon

b) Proctoscope: used to visualize the rectum

c) Anoscope: used to visualize the superficial rectum

d) Bronchoscope: used to visualize the larynx, trachea, and bronchi

e) Otoscope: used to visualize the external and middle ear

f) Cytoscope: used to visualize the urinary bladder

g) Laparoscope: used to visualize the peritoneal and abdominal cavities

III. Sutures and Needles

A. GENERAL

1. Suture: act of stitching or sewing together
2. Material used to stitch or sew
3. May also be used to ligate (tie off)

B. TYPES

1. Absorbable
   a. Dissolves and is absorbed by body's enzymes
   b. Includes:
      1) Surgical catgut (surgical gut)
         a) Used in tissues that heal rapidly
         b) Obtained from sheep, cattle, or pig intestines
         c) Packaged in alcohol to keep it pliable
      2) Chromic
         a) Catgut coated with chromic salts
         b) Delayed absorption of up to 80 days
      3) Vicryl
         a) Synthetic suture made of polyglactin
         b) Takes up to 11 weeks to absorb
2. Nonabsorbable
   a. Left in the body, where it embeds in scar tissue or must be removed when healing is complete
   b. Used frequently in office minor surgeries
   c. Types include:
      1) Silk
         a) Strong
         b) Easy to tie and remove
      2) Cotton: not used much (polyester more common)
      3) Polyester fiber: strongest of all suture material
      4) Stainless steel
         a) Surgical staples
         b) Used on skin, nerves, and blood vessels
         c) Applied with a skin stapler

C. SIZING

1. Diameter of strand determines the size
2. Sized from 6-0 (smallest) to 4 (largest)
3. Lengths of strands are precut (into 18-, 24-, 54-, and 60-inch lengths)
4. 2-0 to 6-0 most common

D. SUTURE REMOVAL

1. Physician determines the length of time sutures remain in place
2. Must always be left in place long enough for proper healing to take place
3. In general
   a. Skin sutures in head and neck: remove in 3 to 5 days
   b. Skin sutures in other areas: 7 to 10 days

E. NEEDLES

1. Chosen according to area used
2. Classified by:
   a. Shape
      1) Straight
      2) Curved (more easily manipulated)
   b. Type of point
      1) Tapered (for delicate tissue)
      2) Cutting (for skin)
   c. Eye
      1) Eyelet (have to thread the needle)
      2) Eyeless (suture material attached to the needle; atraumatic)

F. ADHESIVE SKIN CLOSURES

1. Sterile, nonallergenic tape
2. Available in a variety of widths and lengths
3. Used when not much tension exists on the skin edges
4. Applied transversely across the incision line
5. Eliminate the need for sutures and anesthetic
6. Easily applied and removed
7. Less scarring
8. Example: Steri-Strips

IV. Drapes

A. GENERAL

1. Sterile paper or cloth material placed over or around the operative site
2. Used to maintain sterility

B. TYPES

1. Plain
2. Fenestrated
   a. Contains a precut opening
   b. Opening is placed over the operative site
3. Incisional
   a. Adhesive-backed plastic
   b. Drape adheres directly to skin
   c. Incision is made through the drape

V. Anesthesia

A. GENERAL INFORMATION

1. Injected into the surgical site to prevent the sensation of pain
2. Medications used for anesthesia end in the suffix -*cain(e)*

3. Example of anesthesia medication: Xylocaine, lidocaine, and Novocaine
4. May contain epinephrine
   a. Enhances the effect of the anesthesia
   b. Minimizes bleeding at the operative site
5. Takes effect in from 5 to 15 minutes; will be effective for 1 to 3 hours

B. TYPES OF LOCAL ANESTHESIA

1. Infiltration: solution is injected under the skin to anesthetize nerve endings
2. Nerve block: solution is injected into an accessible main nerve
3. Topical: solution is painted (or sprayed) directly onto the skin or mucous membrane

VI. Surgical Asepsis (see Table 23-1)

A. GENERAL

1. Destruction of organisms before they enter the body
2. Used any time skin or mucous membrane is punctured, pierced, or incised

B. BASIC RULES

1. Clean with clean
2. Dirty with dirty
3. Sterile with sterile
4. When in doubt, throw it out

C. SURGICAL SCRUB

1. Hands and forearms scrubbed for 3 to 10 minutes
2. Use surgical soap with a brush
3. Clean under the fingernails
4. Hands held up; rinsed from fingertips to elbows
5. Dry with sterile towels
6. Glove immediately

D. STERILE GLOVES

1. Used whenever the patient needs to be protected from microorganisms (all surgical procedures)
2. Used when handling sterile instruments or sterile supplies
3. Gloving procedure
   a. Select the proper glove size
   b. Open the package
   c. With the nondominant hand, lift the glove for the dominant hand by the folded edge of the cuff
   d. Put on the glove, keeping it above your waist
   e. Pick up the second glove by placing the gloved fingers under the cuff; insert the hand; adjust the cuffs and fingers
   f. Always keep gloved hands above your waist and away from your body

E. STERILE FIELD

1. Any surface on which sterile items are placed
2. Created by draping sterile towels over a Mayo stand
3. Sterile field is also a draped surgical site after the patient's skin is prepared and draped
4. Any item placed below the waist is considered contaminated
5. The 1-inch edge around the entire sterile field is considered nonsterile
6. Edges of all wrappers, packs, and towels are nonsterile
7. Sides of containers are nonsterile
8. Moisture carries bacteria from nonsterile to sterile surfaces

F. HANDLING INSTRUMENTS AND SUPPLIES

1. Sterile forceps are used to handle sterile instruments or sterile supplies when sterile gloves are not being worn

---

TABLE 23-1   How to Distinguish between Medical and Surgical Asepsis

	Medical Asepsis	Surgical Asepsis
Definition	Destruction of organisms *after* they leave the body	Destruction of organisms *before* they enter the body
Purpose	Prevent reinfection of the patient; avoid cross-infection from one person to another	Care for open wounds; used in surgery
Technique	Universal blood and body-fluid precautions Isolation techniques	Sterile technique
Procedure	Clean objects are kept from contamination	Objects must be sterile
	Clean gloves and clean barriers used	Sterile gloves and articles used
	Objects disinfected as soon as possible after contact with the patient	Objects must be sterilized before contact with the patient
When used	For examinations that do not involve open wounds or breaks in the skin or mucous membranes but do involve patient blood or body fluids; isolating infected persons from others	Surgery, biopsy, wound treatment, insertion of instruments into sterile body cavities
Hand-washing technique	Hands and wrists washed for 1 to 2 minutes; soap, water, and plenty of friction used to remove oil and microorganisms from fingers	Hand and forearms scrubbed for 3 to 10 minutes; surgical soap, running water, friction, and sterile brush used; fingernails must be cleaned
	Hands held downward, running water allowed to drain off fingertips; hands dried with paper towels	Hands held up, under running water, to drain off elbows; hands dried with sterile towels

From Kinn ME, Woods MA: *The medical assistant: administrative and clinical,* ed 8, Philadelphia, 1999, WB Saunders, p 1087.

a. Lift forceps out of the container without touching the sides of the container

b. Touch the tips of the forceps to sterile gauze to dry

c. Always keep forceps tips facing down

2. Lids removed from containers are placed face up on surfaces; hold face down if not placed on surfaces

3. Pour solutions to avoid splashing; avoid touching the rim of a sterile receptacle with the bottle

4. Do not reach over the sterile field

5. Cover the setup with a sterile towel if it is not to be used immediately

G. SKIN PREPARATION

1. Skin cannot be sterilized

2. Resident and transient bacteria must be completely removed

3. Skin preparation is performed by a gloved assistant

4. Make sure that the patient is not allergic to the surgical scrub solution used (examples: Betadine, iodine)

5. Area is cleansed in a circular motion from the inside of the circle out; repeat the cleansing with a new sponge; dry with sterile, dry sponges

VII.   Wounds

A. DEFINITION

1. Interruption in continuity of internal or external body tissues

B. TYPES OF WOUNDS

1. Closed wound
   a. Nonpenetrating
   b. No outward opening
   c. Underlying tissue is damaged

2. Open wound
   a. Skin is broken
   b. Underlying tissue is exposed
   c. Classified according to the appearance of the opening
      1) Laceration: jagged, irregular, breaking or tearing of tissues
      2) Puncture: skin is pierced by a pointed object (e.g., pin, nail, splinter)
      3) Abrasion: superficial wound; scraping of the skin
      4) Avulsion: tissue is torn away or separated
      5) Surgical incision: neat, clean cut
      6) Contusion: closed, nonpenetrating wound; blood from broken vessels accumulates in tissues

C. WOUND HEALING (see Figure 23-13)

1. All wounds go through healing (repair)

2. Three phases:
   a. Lag phase
      1) Blood vessels contract to control bleeding
      2) Platelets form a plug
      3) Fibrin is released to begin clotting (dried clot becomes the scab)
      4) White blood cells arrive at the site to clear away debris
      5) Within 1 to 4 days, fibrin threads contract and pull the edges of the wound together under the scab
   b. Proliferation phase
      1) Lasts from 5 to 20 days
      2) Tissues repair themselves
      3) Wound continues to contract and seal
   c. Remodeling phase
      1) Day 21 on
      2) Scar tissue forms
      3) Scar tissue is not true skin; very strong and nonelastic
      4) Scar tissue is connective tissue without blood or nerve supply

D. CLASSIFICATION OF WOUND REPAIR

1. First intention
   a. Minimal tissue damage and scarring
   b. Wound may be sutured closed

2. Second intention
   a. Wound edges are not sutured or approximated
   b. Heals slowly from bottom up
   c. Large amount of scarring

3. Third intention: infected wound requires reopening

VIII.   Dressings and Bandages

A. DRESSINGS

1. Sterile covering placed over wound

2. Protect wound from injury and/or contamination

3. Maintain constant pressure on the wound

4. Help hold wound edges together

5. Control bleeding

6. Absorb drainage and secretions

7. Hide temporary disfigurement

8. May need to be removed periodically so that the wound can be checked for healing or suture removal

9. Always note drainage in chart
   a. Sanguineous: contains mostly blood
   b. Purulent: contains pus
   c. Serosanguineous: contains blood and serous fluid
   d. Serous: contains no blood
   e. May note amount and odor

B. BANDAGES

1. Nonsterile material used to hold dressings in place
   a. Splints and protects injured tissue
   b. Maintains pressure on the wound
   c. Aids in circulation

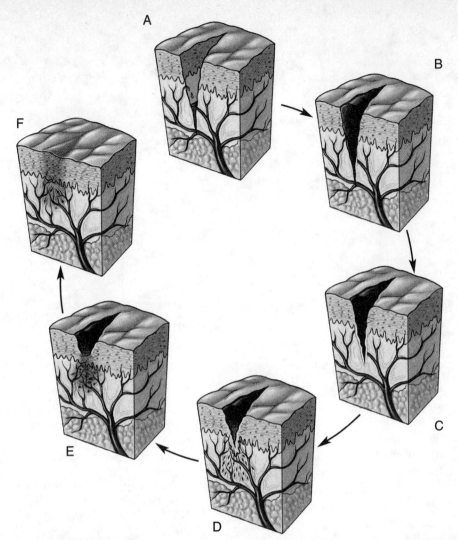

FIGURE 23-13. Steps in tissue repair. **A**, A deep wound to the skin severs blood vessels, causing blood to fill the wound. **B**, A blood clot forms, and as it dries, it forms a scab. **C** and **D**, The process of tissue repair begins. Scar tissue forms in the deep layers. **E**, At the same time, surface epithelial cells multiply and fill the area between the scar tissue and the scab. **F**, When the epithelium is complete, the scab detaches. The result is a fully regenerated layer of epithelium over an underlying area of scar tissue. (From Herlihy B, Maebius N: *The human body in health and illness,* 2 ed, Philadelphia, 2003, Saunders.)

2. Made up of different materials and different sizes
   a. Gauze roller bandage
   b. Kling (self-adhering)
   c. Elastic cloth (Ace)
   d. Adhesive bandage (Band-Aid)
   e. Seamless tubular gauze (Tube-gauze)

IX. Patient Education

A. INSTRUCT THE PATIENT TO CONTACT THE PRACTITIONER IMMEDIATELY TO REPORT:

1. Excessive bleeding at the wound site
2. Fever
3. Redness, swelling, or streaking around the wound site

24 *Office Emergencies*

I. General

A. FIRST AID
1. Immediate care given to a person who has been injured or suddenly taken ill
2. The medical assistant, in emergencies, is covered by Good Samaritan laws at the scene of an accident
3. Keep emergency telephone numbers near telephones in the office
4. As an employee of a medical facility, keep cardiopulmonary resuscitation (CPR) and first-aid cards current
5. Do not provide care beyond your scope of training or beyond your abilities
6. Call for help or 911 when needed

II. Rules for Emergencies

A. STAY CALM
1. Reassure the patient and make the patient as comfortable as possible

B. SURVEY THE SITUATION, AND DECIDE WHETHER THE NEED IS EMERGENT
1. If a true emergency exists, call 911

C. EXAMINE THE SCENE

D. AIRWAY IS FIRST PRIORITY
1. Perform CPR until help arrives

E. IF THE PATIENT IS CONSCIOUS, CONSENT MUST BE OBTAINED; IF THE PATIENT IS UNCONSCIOUS, CONSENT IS IMPLIED

F. CARE FOR LIFE-THREATENING CONDITIONS FIRST

G. AFTER THE EMERGENCY IS UNDER CONTROL, ACCURATELY DOCUMENT THE EVENTS AND MEDICATIONS USED

H. FOLLOW STANDARD PRECAUTIONS AT ALL TIMES

III. Common Emergencies

A. FAINTING (SYNCOPE)
1. Lay the patient with the patient's head lower than the heart
2. Loosen the patient's tight clothing
3. Maintain an open airway
4. Apply a cool cloth to the patient's head
5. Pass aromatic spirits of ammonia under the patient's nose
6. Keep the patient supine for 10 minutes after consciousness is regained

B. CHOKING
1. Do not interfere if the patient can speak, cough, or breathe
2. Use the Heimlich maneuver if the victim cannot speak, cough, or breathe
3. If the patient becomes unconscious, position the patient on his or her back; call for help
4. Begin CPR after removing the foreign body

C. CHEST PAIN
1. Sit the patient down
2. Keep the patient quiet and warm
3. Loosen the patient's tight clothing
4. Take the apical and radial pulse
5. Administer oxygen if the practitioner orders
6. Bring the emergency (*crash*) cart into the room
7. If cardiac arrest occurs, perform CPR

D. CEREBROVASCULAR ACCIDENT (CVA)
1. Call for help
2. Protect the patient against injury while waiting for transport
3. Keep the patient lying down
4. Maintain an open airway
5. Do not give food or water

E. POISONING
1. Ask what was taken, how much was taken, how long ago, and whether vomiting has occurred
2. Call the poison control center
3. Induce vomiting (unless a corrosive had been ingested) or dilute with 1 to 2 cups of water or milk; give 1 tablespoon of syrup of ipecac (or follow specific directions given by the poison control center)

F. ANIMAL BITES
1. Thoroughly wash the wound with soap and water
2. Report the bite to the authorities

G. INSECT BITES AND STINGS
1. Remove the stinger by brushing it off or using tweezers
2. Apply ice to the bite area
3. Be aware of patient allergy to insect bites or stings
4. If the patient is allergic and shows signs of shock or difficulty breathing, a true emergency exists

H. SHOCK
1. Ensure and maintain an open airway
2. Call 911
3. While waiting for transport, place the patient on his or her back with legs elevated above the heart
4. Loosen the patient's tight clothing
5. Cover the patient with a blanket to maintain warmth

I. ASTHMA ATTACK
1. Assist the patient with an inhaler
2. Encourage and assist the patient to relax
3. Patient may breathe into a paper bag if hyperventilating

J. SEIZURES
1. Lay the patient on his or her back
2. Loosen the patient's tight clothing
3. Do not restrain the patient
4. Protect the patient's head from injury
5. Give the patient nothing by mouth
6. Let the patient rest after the seizure subsides

K. SPRAIN
1. Elevate the sprained area
2. Apply mild compression
3. Apply ice

L. FRACTURES
1. Make the patient as comfortable as possible
2. Prevent movement of the injured area
3. Apply ice
4. Control bleeding, if applicable
5. Assist the health care provider

M. BURNS
1. Remove the patient's clothing from the burned area
2. Stay with the patient
3. Assist the health care provider

N. LACERATIONS
1. Keep the patient as calm as possible
2. Cover the area with a sterile dressing using standard precautions
3. Apply direct pressure to the wound to control bleeding using standard precautions
4. Elevate the injured area above the level of the patient's heart
5. Ask the patient about when the last tetanus injection was given
6. Cleanse the wound if it is not bleeding severely
7. Assist the health care provider

O. NOSEBLEEDS (Epistaxis)
1. Keep the patient quiet and in a sitting position
2. Apply direct pressure to the affected nostril by pinching

P. HEMORRHAGE
1. Apply direct pressure over the area; do not remove the original pad when it becomes saturated; add additional pads
2. Elevate the injured part above the patient's heart
3. Apply pressure over the area's pressure point
4. As a last resort, apply a tourniquet as directed by the health care provider
5. Assist the health care provider

Q. HEAD INJURIES
1. Lay the patient flat
2. Do not move the patient if a neck injury is suspected
3. Do not administer the patient anything by mouth
4. Keep the patient warm and quiet
5. Watch the patient's pupils for changes
6. Assist the health care provider

R. DIABETIC EMERGENCIES
1. For hypoglycemia (insulin shock): give juice, candy, or soda (a sugar source)
2. For hyperglycemia (diabetic coma): if the patient is conscious, administer fluids; if you are uncertain whether this is insulin shock or diabetic coma, give the patient a sugar source
3. Assist the health care provider

S. FOREIGN BODY IN THE EYE
1. Place the patient in a darkened room
2. Apply a cool, wet compress to the affected eye; do not apply pressure
3. Assist the health care provider

Post-Test

Directions: Each of the following questions is followed by four or five possible responses. Select the *best* response.

1. Which of the following documents applies to donation of anatomical gifts?
   A. Advanced directive
   B. Uniform Anatomical Gift Act
   C. Living will
   D. Durable power of attorney

2. Which endocrine gland produces calcitonin?
   A. Pituitary
   B. Thyroid
   C. Pineal
   D. Adrenal

3. In which of the following situations can a patient's medical record be released without a signed authorization?
   A. The patient's attorney requests them
   B. The patient is human immunodeficiency virus (HIV) positive
   C. An insurance company requests them
   D. Another physician requests them

4. Which of the following health care workers is licensed to practice?
   A. Medical assistant
   B. Histotechnologist
   C. Registered nurse
   D. Laboratory assistant

5. Which of the following would be the most appropriate first step when dealing with a patient who is distraught and angry?
   A. Escort the patient to a private area
   B. Ask the patient to calm down
   C. Inform the patient that the physician will see him or her shortly
   D. Ask the patient to have a seat in the waiting room

6. Hematopoiesis is
   A. The formation of new fingernails
   B. The production of new blood cells
   C. State of equilibrium within the body
   D. The formation of scar tissue

7. A 75-year-old woman with emphysema continues to smoke and to miss appointments against the orders of her physician. What is the most appropriate next step?
   A. Notify the patient that her medical care is being terminated
   B. Instruct her family how to change her behavior
   C. Accept her behavior and adjust her treatment
   D. Refer her to a psychiatrist

8. Which of the following would be the most appropriate action for the medical assistant to take when the physician is running behind schedule?
   A. Tell the patients that the physician will be with them soon
   B. Show a video in the waiting room
   C. Explain the delay and offer another appointment if the patient requests one
   D. Tell the physician to not spend as much time with the patients

9. Which of the following agencies regulates licensure for physicians?
   A. Local hospital boards
   B. Federal government
   C. Medical colleges
   D. State government

10. This document allows a patient to grant her husband legal authority to act on her behalf?
    A. A living will
    B. A deposition
    C. Informed consent
    D. Durable power of attorney

11. "Have you had this problem in the past?" is an example of which of the following types of questions?
    A. Leading
    B. Open-ended
    C. Closed-ended
    D. Nonleading

12. An 18-year-old woman comes into the office for a sexually transmitted disease (STD) test. The next day, her mother calls and asks for the results. Which of the following prevents disclosure of this information?
    A. Health Insurance Portability and Accountability Act (HIPAA)
    B. Health Care Improvement Act
    C. Patient Self-Determination Act
    D. Durable power of attorney

13. Which of the following developmental stages is characterized by the desire to belong to a group and a need for independence and privacy?
    A. Infancy
    B. Adolescence
    C. Adulthood
    D. Old age

14. A lateral curvature of the spine is known as
    A. Spondylosis
    B. Scoliosis
    C. Kyphosis
    D. Lordosis

15. The best method for transmitting confidential information from one medical practice to another is by
    A. Fax
    B. E-mail
    C. Cellular telephone
    D. Answering machine

16. The best method for communicating with an elderly patient would be to
    A. Speak loudly
    B. Avoid eye contact
    C. Use medical terminology to explain information
    D. Encourage questions

17. Ischemia is
    A. An irregular heartbeat
    B. Dilation of the aorta
    C. Lack of blood flow to tissue
    D. Infection of the myocardium

18. The correct term that describes fluid that drains from a wound is
    A. Cirrus
    B. Serious
    C. Serous
    D. Sclerotic

19. A patient whose husband recently passed away comes into the office because of malaise. She is unkempt and weepy. She tells the medical assistant that she wishes she were dead. Which of the following would be the most sensitive response to this patient?
    A. "Please tell me more about those feelings."
    B. "Why is that?"
    C. "You need to talk to the doctor about this."
    D. "That's natural to feel that way after the death of a spouse."

20. Which of the following would most likely be the cause of the revocation of a physician's license?
    A. Self-teaching a new surgical procedure
    B. Failing to obtain continuing education units
    C. Failing to produce medical records that have been subpoenaed by the court
    D. Committing active euthanasia
    E. Performing medical research without the consent of the patient

21. Tingling in the hands, numbness in the arm, and frequent episodes of blurred vision are characteristic of
    A. An aneurysm
    B. Epilepsy
    C. Tourette's syndrome
    D. Lou Gehrig's disease
    E. Transient ischemic attack

22. A woman patient with advanced breast cancer refuses to allow her mother to care for her. She becomes extremely upset when her family members talk about her maternal grandmother who died of the disease. Which of the following defense mechanisms is this patient using?
    A. Sublimation
    B. Denial
    C. Projection
    D. Displacement
    E. Rationalization

23. Which of the following punctuation marks is used to indicate the exact words of the patient?
    A. Semicolon
    B. Comma
    C. Quotation marks
    D. Colon

24. The suffix that means *deficiency* is
    A. -penia
    B. -plasia
    C. -plegia
    D. -plexy

25. A mucous membrane
    A. Lines closed cavities of the body
    B. Covers the lungs
    C. Lines the abdominal cavity
    D. Lines body cavities that open to the outside of the body

26. Which of the following demonstrates proper grammar?
    A. There was no recurrence of the tumor
    B. Review of systems were negative
    C. She neither drinks or smokes
    D. He was scheduled for replacement of his aorta valve

27. Which of the following is the most effective way of communicating with a patient who does not speak English?
    A. Speaking slowly and loudly
    B. Encouraging nonverbal communication
    C. Maintaining eye contact with the patient
    D. Putting messages in writing

28. Which of the following is a fungal infection of the skin?
    A. Scabies
    B. Ringworm
    C. Impetigo
    D. Psoriasis

29. The term that refers to the back of the body is
    A. Frontal
    B. Distal
    C. Dorsal
    D. Proximal

30. An x-ray study to confirm the diagnosis of a break in the bone of the thigh would be ordered on which of the following?
    A. Femur
    B. Radius
    C. Tibia
    D. Humerus

31. Spermatozoa are produced in the
    A. Epididymis
    B. Seminiferous tubules
    C. Prostate gland
    D. Vas deferens

32. An acute infectious skin disease caused by streptococci or staphylococci is
    A. Impetigo
    B. Psoriasis
    C. Athlete's foot
    D. Eczema

33. The bone located in the posterior of the skull is the
    A. Frontal
    B. Ethmoid
    C. Temporal
    D. Occipital

34. Bile is produced in which of the following organs?
    A. Gallbladder
    B. Liver
    C. Pancreas
    D. Stomach

35. According to Maslow's hierarchy of needs, which of the following is the primary motivation for human behavior?
    A. Survival
    B. Safety
    C. Love
    D. Self-actualization

36. Oxygen that has been inspired enters the circulatory system through which of the following structures of the respiratory system?
    A. Pharynx
    B. Trachea
    C. Bronchi
    D. Alveoli

37. A failure of bone marrow to produce red blood cells results in which type of anemia?
   A. Aplastic
   B. Hemolytic
   C. Pernicious
   D. Microcytic

38. Protrusion of a part of the stomach through the esophageal opening in the diaphragm is a(n)
   A. Esophageal aneurysm
   B. Esophageal varices
   C. Hiatal hernia
   D. Pyloric stenosis

39. Which of the following is an example of an open-ended question?
   A. "Have you been staying on your diet?"
   B. "Did you have a nice trip?"
   C. "Are you single or married?"
   D. "Can you tell me more about that?"

40. The suffix -iasis means
   A. Surgical puncture
   B. Abnormal condition
   C. Inflammation
   D. Artificial opening

41. Res ipsa loquitur is best illustrated by which of the following?
   A. A physician accidentally amputates the wrong finger from a patient
   B. A physician diagnoses lung cancer but the patient continues to smoke
   C. A physician prescribes the wrong medication for a patient
   D. A physician terminates care of a patient but does notify him or her in writing

42. A physician accepts payment from another physician for the referral of a patient. This practice is known as
   A. Fee for service
   B. Fee splitting
   C. Professional courtesy
   D. Referral

43. Which of the following demonstrates an involuntary muscle action?
   A. Heartbeat
   B. Breathing
   C. Peristalsis
   D. Pupil dilation
   E. All of the above

44. Which of the following combining forms means tongue?
   A. Gloss/o
   B. Goni/o
   C. Gingiv/o
   D. Galact/o

45. Release of a patient's medical records without proper authorization might result in charges of
   A. Abandonment
   B. Invasion of privacy
   C. Defamation of character
   D. Negligence

46. Which of the following federal acts regulates the dispensing of a controlled substance?
   A. Drug Enforcement Act
   B. Food, Drug and Cosmetic Act
   C. Occupational Safety and Health Act
   D. Controlled Substance Act

47. The alpha cells in the pancreas are responsible for the production of
   A. Insulin
   B. Glucagon
   C. Hydrochloric acid
   D. Pepsin

48. The surgical removal of the gallbladder is a
   A. Cholectomy
   B. Colostomy
   C. Cholecystectomy
   D. Laparoscopy

49. These tiny projections on the surface of the small intestines increase the surface area and allow for greater absorption of nutrients.
   A. Rugae
   B. Villi
   C. Diverticula
   D. Omenta

50. The substances produced by the body to counteract viruses, bacteria, and toxins are
   A. Antigens
   B. Antibodies
   C. Agranulocytes
   D. Antibiotics

51. Legally, a physician
    A. May not refuse treatment in an emergency situation
    B. May refuse to provide follow-up care after initial treatment
    C. Must provide a diagnosis to a patient's employer if requested
    D. Must provide a medical history to the patient's insurance company if the insurance company requests it
    E. May refuse to accept a patient if he or she chooses

52. An itinerary
    A. Is a yearly schedule
    B. Is a travel guide
    C. Contains tickets
    D. Is a detailed outline of a trip
    E. Makes travel arrangements

53. Professionalism may best be displayed by
    A. Keeping emotions to self
    B. Staying calm when dealing with angry patients
    C. Showing no consideration for other members of the team
    D. Referring all problems to the physician
    E. Arriving late or leaving early

54. The ability to imagine taking the place of the patient and accepting the patient's behavior is
    A. Objectivity
    B. Empathy
    C. Sympathy
    D. Industry
    E. Subjectivity

55. The combining form for *uterus* is
    A. Vagin/o
    B. Hyster/o
    C. Salping/o
    D. Oophor/o

56. A breast mass is found in a woman whose mother and sister have died from breast cancer. She cancels her next three follow-up appointments. Which defense mechanism is she using?
    A. Denial
    B. Anxiety
    C. Acceptance
    D. Isolation
    E. Suppression

57. Personality differences are due to
    A. Age
    B. Experience
    C. Heredity
    D. Environment
    E. All of the above

58. Which is *not* a characteristic desirable in a medical assistant?
    A. Appreciation
    B. Impatience
    C. Flexibility
    D. Friendliness
    E. Concern

59. Which of the following is a segment of the large intestine?
    A. Pylorus
    B. Cecum
    C. Duodenum
    D. Jejunum

60. To release medical information,
    A. The physician must sign a waiver
    B. The insurance company must make the request in writing
    C. The patient must sign a release form
    D. A certified record technician must be employed by the office

61. Blood that is low in oxygen exits the heart through the
    A. Aorta
    B. Pulmonary artery
    C. Pulmonary vein
    D. Inferior vena cava

62. Which of the following is considered to be part of objective data?
    A. Vital signs
    B. Surgical history
    C. Last menstrual period (LMP)
    D. Insurance information

63. Which of the following telephone calls should be given immediately to the physician?
    A. Another physician
    B. An angry patient
    C. A patient's family member
    D. An insurance company

64. The combining form *enter/o* means
    A. Trachea
    B. Small intestines
    C. Stomach
    D. Rectum

65. If a patient refuses to consent to treatment, the medical assistant should
    A. Schedule the patient for another appointment
    B. Force treatment on the patient
    C. Force the patient to consent
    D. Delay treatment and inform or consult with the physician

66. An enforceable contract contains
    A. An offer
    B. An acceptance
    C. A consideration
    D. A capacity
    E. All of the above

67. Which of the following suffixes means *cutting into?*
    A. -ectomy
    B. -ostomy
    C. -plasty
    D. -itis

68. Informed consent should include which of the following elements?
    A. Benefits and risks of the treatment
    B. Purpose of treatment
    C. Nature of the patient's condition
    D. Assessment of the patient's understanding of the treatment
    E. All of the above

69. Contraction of the smooth muscles of the walls of the small intestines that facilitates the movement of food is called
    A. Deglutition
    B. Mastication
    C. Peristalsis
    D. Eructation

70. The tube that leads from the kidney to the urinary bladder is the
    A. Vas deferens
    B. Ureter
    C. Urethra
    D. Epididymis

71. Which of the following mandates identifies the need for patient privacy in medical facilities?
    A. Occupational Safety and Health Administration (OSHA)
    B. Americans with Disabilities Act (ADA)
    C. Health Insurance Portability and Accountability Act (HIPAA)
    D. Clinical Laboratory Improvement Amendments of 1988 (CLIA '88)

72. Which is *not* a bone of the lower extremity?
    A. Femur
    B. Humerus
    C. Tibia
    D. Fibula

73. The muscle in the upper extremity that is used as an injection site is the
    A. Deltoid
    B. Biceps brachii
    C. Triceps brachii
    D. Gluteus medius

74. The disease characterized by an abnormal hardening and thickening of the walls of the arteries is
    A. Atherosclerosis
    B. Arteriostenosis
    C. Atheronecrosis
    D. Atheromatosis

75. Which of the following suffixes means *to crush?*
    A. -tomy
    B. -tripsy
    C. -tropic
    D. -tresia

76. The liver
    A. Makes bile
    B. Detoxifies harmful substances
    C. Produces heparin
    D. Stores glycogen
    E. All of the above

77. A patient's medical information can be released without written consent to which of the following?
    A. A member of the patient's family
    B. A referring physician when it pertains directly to the course of treatment
    C. A private insurance company
    D. A physician who has treated the patient in the past

78. This type of tissue forms the outer surface of the body.
    A. Adipose
    B. Connective
    C. Epithelial
    D. Mucosa

79. Which of the following medical terms is in plural form?
    A. Apex
    B. Bacteria
    C. Epiphysis
    D. Nucleus

80. The best way to interview a 9-year-old child who has severe bruising on his upper arms is to
    A. Finish the child's sentences
    B. Ask leading questions
    C. Allow the parent to answer the questions
    D. Allow the child to answer the questions in his own words

81. The Occupational Safety and Health Act is designed primarily to protect which of the following individuals?
    A. The employee
    B. The employer
    C. The patient
    D. The drug salesman

82. Insulin
    A. Is produced by the liver
    B. Increases blood sugar levels
    C. Decreases blood sugar levels
    D. Controls blood calcium levels

83. A decrease in the total number of white blood cells is
    A. Leukocyte
    B. Leukocytosis
    C. Anemia
    D. Leukopenia

84. The abbreviation meaning *immediately* is
    A. prn
    B. stat
    C. qod
    D. ad lib

85. The physician is legally obligated to report
    A. Deaths
    B. Births
    C. Communicable diseases
    D. Abuse
    E. All of the above

86. The prefix *brady-* denotes
    A. Slow
    B. Fast
    C. Hard
    D. Difficult

87. The opposite of superficial is
    A. Ventral
    B. Proximal
    C. Deep
    D. Distal

88. An authorization in advance to withdraw artificial life support is
    A. Battery
    B. An advanced directive
    C. Uniform Anatomical Gift Act
    D. Good Samaritan Act

89. Unconsciously avoiding the reality of an unpleasant event is
    A. Regression
    B. Denial
    C. Repression
    D. Suppression

90. Excess carbohydrates are stored in muscles and the liver in the form of
    A. Glucagon
    B. Glucose
    C. Glucoside
    D. Glycogen

91. The study of the cause of disease is
    A. Epidemiology
    B. Pathology
    C. Etiology
    D. Risk management

92. Nonverbal communication may be conveyed by
    A. Touch
    B. Eye contact
    C. Body position
    D. Silence
    E. All of the above

93. Bulimia is
    A. A mass of food
    B. An eating disorder
    C. Loss of appetite
    D. A blood condition

94. A cerebral vascular accident can also be called a(n)
    A. Arrhythmia
    B. Heart attack
    C. Aneurysm
    D. Stroke

95. Rubeola is another name for
    A. Herpes simplex I
    B. Whooping cough
    C. Measles
    D. Chicken pox

96. A sexually transmitted disease caused by a protozoal infestation is
    A. Herpes
    B. Gonorrhea
    C. Trichomoniasis
    D. Syphilis

97. An electrolyte that has an important influence of the activity of the heart muscles is
    A. Chloride
    B. Magnesium
    C. Phosphorus
    D. Potassium

98. Which of the following respiratory disorders is characterized by a loss of lung capacity?
    A. Asthma
    B. Emphysema
    C. Bronchitis
    D. Tuberculosis

99. Which of the following specialists would treat patients with disorders of the larynx?
    A. Cardiologist
    B. Dermatologist
    C. Neurologist
    D. Otorhinolaryngologist

100. When a visually impaired patient comes into the medical office, which of the following actions would be the *least* appropriate?
    A. Taking the patient's arm to guide him or her without speaking
    B. Asking what assistance he or she may prefer to receive
    C. Respecting him or her refusal of assistance
    D. Waiting until he or she gives a cue for assistance

Administrative Content

101. Which of the following is most likely to reduce patient satisfaction with a medical practice?
    A. Explaining the risks and benefits of a procedure
    B. Discussing fees
    C. Overbooking
    D. Taking notes while interviewing the patient

102. Which of the following documents contains information about hotel reservations and travel arrangements?
    A. Agenda
    B. Minutes
    C. Memorandum
    D. Itinerary

103. Which of the following devices has the ability to digitize and convert images into an electronic format?
    A. A keyboard
    B. A monitor
    C. A printer
    D. A scanner

104. This type of agreement is designed to prevent excessive costs for equipment repairs.
    A. Service contract
    B. Factory warranty agreement
    C. Extended warranty agreement
    D. A lease

105. What is the monthly net income for a medical practice whose expenses are $8,500, revenue is $14,130, total assets are $263,000, and liabilities are $53,000?
    A. $5,630
    B. $22,630
    C. $39,000
    D. $210,000

106. Which of the following letter styles has all lines beginning flush with the left margin?
    A. Full block
    B. Simple
    C. Standard modifies block
    D. Indented modified block

107. The file folder label for Jennie Holmes-Mathis should be
    A. Jennie, Holmes-Mathis
    B. Mathis, Jennie Holmes
    C. Holmes-Mathis, Jennie
    D. Mathis, Jennie (nee Holmes)

108. A fee schedule can also be known as a(n)
    A. Encounter form
    B. Patient ledger card
    C. Price list
    D. Inventory

109. The date must be changed daily on which of the following?
    A. Computer
    B. Transcriber
    C. Fax machine
    D. Postage meter

110. The practice of leaving two appointment times open in the daily schedule is known as
    A. Triage
    B. Buffer time
    C. Offering flexible office hours
    D. Modified-wave scheduling

111. When the word *Confidential* is to be typed on the envelope, it should be placed
    A. In the lower right corner
    B. In the lower left corner
    C. Below the return address
    D. Both B and C

112. What will happen when the fourth and fifth digits of an ICD-9-CM code are omitted?
    A. The claim will be denied
    B. The claim will be paid faster
    C. The payment amount will be increased
    D. Third-party downcoding will take place

113. Which of the following may be used to replace a medical record that has temporarily been removed from the filing cabinet?
    A. 3 × 5 card
    B. An OUTguide
    C. A yellow Post-it note
    D. An empty file folder

114. Which of the following coding systems is used for morbidity coding?
    A. *Physicians' Desk Reference* (PDR)
    B. *Current Procedural Terminology* (CPT)
    C. *International Classification of Diseases*, ninth edition, Clinical Modification (ICD-9-CM)
    D. Health Care Financing Administration Common Procedure Coding System (HCPCS)

115. When is the most appropriate time to discuss payment arrangements with a new patient?
    A. When the patient calls to make an appointment
    B. When the insurance form is processed
    C. When statements are sent out
    D. At the time of the first visit

116. A tickler file is
    A. A guide for processing insurance claims
    B. A list of procedures for equipment maintenance
    C. A type of color-coding
    D. Future events arranged in chronologic order

117. All of the following would require a CPT code *except*
    A. Diarrhea
    B. Mastectomy
    C. Hysterectomy
    D. Sigmoidoscopy

118. In a medical record that uses the POMR method, where would management, workup, and therapy be located?
    A. Database
    B. Progress notes
    C. Problem list
    D. Treatment plan

119. A patient has had a left thyroid lobectomy performed. In preparing the insurance claim form, coding for which of the following body systems should be selected?
    A. Sensory
    B. Integumentary
    C. Endocrine
    D. Nervous

120. When preparing a purchase order, which of the following should be calculated first?
    A. Shipping costs
    B. Sales tax
    C. Cost of items
    D. Delivery charges

121. The amount of federal tax withheld is based on the employee's exemptions, pay period, and
    A. State income tax
    B. Employee's marital status
    C. Benefits offered by the employer
    D. Disability of the employee

122. Which of the following are Evaluation and Management (E&M) descriptors?
    A. Physical examination
    B. School physical
    C. Well-baby check-up
    D. Preoperative physical
    E. All of the above

123. Which of the following is an example of an indirect filing system?
    A. Alphabetic
    B. Chronologic
    C. Numeric
    D. Subject

124. What is the primary purpose of a patient medical record filing system?
    A. To protect the confidentiality of the patient
    B. To make document retrieval easier
    C. To organize documents for physician review
    D. To make documents available to all staff members

125. When creating an office policy manual, it should begin with
    A. The dress code
    B. The hierarchy chart
    C. Office hours
    D. The mission statement

126. When adding information to the medical record, new notes are added
  A. In alphabetic order
  B. In subject order
  C. Newest to the front
  D. Newest to the back

127. Which of the following telephone calls require immediate transfer to the physician?
  A. A young child with a high fever
  B. A patient with a possible medical allergy
  C. Another physician
  D. An adult with a low-grade fever

128. An example of an expendable item is a(n)
  A. Syringe
  B. Computer
  C. Autoclave
  D. Otoscope

129. In the double-entry accounting system, an asset would be
  A. The amount owed to a creditor
  B. Properties owned by the business
  C. Money owed to the practice by patients
  D. The amount by which liabilities exceed the equity

130. Standard size paper and envelope for business correspondence is
  A. 8½ × 11; no. 10 envelope
  B. 7¼ × 10½; no. 7¾ envelope
  C. 5½ × 8½; 3½ × 6 envelope
  D. 6¼ × 9¼; no. 6¾ envelope

131. Which of the following forms indicates an employee's withholding allowance?
  A. 1099
  B. W-2
  C. W-3
  D. W-4

132. Which of the following guarantees overnight delivery?
  A. Certified mail
  B. Express mail
  C. Priority mail
  D. Registered mail

133. The record of the proceedings of a meeting is the
  A. Agenda
  B. "Robert's Rules"
  C. Itinerary
  D. Minutes

134. In an ICD-9-CM code, how many digits are contained in the code that is listed at the highest level of specificity?
  A. two
  B. three
  C. four
  D. five
  E. six

135. The scheduling system based on scheduling similar appointments or procedures together is called
  A. Wave
  B. Modified wave
  C. Grouping
  D. Double-booking
  E. Open scheduling

136. Which of the following should be included in the subjective information section of a SOAP note?
  A. Blood pressure reading
  B. Rash
  C. Medications the patient has taken
  D. X-ray reports

137. Which of the following is considered to be capital equipment?
  A. Coffee maker
  B. Laboratory coats
  C. Photocopier
  D. Trash cans

138. Which of the following abbreviations is *not* correct?
  A. pH
  B. mEq
  C. PKU
  D. HGB

139. According to CPT, E&M codes begin with which of the following two digits?
  A. 93
  B. 95
  C. 97
  D. 99

140. This type of insurance policy covers the medical expenses for persons who are injured on the physician's property.
  A. Liability
  B. Overhead
  C. Special risk
  D. Workers' compensation

141. Which of the following circumstances would waive the need for a written release of medical records?
    A. A subpoena
    B. Attorney request
    C. Hospital request
    D. Insurance company request

142. When using a terminal digit filing system, which of the following records should be filed first?
    A. 033233
    B. 044556
    C. 090432
    D. 101986

143. The correct way to indicate an enclosure notation is
    A. encl:
    B. Enclosure
    C. enclosure
    D. enc
    E. encl

144. Which of the following agencies would be the most appropriate to refer a patient with a multiple personality disorder?
    A. Centers for Disease Control and Prevention (CDC)
    B. Centers for Medicare and Medicaid Services (CMS)
    C. Department of Family and Children Services
    D. Substance Abuse and Mental Health Services Administration

145. Which of the following is the purpose of records management?
    A. Storage
    B. Arranging
    C. Accessibility
    D. Classifying
    E. All of the above

146. Which coding system is *not* associated with medical procedures?
    A. CPT
    B. ICD-9-CM
    C. HCPCS
    D. RVS
    E. RBRVS

147. Which is *not* an indexing rule?
    A. Unit 1 is the surname
    B. A hyphen is disregarded
    C. Initials come after complete names
    D. Apostrophes are disregarded
    E. Names are divided into units

148. ICD-9-CM codes that refer to factors that may influence the patient's health status are
    A. Volume I codes
    B. Volume II codes
    C. E-codes
    D. V-codes

149. When selecting the E&M code for CPT coding, which of the following elements is required for all levels of the history?
    A. Chief complaint
    B. Family history
    C. Social history
    D. Medical history
    E. Review of systems

150. Which of the following filing systems would be the most appropriate for storing and organizing medical research material?
    A. Alphabetic
    B. Chronologic
    C. Numeric
    D. Subject

151. Which of the following taxes are paid entirely by the employer?
    A. Social security
    B. Health insurance
    C. Federal income tax
    D. State income tax
    E. Unemployment tax

152. When using a source-oriented medical records system, documents should be arranged
    A. By subject
    B. In alphabetic order
    C. In numeric order
    D. By geographic location
    E. In reverse chronologic order

153. A spreadsheet would be commonly used for which of the following?
    A. Word processing
    B. Appointment scheduling
    C. Electronic mailings
    D. Accounting
    E. Desktop publishing

154. Which of the following would be the first step in arranging plans for the physicians' out-of-state conference?
    A. Research the city where the conference will be held
    B. Contact a travel agency
    C. Obtain preferences from the physician
    D. Call the physician's spouse
    E. Delegate the task to the office manager

155. An illness that existed before an insurance policy is written is known as a(n)
     A. Special risk
     B. Exclusion
     C. Preexisting condition
     D. Waiting period
     E. Prior authorization required

156. The ICD-9-CM is a coding system for
     A. Determining office charges
     B. Determining relative value scale (RVS)
     C. Determining the amount of payment from the insurance company
     D. Identifying and reporting diagnoses
     E. Providing a universal language for designating clinical procedures

157. Medical assistants in the clinic are paid biweekly at the regular rate of $13.00/hour. The clinic pays 1.5 times the regular rate for any hours exceeding 80 hours within the 2-week pay period. What would be the gross pay if a medical assistant worked 85 hours during the pay period?
     A. $1150.00
     B. $1200.00
     C. $1137.50
     D. $1040.00
     E. $1000.00

158. "Radial pulses are present bilaterally."
     When entering the above information in the medical record, under which of the following headings should it be entered?
     A. Reflexes
     B. Head and neck
     C. Extremities
     D. Chest
     E. Axilla

159. Which of the following allows data that are saved on a floppy disk or compact disk to be read but not altered?
     A. Clipboard
     B. *Save As*
     C. Write protect
     D. Read-only memory
     E. Random-access memory

160. This computer component allows the computer to perform operations.
     A. Read-only memory
     B. The keyboard
     C. The central processing unit
     D. The modem
     E. The disk drive

161. In an alphabetic filing system, which of the following records would be filed first?
     A. Holmes, Jennifer
     B. Holmes, Jen
     C. Holmes, Jennie
     D. Holmes, Jenna
     E. Holmes-Mathis, Jennifer

162. Which of the following is the most appropriate first step in correcting a misspelled word in a patient's medical record?
     A. Apply a thin covering of correction fluid over the error
     B. Circle the misspelled word in red
     C. Draw a single line through the misspelled word
     D. Completely erase the misspelled word
     E. Mark a red X through the misspelled word

163. How often must employee payroll taxes be reported to the Internal Revenue Service?
     A. Weekly
     B. Monthly
     C. Annually
     D. Biannually
     E. Quarterly

164. Which of the following filing systems is best for protecting the confidentiality of the patient?
     A. Subject
     B. Numeric
     C. Alphabetic
     D. Color-coded
     E. Geographic

165. An elderly patient wishes to move into a facility where she can remain autonomous. To which of the following might the medical assistant refer this patient?
     A. An assisted living community
     B. A retirement complex with individual apartments
     C. An extended care facility
     D. A nursing home
     E. A rehabilitation hospital

166. Which of the following types of mail ensures immediate delivery?
     A. Certified
     B. Insured
     C. First class
     D. Registered
     E. Special delivery

167. Which of the following is available to the medical office only through a lease agreement?
    A. A scanner
    B. A modem
    C. A copier
    D. A fax machine
    E. A postage meter

168. How many digits are used for modifiers when added to a five-digit CPT code?
    A. One
    B. Two
    C. Three
    D. Five
    E. Seven

169. A memorandum should include
    A. A subject line
    B. A signature
    C. A salutation
    D. An inside address
    E. A complimentary close

170. When removing characters to the right of the cursor, which of the following computer keys would be used?
    A. The backspace key
    B. The delete key
    C. The control key
    D. The escape key
    E. The insert key

171. This type of software application is used to manage large quantities of information such as inventory or an employee directory.
    A. Word processing
    B. Database
    C. Spreadsheet
    D. Graphics
    E. Spam protection

172. When determining a realistic time frame for scheduling appointments, which of the following would be the most useful?
    A. Adding slack time to the schedule
    B. Developing a realistic mission statement for the office
    C. Doing a patient flow analysis
    D. Using a computerized scheduling system
    E. Mailing reminder cards for appointments and immunizations

173. Which of the following is most characteristic of an alphabetic filing system?
    A. It is indexed by only one letter
    B. It is only effective when used with a color-coding system
    C. It requires less space than any other system
    D. It is a direct filing system
    E. It is an indirect filing system

174. Which of the following is used to analyze 60-, 90-, and 120-day delinquencies on accounts receivables?
    A. Aging accounts
    B. Extending credit
    C. Skip tracing
    D. Cycle billing
    E. Posting transactions

175. Which of the following software applications can be used to locate and display a web page?
    A. Motherboard
    B. Browser
    C. Clipboard
    D. Keyboard
    E. Jump drive

176. The clinic used 10 reams of copy paper every 2 weeks. How many reams will be used in 12 months?
    A. 120
    B. 180
    C. 200
    D. 260
    E. 300

177. When reconciling a bank statement, outstanding checks are
    A. Added to the bank statement balance
    B. Added to the checkbook balance
    C. Added to the deposits not shown on the statement
    D. Subtracted from the bank statement balance
    E. Subtracted from the checkbook balance

178. This type of employee compensation is a set sum each pay period, regardless of the amount of time worked.
    A. Commission
    B. Minimum wage
    C. Hourly wage
    D. Salary
    E. Overtime pay

179. Which of the following dates is correctly written for the heading of a business letter?
    A. 06/15/06
    B. June 15th, 2006
    C. June 15, 2006
    D. June 15, '06
    E. 15/06/06

180. Which of the following refers to the balance owed to a creditor on a current account?
A. Accounts payable
B. Accounts receivable
C. Cash receipts
D. Cash disbursements
E. Asset

181. The most effective way to convey instructions to a patient who is scheduled to have a surgical procedure would be to
A. Give the patient a video to watch at home
B. Give the patient detailed oral instructions
C. Give the patient medical literature about the procedure
D. Give the patient written instructions on the procedure
E. Tell the patient to ask the physician about the preparation

182. This insurance program provides for the medically indigent.
A. TRICARE
B. Medicaid
C. Medicare
D. Blue Cross/Blue Shield
E. CHAMPUS

183. The most appropriate source for locating a code for pharyngitis is
A. CPT
B. HCPCS
C. ICD-9-CM
D. RVS
E. Resource-based RVS

184. In the medical office, patients who require more examination time are scheduled at the beginning of each hour. Patients who require less examination time are scheduled 30 minutes after the hour. Patients who call at the last minute are scheduled at the end of each hour. This arrangement is an example of which of the following types of scheduling?
A. Wave
B. Clustering
C. Stream
D. Modified wave
E. Open booking

185. Which of the following describes a physician who accepts a check from Medicare for payment?
A. Sponsoring
B. Eligible
C. Registered
D. Accepting
E. Participating

186. Which of the following sections of the CPT book refers to surgery?
A. 00100-01999
B. 10040-69979
C. 70010-79999
D. 80000-89399
E. 90701-99199

187. If a patient with a balance on the account files for bankruptcy, which of the following would be the most appropriate initial step to be taken by the medical office?
A. Stop sending statements to the patient
B. File a claim with small-claims court
C. File an objection with a judge
D. Give the account to a collection agency
E. Write off the balance due

188. This type of scheduling system posts the office hours, and patients are seen in the order that they arrive at the office.
A. Wave
B. Clustering
C. Modified wave
D. Open hours
E. Double booking

189. Which of the following acts requires the health care provider to specify charges in writing and to identify the interest to be charged as an annual rate?
A. Truth in Lending Act
B. Tax Equity and Fiscal Responsibility Act
C. Fair Debt Collection Practices Act
D. Fair Credit Practices Act
E. Equal Credit Opportunity Act

190. Which of the following is an appropriate telephone technique for collecting payments owed the practice?
A. Allow the patient time to offer explanations
B. Threaten further action if payment is not made
C. Describe the financial status of the practice
D. Suggest alternative methods of payment
E. Review the value of the medical treatment the patient has received

191. A 67-year-old person who receives Social Security payments is also entitled to receive which of the following at no cost?
A. TRICARE
B. Medicaid
C. Medicare Part A
D. Medicare Part B
E. Workers' Compensation

192. Which of the following forms can provide demographic information about a patient?
  A. Physical examination form
  B. Patient referral form
  C. Patient encounter form
  D. Patient information form
  E. Patient health questionnaire

193. Which of the following should be saved indefinitely?
  A. Fee schedules
  B. Announcements of inservices
  C. Letters of acknowledgment
  D. Receipts for business equipment
  E. Professional liability insurance policies

194. In addition to the patient's name, which of the following is most important to record when scheduling an appointment for a new patient?
  A. The name of the referring physician
  B. The name of the patient's insurance company
  C. The home address of the patient
  D. The daytime telephone number of the patient
  E. The patient's date of birth

195. The amount of income tax withheld from an employee's salary is based on
  A. The employee's age
  B. The employee's gender
  C. The number of employees
  D. The number of exemptions the employee has claimed
  E. The number of years of employment

196. Which of the following coding systems utilizes a V code?
  A. CPT
  B. DRGs
  C. HCPCS
  D. ICD-9-CM
  E. RVS

197. The mother of a 6-week-old infant calls the office because she is concerned that the infant is not getting enough milk. She is breast-feeding the infant. Which of the following questions would evaluate the mother's milk supply?
  A. "How many wet diapers do you change in a day?"
  B. "Is the baby running a fever?"
  C. "Does the baby's skin look yellow?"
  D. "Is the baby lethargic?"
  E. "Do you also feed the baby formula?"

198. Which of the following is *not* a correct technique when performing data entry?
  A. Keep eyes on the source copy
  B. Strike the keys with a smooth flowing stroke
  C. Keep feet flat on the floor
  D. Sit with back curved and with the keyboard on the lap
  E. Keep the fingers curved over the home row keys

199. Third-party participation in an office indicates the relationships among the
  A. Physician, patient, and medical assistant
  B. Physician, medical assistant, and insurance company
  C. Physician, patient, and insurance company
  D. Physician, hospital, and insurance company
  E. Physician, patient, and hospital

200. A claim may be rejected by an insurance company because of the omission of
  A. Complete diagnosis
  B. Policy number
  C. Patient birth date
  D. Itemization of charges
  E. All of the above

Clinical Content

201. An agent that prevents the growth, development or proliferation of malignant cells is an
  A. Antitussive
  B. Antineoplastic
  C. Anticoagulant
  D. Antidepressant

202. Which of the following needle length and gauge would the medical assistant choose to administer an intramuscular injection?
  A. 1 inch, 25 gauge
  B. 1½ inch, 22 gauge
  C. 1 inch, 18 gauge
  D. ½ inch, 22 gauge

203. A type of drug that increases urinary output is a(n)
  A. Emetic
  B. Diuretic
  C. Miotic
  D. Cathartic

204. The physician orders 1000 mg amoxicillin intramuscularly. The vial reads *500 mg per 1 mL*. How many milliliters would be administered to the patient?
  A. 0.5 mL
  B. 1 mL
  C. 2 mL
  D. 3 mL
  E. 5 mL

205. The purpose of pouring off a small amount of a sterile solution from a container with a single cap is to
   A. Rinse contaminants from the lip of the bottle
   B. Avoid staining the label of the bottle
   C. Generate an even flow so the solution does not splash
   D. Expel air bubbles from the solution

206. Before transferring a sterile solution from a bottle to a container on a sterile field
   A. Clean the outside of the bottle
   B. Rest the lip of the bottle on the edge of the sterile container
   C. Read the label on the bottle, and check the expiration date
   D. Remove the cap from the bottle, and place it face down on the counter

207. A postprandial blood glucose level is measured after
   A. Drinking water
   B. Exercising
   C. Fasting
   D. Eating

208. The normal range for specific gravity is usually between
   A. 1.000 and 1.005
   B. 1.010 and 1.025
   C. 1.025 and 1.500
   D. 1.005 and 1.050

209. When assisting with a sigmoidoscopy, which of the following would be most appropriate to wear?
   A. Laboratory coat and goggles
   B. Nonsterile gloves and goggles
   C. Nonsterile gloves, laboratory coat, and goggles
   D. Nonsterile gloves, laboratory coat, and mouth barrier

210. Which of the following procedures would require surgical asepsis?
   A. Digital rectal examination
   B. Bimanual pelvic examination
   C. Aspiration of a breast cyst
   D. Auscultation of the chest

211. A cholecystogram is used to view the
   A. Urinary bladder
   B. Liver
   C. Gallbladder
   D. Kidneys

212. Which of the following instruments is used to measure a patient's hearing acuity?
   A. Audiometer
   B. Refractometer
   C. Otoscope
   D. Ophthalmoscope

213. 1 cc is equivalent to
   A. 1 mL
   B. 5 mL
   C. 10 mL
   D. 20 mL

214. Which of the following medications may be used to treat duodenal ulcers?
   A. Prempro (conjugated estrogen/medroxyprogesterone acetate)
   B. Prilosec (omeprazole)
   C. Paxil (paroxetine)
   D. Pravachol (pravastatin sodium)

215. Which of the following laboratory values might indicate cardiac muscle injury?
   A. Alanine aminotransferase (ALT)
   B. Blood urea nitrogen (BUN)
   C. Creatine kinase (CK)
   D. Bilirubin

216. Hematemesis should be recorded under which of the following body systems?
   A. Respiratory
   B. Gastrointestinal
   C. Genitourinary
   D. Reproductive

217. To cauterize a small lesion on the oral mucosa, the physician might use an applicator with
   A. Silver nitrate
   B. Alcohol
   C. Formalin
   D. Betadine

218. A common laboratory test that may be ordered for a patient receiving Coumadin therapy is a
   A. Prothrombin time
   B. Erythrocyte sedimentation rate
   C. Complete blood count
   D. Hematocrit

219. This type of microorganism appears as grapelike clusters when stained and viewed microscopically.
   A. Bacilli
   B. Cocci
   C. Staphylococci
   D. Streptococci

220. The most appropriate site for an intramuscular injection in an infant is
   A. Deltoid
   B. Rectus femoris
   C. Vastus lateralis
   D. Dorsogluteal

221. A hemoglobin value of 10 g/dL is approximately equivalent to a hematocrit of
   A. 10%
   B. 20%
   C. 30%
   D. 40%

222. Which of the following describes an agent that eases or alleviates a condition but does not cure the patient?
   A. Homeopathic
   B. Idiopathic
   C. Palliative
   D. Prophylactic

223. The physician orders an intramuscular injection of meperidine (Demerol) 50 mg for pain relief. On hand is a 30-mL, multiple-dose vial of Demerol that contains 50 mg/mL. The medical assistant would administer
   A. 0.5 mL
   B. 1.0 mL
   C. 1.5 mL
   D. 2.0 mL

224. Which of the following laboratory tests is a screening test for kidney function?
   A. Alpha-fetoprotein (AFP)
   B. Amylase
   C. Blood urea nitrogen (BUN)
   D. High-density lipoprotein cholesterol (HDL)

225. Sanitization
   A. Destroys all pathogenic microorganisms
   B. Destroys most pathogenic organisms
   C. Reduces the number of contaminants to a safe level
   D. Replaces defective instruments with new instruments

226. The reason for removing jewelry from the hands and wrists before a surgical scrub is
   A. The solution may damage the jewelry
   B. The jewelry can harbor microorganisms
   C. The jewelry may tear the sterile gloves
   D. The jewelry might injure the patient

227. During manual audiometry, the patient should be positioned
   A. Facing away from the examiner
   B. Behind the examiner
   C. Facing the examiner
   D. Next to the examiner

228. The material used to wrap instruments for autoclaving must be
   A. Permeable to steam but protective against airborne contaminants
   B. Easily opened to check the indicator
   C. Made of cotton
   D. Permeable to steam, as well as allowing good ventilation during storage

229. Which of the following injuries is classified as a closed wound?
   A. Puncture
   B. Laceration
   C. Ecchymosis
   D. Avulsion

230. Which of the following types of casts found in urine sediment is the most benign?
   A. Red blood cell
   B. Fatty
   C. Hyaline
   D. White blood cell

231. Proventil (albuterol) is classified as a(n)
   A. Antiinflammatory
   B. Antihistamine
   C. Antihypertensive
   D. Bronchodilator

232. On a patient's chart, the temperature is noted as T: 99.4° F (A). The (A) in the chart note indicates
   A. Accurate
   B. Adjusted
   C. Aural
   D. Axillary

233. Controlled substances that are considered to be illegal and of no medical use are classified as
   A. Schedule I
   B. Schedule II
   C. Schedule III
   D. Schedule IV
   E. Schedule V

234. Which of the following positions would be the most appropriate for a patient undergoing a pelvic examination?
   A. Prone
   B. Fowler's
   C. Sims'
   D. Lithotomy

235. Which of the following instructions should be given to a patient who needs to collect stool specimens for occult blood screening?
    A. Eat a high-carbohydrate diet for 48 hours before collection
    B. Fast for 12 hours before the collection
    C. Do not eat red meat for 48 hours before the collection
    D. Do not eat fats for 12 hours before the collection

236. The correct dilution of bleach (sodium hypochlorite) and water used to disinfect a contaminated work area is
    A. 1:5
    B. 1:10
    C. 1:20
    D. 1:50

237. This term is used to describe a variation in the size of erythrocytes.
    A. Anisocytosis
    B. Poikilocytosis
    C. Polychromic
    D. Leukocytosis

238. The physician advises a patient to increase her daily intake of carbohydrates. Which of the following foods should be increased in her diet?
    A. Meat
    B. Cheese
    C. Bread
    D. Fruit

239. Which of the following substances in urine may indicate liver dysfunction?
    A. Albumin
    B. Glucose
    C. Ketones
    D. Urobilinogen

240. Which of the following medications may be used in the treatment of seasonal allergies?
    A. Keflex (cephalexin)
    B. Cipro (ciprofloxacin)
    C. Claritin (loratadine)
    D. Coumadin (warfarin)

241. On a Gram stain, gram-negative bacteria will appear
    A. Blue
    B. Pink or red
    C. Green
    D. Purple

242. When instilling drops in an adult patient's ear, the ear canal should be straightened by gently pulling the pinna
    A. Down and back
    B. Up and back
    C. Straight back
    D. Up and forward

243. The abbreviation for *both ears* is
    A. AS
    B. AD
    C. AU
    D. BE

244. The correct injection technique used to place a tuberculin (Mantoux) skin test is
    A. Intradermal
    B. Intramuscular
    C. Intravenous
    D. Transdermal

245. Which of the following terms describes *the removal of infectious agents on a surface or object using physical and/or chemical means?*
    A. Decontamination
    B. Disinfection
    C. Sanitization
    D. Sterilization

246. An adult blood pressure is measured at which of the following arteries?
    A. Brachial
    B. Radial
    C. Carotid
    D. Dorsalis pedis

247. A patient in the medical office has a nosebleed. Which of the following would be the most appropriate action to be taken first by the medical assistant?
    A. Apply ice to the patient's nose
    B. Call 911
    C. Tell the patient to lie down
    D. Tilt the patient's head forward

248. The first group of leads to be recorded on an electrocardiogram are the
    A. Augmented leads
    B. Leads I, II, and III
    C. aVR, aVL, and aVF
    D. Leads V_1 through V_3
    E. Leads V_1 through V_6

249. Which of the following is the most effective method to clean a drop of blood from a countertop?
   A. Iodine and sterile gauze
   B. 1:10 bleach solution
   C. Alcohol and sterile cotton ball
   D. Surgical soap and water

250. When recording an electrocardiogram, depressing the standardization button will move the stylus upward how many small squares?
   A. 5
   B. 10
   C. 15
   D. 20

251. The drug order *2 gtt AD q4h prn* is translated as
   A. Two drops in both ears every 4 hours as needed
   B. Two drops in both eyes every 4 hours as desired
   C. Two drops in both ears four times a day
   D. Two drops in the left eye every 4 hours if needed

252. Which of the following injection techniques is most appropriate for the administration of an antibiotic?
   A. Intradermal
   B. Intramuscular
   C. Intravenous
   D. Subcutaneous

253. Which of the following additives should be used when drawing a specimen for a differential smear?
   A. EDTA
   B. Heparin
   C. Potassium oxalate
   D. Sodium citrate

254. An x-ray study of the spinal cord is known as a(n)
   A. Angiogram
   B. Arthrogram
   C. Myelogram
   D. Urogram

255. Which of the following results on a urinalysis is abnormal?
   A. Color: yellow
   B. pH: 5.2
   C. Specific gravity: 1.005
   D. Leukocytes: ++

256. Which of the following agencies mandates the use of standard precautions?
   A. American Association of Medical Assistants
   B. American Medical Association
   C. Centers for Disease Control and Prevention
   D. Occupational Safety and Health Administration

257. A sphygmomanometer is used to perform which of the following procedures?
   A. Assess hearing
   B. Examine the rectum
   C. Evaluate vision
   D. Measure blood pressure

258. Which of the following nutrients provides the best source of energy for the body?
   A. Carbohydrates
   B. Fats
   C. Proteins
   D. Vitamins

259. Which of the following methods is used to listen to heart, lung, and bowel sounds?
   A. Manipulation
   B. Auscultation
   C. Mensuration
   D. Percussion

260. Which of the following is the route of administration for parenteral medications?
   A. Oral
   B. Inhalation
   C. Injection
   D. Transdermal

261. Which of the following terms refers to the total amount of air that is exhaled from fully inflated lungs?
   A. Forced vital capacity
   B. Forced expiratory flow
   C. Forced expiratory volume in 1 second
   D. Tidal volume

262. Which of the following abbreviations is correctly defined?
   A. bid (twice a day)
   B. tid (every day)
   C. OD (left eye)
   D. ac (after meals)

263. During a Snellen visual acuity test, the patient should stand how many feet from the chart?
   A. 5
   B. 10
   C. 15
   D. 20

264. How many minutes should a urine specimen be centrifuged before preparing the sediment for microscopic examination?
   A. 1
   B. 5
   C. 7
   D. 10

265. When performing an electrocardiogram, which of the following chest leads would be placed on the fifth intercostals space at the midclavicular line?
    A. V_1
    B. V_2
    C. V_3
    D. V_4
    E. V_5

266. The most appropriate method of establishing an airway in a conscious adult who is choking and unable to breathe would be to
    A. Deliver blows to the back
    B. Perform the Heimlich maneuver
    C. Sweep the back of the throat
    D. Perform the head tilt, chin lift maneuver

267. A blood sample that requires serum would be collected in an evacuated tube with which color stopper?
    A. Gray
    B. Green
    C. Lavender
    D. Red

268. A decrease in bone density may indicate
    A. Osteolysis
    B. Osteoclasis
    C. Osteoporosis
    D. Crepitus

269. Which of the following terms describes the destruction of all living microorganisms before possible entry into the body?
    A. Decontamination
    B. Disinfection
    C. Sanitization
    D. Sterilization

270. A child's head circumference should be measured during a routine pediatric examination until a child reaches how many months of age?
    A. 12
    B. 24
    C. 36
    D. 48

271. Lead I of the electrocardiograph measures the heart's voltage between which of the following limbs?
    A. Left arm and left leg
    B. Left arm and left leg
    C. Right arm and left arm
    D. Right arm and left leg

272. The medical assistant usually performs which of the following types of injections?
    A. Intradermal
    B. Intralesional
    C. Intrathecal
    D. Intravenous

273. The terms *colicky, stabbing, excruciating*, and *intractable* best describe
    A. Congestion
    B. Pain
    C. Contractions
    D. Heart murmurs

274. Which of the following methods of examination is used to assess range of motion of a joint?
    A. Manipulation
    B. Mensuration
    C. Palpation
    D. Inspection

275. Which of the following immunizations is routinely administered to a newborn?
    A. Diphtheria-tetanus-pertussis (DTaP)
    B. *Haemophilus influenza* type B
    C. Hepatitis B
    D. Mumps, measles and rubella (MMR)

276. Which of the following is used to screen for occult blood in stool?
    A. Blood smear
    B. Guaiac test
    C. Prothrombin time
    D. Red blood cell count

277. When recording a patient's history, which of the following should be written with quotation marks (" ") indicating the patient's own words?
    A. Chief complaint
    B. Personal data
    C. Review of systems
    D. Social history

278. The patient's skin is cleansed and prepped with an antiseptic before a minor surgical procedure to
    A. Increase the effectiveness of the local anesthetic agent
    B. Prevent the entry of microorganisms into the patient's body
    C. Protect the physician from becoming infected by a pathogen
    D. Restore the function of the damaged tissue

279. Which of the following should be included on the label of a specimen to be sent to the laboratory?
- **A.** Patient's name, date of birth, and address
- **B.** Patient's name, address, and date of collection
- **C.** Patient's name, date of birth, and physician's name
- **D.** Patient's name, date of collection, and source of the specimen

280. A woman who has given birth to two or more children may be called
- **A.** Nullipara
- **B.** Multipara
- **C.** Unipara
- **D.** Multigravida

281. Which of the following describes the action of acetaminophen?
- **A.** Anesthetic
- **B.** Antiinflammatory
- **C.** Antipyretic
- **D.** Antitussive

282. A patient with diabetes mellitus would be most likely to develop
- **A.** Hyperglycemia
- **B.** Hemoglobinuria
- **C.** Hyperlipidemia
- **D.** Phenylketonuria

283. Which of the following are ways in which pathogens can be spread?
- **A.** Transmission by a vector
- **B.** Person-to-person contact
- **C.** Environmental contact
- **D.** Object-to-person contact
- **E.** All of the above

284. The physician writes the following prescription:
Patient: Mary Smith
Rx: Synthroid 0.3 mcg
Sig: ii tabs po qd
#30
Refills: 60 (six)
Before explaining the prescription to the patient, the medical assistant should ask the physician to do which of the following?
- **A.** Clarify the route of administration
- **B.** Correct the dosage
- **C.** Verify the number of refills
- **D.** Verify the number of tablets to be dispensed

285. Which of the following dietary fat sources would be most beneficial for a patient who is trying to maintain a healthy diet?
- **A.** Fish oil
- **B.** Corn oil
- **C.** Butter
- **D.** Bacon

286. Squeezing the site of a capillary puncture can result in
- **A.** Coagulation of the blood sample
- **B.** Increased hemolysis of the blood sample
- **C.** Dilution of the blood sample with tissue fluid
- **D.** Increased number of red blood cells in the sample

287. Which of the following actions is most appropriate when a patient is in shock?
- **A.** Apply cold packs to the patient's forehead
- **B.** Place the patient in a supine position with legs elevated
- **C.** Place the patient on his or her side
- **D.** Place the patient on his or her stomach

288. The most common way for spreading infectious agents in the medical office is
- **A.** Air conditioning ducts
- **B.** Contaminated supplies and instruments
- **C.** Hands of employees
- **D.** Improper sterilization of supplies and instruments

289. According to the childhood immunization schedule, children should receive a total of how many doses of inactivated poliovirus (IPV) vaccine?
- **A.** 2
- **B.** 3
- **C.** 4
- **D.** 5

290. An endoscopic examination of the rectum is charted as a(n)
- **A.** Sigmoidoscopy
- **B.** Proctoscopy
- **C.** Endoscopy
- **D.** Barium enema

291. The Ishihara test is used to evaluate
- **A.** Color vision
- **B.** Intraocular pressure
- **C.** Visual acuity
- **D.** Farsightedness

292. Which of the following instruments would be used to incise and drain an abscess?
    A. Bandage scissors
    B. Needle holder
    C. Scalpel
    D. Tissue forceps

293. *Sig* on a prescription represents which of the following?
    A. The name of the drug
    B. Instructions to the patient
    C. Number of refills allowed
    D. Quantity to dispense

294. The hemoglobin level multiplied by three is approximately equal to which of the following?
    A. Hematocrit
    B. Platelet count
    C. Red blood cell count
    D. White blood cell count

295. Which of the following methods of taking a temperature is *not* appropriate for a patient with dyspnea?
    A. Rectal
    B. Axillary
    C. Aural
    D. Oral

296. The region between the vagina and anus is termed the
    A. Perimetrium
    B. Perineum
    C. Placenta
    D. Peritoneum
    E. Puerpera

297. An increase in the serum level of which of the following is *not* an independent risk factor for cardiovascular disease?
    A. Triglycerides
    B. Low-density lipoprotein (LDL)
    C. High-density lipoprotein (HDL)
    D. Cholesterol

298. To set up for an examination of a patient with vaginitis, all of the following would be used *except*
    A. Vaginal speculum
    B. Microscope slide
    C. KOH (potassium hydroxide)
    D. Cytologic fixative

299. Standard precautions should be used when handling each of the following specimens *except*
    A. Sweat
    B. Blood
    C. Semen
    D. Vaginal secretions

300. An antipyretic agent works against
    A. Fever
    B. Rash
    C. Poison
    D. Acne

Pre-Test 1 Answer Key

1. B Atrophy

RATIONALE: The prefix *a-* means without, lack of. The suffix *-trophy* means development.

2. C Myoblast

RATIONALE: The root word *myo-* means muscle. The suffix *-blast* means immature cell, form.

3. A AD

RATIONALE: *AD* is the abbreviation for right ear (auris dextra). *AS* is the abbreviation for left ear, *AU* for both ears, *OD* for right eye, and *OS* for left eye.

4. B Inspect the exterior ear canal

RATIONALE: An otoscope is a lighted instrument used to visually examine the outer ear and tympanic membrane.

5. D Thoracentesis

RATIONALE: A thoracentesis is the surgical puncture of the chest wall and pleural space. Fluid or air can then be withdrawn.

6. B Hematocrit and hemoglobin

RATIONALE: Anemia is a disorder characterized by a decrease in hemoglobin or a decrease in the total number of red blood cells.

7. C Endocrinologist

RATIONALE: Hyperparathyroidism is an abnormal endocrine condition in which an excess of parathyroid hormone is secreted. An endocrinologist diagnoses and treats diseases and disorders of the endocrine system.

8. D Leukocytosis

RATIONALE: Leukocytosis is an increase in the total number of circulating white blood cells. *Leuko-* refers to white, *-cyt* refers to cells, and *-osis* is an abnormal condition.

9. A Hyperpnea

RATIONALE: Hyperpnea is deep or rapid breathing. The prefix *hyper-* means above. The root word *-pnea* refers to breathing.

10. D -algia

RATIONALE: The suffix *-algia* means pain or painful condition.

11. C -plasty

RATIONALE: The suffix *-plasty* means surgical repair.

12. C Breast

RATIONALE: A mammogram is an x-ray film of the soft tissue of the breast. The root word *mammo-* refers to breast. The suffix *-gram* refers to a record (x-ray).

13. D Baldness

RATIONALE: Alopecia is the partial or complete lack of hair, which can be caused by normal aging, an endocrine disorder, chemotherapy, or a skin disease.

14. A Mastication

RATIONALE: Mastication is the chewing, tearing, or grinding of food with the teeth while it becomes mixed with saliva.

15. E Mole on the inside of the elbow

RATIONALE: A nevus is a mole. The antecubital area is located on the inner aspect of the elbow.

16. D Arthritis

RATIONALE: The root word *arth-* means joint. The suffix *-itis* means inflammation.

17. B Adipose tissue

RATIONALE: Adipose tissue is made up of fat cells arranged in globules. It is found under the skin and serves as a reserve energy source and for insulation.

18. C Pathology

RATIONALE: Pathology is the study of the characteristics, causes, and effects of disease on the structure and function of the body.

19. C Smelling

RATIONALE: The olfactory nerve, cranial nerve I, is one of two pairs of nerves associated with the sense of smell.

20. B Ovaries
RATIONALE: An oophorectomy is the surgical removal of one or both ovaries. The root word *oophor-* means ovary. The suffix *-ectomy* means surgical removal.

21. C Urology
RATIONALE: Urology is the branch of medicine concerned with the urinary tract in men and women, as well as the male genital tract. The physician who specializes in urology is a urologist.

22. D Cystoscopy
RATIONALE: Cystoscopy is the direct visualization of the urinary tract and/or bladder by means of a cystoscope inserted into the urethra.

23. A Urticaria
RATIONALE: Urticaria is a pruritic skin eruption characterized by wheals (hives) of various shapes and sizes. This condition can be caused by allergic reactions to drugs, insect bites, and foods.

24. C Pericardium
RATIONALE: The pericardium is the serous membrane that surrounds the heart.

25. D Lines body cavities that open to the outside
RATIONALE: A mucous membrane lines body cavities or spaces of the body that open to the outside, including the mouth, digestive tract, respiratory tract, and genitourinary tract.

26. D Anterior
RATIONALE: The ventral area of the body is toward the front of the body (anterior).

27. C Abdominal
RATIONALE: The abdominal cavity is part of the ventral cavity of the body. It contains the stomach, small and large intestines, spleen, liver, gallbladder, and pancreas.

28. C Adduction
RATIONALE: Adduction is the movement of a limb or body part toward the body.

29. A Frontal
RATIONALE: The frontal plane is the vertical plane that divides the body or a structure into anterior and posterior portions.

30. A Can follow a viral illness in children
RATIONALE: Reye's syndrome is an acute and sometimes fatal illness characterized by fatty invasion of internal organs and swelling of the brain. The cause is unknown, but the condition has been linked to the use of aspirin and viral illnesses in children.

31. C Lumbar
RATIONALE: The vertebral column is divided into five sections: (1) cervical (neck), (2) thoracic (chest), (3) lumbar (lower back), (4) sacral (below the lumbar), and (5) coccygeal (tailbone).

32. A Impetigo
RATIONALE: Impetigo is an infection of the skin caused by staphylococci, streptococci, or a combination of the two. The lesions usually begin around the mouth and nose and spread locally. The lesions blister and crust.

33. D Occipital
RATIONALE: The occipital bone of the skull is located at the back of the skull. It articulates with the two parietal bones and contains the foramen magnum (opening for the spinal cord).

34. C Greenstick fracture
RATIONALE: A greenstick fracture is an incomplete fracture. The bone is bent but fractured only on the outer arc of the bend.

35. E 31
RATIONALE: The peripheral nervous system is made up of the motor and sensory nerves and ganglia located outside the brain and spinal cord. It consists of 12 pairs of cranial nerves and 31 pairs of spinal nerves.

36. A Brainstem
RATIONALE: The brainstem is the portion of the brain made up of the midbrain, pons, and medulla. It performs sensory, motor, and reflex functions. Vital centers that regulate internal body functions are located here.

37. A Aplastic
RATIONALE: Aplastic anemia results from a failure of blood cell production resulting from the failure of bone marrow to produce cells. The cause is unknown.

38. C Hiatal hernia
RATIONALE: A hernia is the abnormal protrusion of an organ or tissue through the structures that normally contain it. A hiatal hernia is the protrusion of the upper portion of the stomach upward through the esophageal opening in the diaphragm.

39. D Eardrum
RATIONALE: The tympanic membrane is the membrane between the external and middle ear. It is commonly called the eardrum.

40. D Aorta
RATIONALE: The aorta is the main trunk of the systemic arterial circulation. Blood is pumped out of the left ventricle through the aortic valve into the aorta. The aorta then branches and carries blood throughout the body.

41. C Is the pacemaker of the heart
RATIONALE: The sinoatrial node of the heart is located in the right atrium. The electrical impulse that initiates the heartbeat originates here.

42. B Radius and ulna
RATIONALE: The radius is the lateral lower arm bone on line with the thumb. The ulna is the medial lower arm bone.

43. E All of the above

RATIONALE: Involuntary (smooth) muscle is muscle that is not under a person's conscious or voluntary control. These muscles actions include muscles of the heart and muscles of the intestines, stomach, and other visceral organs.

44. A Liver

RATIONALE: The right upper quadrant of the abdominopelvic area contains the liver, gallbladder, part of the pancreas, and parts of the small and large intestines.

45. D Phrenic

RATIONALE: The diaphragm is stimulated by the phrenic nerve from the cervical plexus. The diaphragm aids in respiration by moving up and down.

46. C Scoliosis

RATIONALE: Scoliosis is a lateral curvature of the spine commonly seen in children. Unequal heights of hips and shoulders may be a sign of this condition.

47. B Glucagon

RATIONALE: Glucagon is a hormone produced by the alpha cells in the islets of Langerhans in the pancreas. It stimulates the conversion of glycogen to glucose in the liver.

48. C Cholecystectomy

RATIONALE: The root word *cholecyst*- means gallbladder. The suffix *-ectomy* means surgical removal.

49. E Optic

RATIONALE: The optic nerve (cranial nerve II) is a sensory nerve that is involved with the sense of vision.

50. D 32

RATIONALE: The deciduous (baby) teeth are replaced by 32 adult (permanent) teeth. These adult teeth include four central incisors, lateral incisors, cuspids, first and second premolars, first molars, second molars, and third molars (wisdom teeth).

51. E May refuse to accept a patient if he or she chooses

RATIONALE: Physicians have the right to determine whom they will accept as patients. Patient load may be as large as one person can adequately care for, and the decision may be made to limit new patients.

52. D Is a detailed outline of a trip

RATIONALE: An itinerary is detailed information about a trip. It includes the date and time of departure; flight numbers; mode of transportation to hotel; name, address, and telephone number of hotel; and the date and time of return.

53. B Staying calm when dealing with angry patients

RATIONALE: Professional qualities that a medical assistant must have include a friendly and pleasant attitude, ability to maintain confidentiality, courtesy, ability to control temper, consideration, respect and kindness, dependability, and accuracy.

54. B Empathy

RATIONALE: Empathy is the ability to recognize the emotions and state of mind of another person.

55. B The physician

RATIONALE: The physician owns the medical record, but the patient owns the information contained in the record.

56. A Denial

RATIONALE: Denial is the unconscious avoidance of the reality of an unpleasant or disturbing situation.

57. E All of the above

RATIONALE: Personality is the pattern of behavior each person develops as a means of adapting to a particular environment and its standards. Age, life experiences, heredity, and environment all play a part in this development.

58. B Impatience

RATIONALE: The professional services of a medical assistant are extremely personal, and the manner in which these services are performed can affect the health and well being of the patient. An impatient person might negatively affect the patient.

59. E Young children react differently to stressful situations

RATIONALE: Stereotyping is a preconceived generalized belief. Young children do react differently to stressful situations than adults react.

60. C The patient must sign a release form

RATIONALE: The patient must sign a release of information form before information from the medical record can be released to anyone. This precaution preserves the patient's confidentiality.

61. E Human immunodeficiency virus

RATIONALE: The physician has a legal duty to report communicable diseases to the county health department. This requirement helps the state provide for the public's health, safety, and welfare.

62. B Vital signs

RATIONALE: Objective data is data determined in some way by someone other than the patient, such as the physician or medical assistant. Vital signs are considered to be objective.

63. A Another physician

RATIONALE: A call from another physician or professional colleague should be transferred to the physician immediately.

64. C Social need

RATIONALE: Maslow believed that lower-level needs must be satisfied before higher-level needs can be satisfied. These levels, from lowest to highest, include physiologic needs, safety needs, social needs, self-esteem needs, and self-actualization needs.

65. D Delay treatment and inform or consult with the physician

RATIONALE: A physician must have consent to treat a patient even though this consent is usually implied. A physician who fails to secure some formal type of consent might be charged with assault and battery or trespass.

66. E All of the above

RATIONALE: A contract is an agreement that creates an obligation. To be valid or enforceable, the contract must have four basic elements: (1) an offer and acceptance, (2) consideration, (3) capacity, and (4) legality.

67. D Posterior

RATIONALE: The anterior of a structure is the front of the structure. The posterior of a structure is the back of the structure.

68. E All of the above

RATIONALE: Informed consent must be obtained from the patient when a complex procedure is to be performed. Informed consent implies an understanding of what is to be done, why it should be done, the risks involved, the expected outcomes, and alternative treatments, including consequences of failure to treat.

69. E Providing atypical care

RATIONALE: The license to practice medicine may be revoked or suspended under certain circumstances. Grounds for revoking or suspending a license generally falls within one of three categories: (1) conviction of a crime, (2) unprofessional conduct, and (3) personal and professional incapacity.

70. C Nucleus

RATIONALE: The nucleus is the control center of every cell. It contains DNA, which is the genetic material.

71. E All of the above

RATIONALE: The subcutaneous tissue is a layer of connective tissue found between the skin and the deep fascia. It contains a fatty layer. Hypodermic injections into this tissue are usually on the upper arm, thigh, or abdomen.

72. B Humerus

RATIONALE: The humerus is the largest bone of the upper arm. The femur is the bone of the thigh; the tibia and fibula make up the lower leg; the metatarsals form the arch of the foot.

73. A Deltoid

RATIONALE: The deltoid is a large, thick, triangular muscle that covers the shoulder.

74. B Sinoatrial node

RATIONALE: The sinoatrial node is a cluster of specialized cells located in the right atrial wall of the heart. It generates impulses that travel throughout the muscle fibers of the atria and cause them to contract.

75. E Alveoli

RATIONALE: The alveoli are small saclike structures at the terminal ends of the bronchioles. They are the functional units of respiration and are composed of a single layer of epithelium, which allows oxygen and carbon dioxide to be easily exchanged with the surrounding capillaries.

76. E All of the above

RATIONALE: The liver is the largest gland of the body. Its main functions include production of bile, detoxification of toxins and wastes, metabolism of proteins and carbohydrates, storage of vitamins and glycogen, production of heparin, and recycling of worn-out red blood cells.

77. B Endometrium

RATIONALE: The endometrium is the innermost layer of the uterus. The fertilized ovum implants into this layer where it develops until delivery.

78. B Testes

RATIONALE: Testosterone, the male hormone, is manufactured in the interstitial cells of the testes.

79. A Cerebrum

RATIONALE: The cerebrum is the largest portion of the brain. It is divided into two hemispheres, which are further divided into lobes. Its outer surface (cortex) is made up of gray matter.

80. E 31

RATIONALE: There are 31 pairs of spinal nerves that are connected to the spinal cord. They are numbered according to the vertebra from which they emerge.

81. A Mouth

RATIONALE: The gustatory sense is the sense of taste. The receptors are located on the tongue within papillae (taste buds).

82. D Decreases blood sugar levels

RATIONALE: Insulin is a hormone manufactured by the beta cells in the pancreas. Its main function is to metabolize glucose and thus reduce blood sugar levels.

83. E Leukopenia

RATIONALE: Leukopenia is an abnormal decrease in the number of white blood cells to fewer than 5000 cells/mm³ of blood. The root word *leuko-* means white, or white blood cell. The suffix *-penia* means a decrease.

84. B stat

RATIONALE: The term *stat* is the abbreviation for *statim,* meaning immediately.

85. E All of the above

RATIONALE: The physician has a legal duty to report information that may have an effect on the health, safety, or welfare of the public. This information includes births, deaths, communicable diseases, abuse, criminal acts, and professional misconduct.

86. A Slow

RATIONALE: The prefix *brady-* means slow.

87. C Deep

RATIONALE: Superficial pertains to the skin or another surface. Deep refers to away from the surface.

88. C An advanced directive

RATIONALE: An advanced directive is a legal document that gives persons the right to determine what medical procedures they want provided if they become unable to make those decisions.

89. B Denial

RATIONALE: Unconscious defense mechanisms help protect the mind from guilt or anxiety. Denial is the unconscious avoidance of the reality of an unpleasant or disturbing feeling, thought, or event.

90. A An open-ended statement

RATIONALE: An open-ended statement or question helps the patient decide what is relevant. It also encourages the patient to continue the discussion.

91. C Etiology

RATIONALE: Etiology is the study of all factors that may be involved in the development of a disease. This area can include the susceptibility of the patient, the nature of the disease-causing agent, and the way agent invades the patient's body.

92. E All of the above

RATIONALE: Nonverbal communications are messages conveyed without the use of words. They are transmitted by body language. Body language involves grooming, dress, eye contact, facial expression, hand gestures, space, tone of voice, posture, and touch.

93. B An eating disorder

RATIONALE: Bulimia is an insatiable craving for food characterized by binge eating and self-induced vomiting.

94. D Stroke

RATIONALE: A cerebrovascular accident, or brain attack, is an abnormal condition of the blood vessels of the brain characterized by an occlusion that results in an ischemia of the brain tissue. Paralysis, weakness, speech defect, aphasia, or death may occur.

95. D Measles

RATIONALE: Measles (rubeola) is an acute, highly contagious viral infection. It involves the respiratory tract and is characterized by a spreading cutaneous rash. It is caused by the paramyxovirus and is transmitted by droplets.

96. C Trichomoniasis

RATIONALE: Trichomoniasis is a vaginal infection caused by the protozoan *Trichomonas vaginalis*. It is transmitted by sexual intercourse.

97. E Potassium

RATIONALE: Potassium is necessary to the life of all animals. It is the major intracellular cation and helps regulate neuromuscular excitability and muscle contraction.

98. B Emphysema

RATIONALE: Emphysema is an abnormal condition of the pulmonary system. It is characterized by overinflation and destructive changes of the alveoli, which results in a loss of lung elasticity and a decreased gas exchange.

99. C Mucous

RATIONALE: A mucous membrane is a major kind of body membrane that covers or lines cavities or canals that open to the outside of the body.

100. E Compound fracture

RATIONALE: An open or compound fracture is one in which the broken end of the bone tears open the skin.

Pre-Test 2 Answer Key

1. E Grouping

RATIONALE: Grouping is the practice of scheduling patients with the same type of examination (e.g., complete physicals), conditions (e.g., pregnancy), or procedures (e.g., Papanicolaou [Pap] smears) within a certain time frame.

2. C Envelope marked *Personal*

RATIONALE: Incoming mail should be sorted according to importance and urgency. The order of importance is the physician's personal mail, ordinary first-class mail, periodicals and newspapers, and lastly, all other pieces.

3. B Absence of punctuation after the salutation and a comma after the complimentary close

RATIONALE: Open punctuation style uses no punctuation at the end of any line outside of the body of the letter unless the line ends with an abbreviation. This type of punctuation is used with the simplified block letter style.

4. D Medicaid

RATIONALE: Medicaid is a federally funded insurance program that was set up by the federal government in 1965 to provide for the medically indigent. It is regulated by each state.

5. C Posting

RATIONALE: Posting is the transfer of information from one record to another. Transactions are posted from the day sheet to the ledger.

6. B An alphabetical cross-reference

RATIONALE: Numeric filing involves filing records, correspondence, or cards by number. It is an indirect filing system and requires the use of an alphabetical cross-reference to find a given file.

7. D Holmes-Mathis, Jennie

RATIONALE: Hyphenated elements of a name, whether first name, middle name, or surname, are considered as one unit.

8. C Physician, patient, and insurance company

RATIONALE: A third-party payor is some entity other than the patient, spouse, or parent who is responsible for paying all or part of the patient's medical costs.

9. E All of the above

RATIONALE: If a claim form is not sufficiently detailed, complete, and accurate, then the insurance company may reject the claim. Reasons for claim rejection might include missing or incomplete diagnosis; incorrectly coded diagnosis; charges not itemized; patient's group, member, or policy number missing; patient signature missing; patient's date of birth missing; dates missing or incorrect; and physician's signature missing.

10. D $0.84

RATIONALE: The first ounce would cost $0.34, and the two additional ounces would total $0.50 ($0.34 + $0.50 = $0.84).

11. D Below the return address

RATIONALE: Any notation on the envelope directed toward the addressee, such as *Personal* or *Confidential*, should be typed and underlined on the third line below the return address. It should be aligned with the return address on the left edge of the envelope.

12. A Very truly yours

RATIONALE: The complimentary close is the writer's way of saying good-bye. The words used are determined by the formality used in the salutation.

13. D Insurance information

RATIONALE: The patient's insurance information is obtained at the time of the first visit to the office. Necessary information includes the patient's name, telephone number, reason for coming to the office, and times available for the appointment.

14. B Conference call

RATIONALE: A conference call allows more than two people to participate in a conversation at one time. Each person can hear or talk to all others who are participating.

15. C   Backing up

RATIONALE: A back up is a tape or disk for storage of files to prevent their loss in the event of hard drive failure.

16. E   Future events arranged in chronologic order

RATIONALE: A tickler file is a chronologic file used as a reminder that something must be done on a certain date. This type of file is frequently used as a follow-up method.

17. A   Diarrhea

RATIONALE: CPT is a listing of descriptive terms and identifying codes used for reporting medical services and procedures performed by the physician. All of the choices are procedures except diarrhea.

18. E   All of the above

RATIONALE: The receptionist is usually the first person in the medical office with whom the patient has contact. The appearance, professionalism, attitude, and manners of the receptionist, as well as the appearance of the reception area as a whole, can influence the patient's perception of the entire practice.

19. C   See also

RATIONALE: *See also* is the coding convention that gives the direction to the coder to consider another code.

20. C   Refers to factors that influence health status

RATIONALE: V-codes (V01 through V82) are codes referring to factors that influence health status. A definite diagnosis is not stated, but a valid reason for seeking medical care exists. Reasons can include annual physical examinations, well-baby checks, and preoperative physicals. These codes are part of the ICD-9-CM coding system.

21. D   Resealed with tape and noted as *opened in error*

RATIONALE: All offices should have a procedure to follow regarding incoming mail. Personal mail should be left unopened. Should it be opened in error, fold and replace it inside the envelope, reseal the envelope, and write across the outside *opened in error* followed by the opener's initials.

22. E   All of the above

RATIONALE: E&M descriptors include basic diagnostic and treatment services such as office visits and physical examinations. These descriptors are part of the CPT coding system.

23. B   Medicare

RATIONALE: A third-party payor is any person, insurance company, or government agent other than the patient or the patient's family who pays the patient's account.

24. C   A numbered list of present problems

RATIONALE: The POMR system is designed to organize the patient's medical record and the information it contains. The system uses four parts: (1) the database, (2) the problem list, (3) the treatment plan, and (4) the progress notes. The database includes the chief complaint, present illness or illnesses, and the patient profile.

25. D   Ledger card totals and account-receivable balance

RATIONALE: A trial balance is a method of checking the accuracy of accounts. It should be done once a month after all posting has been completed and before preparing monthly statements. The purpose of a trial balance is to disclose any discrepancies between the ledger cards and accounts receivable. It does not prove the accuracy of the accounts.

26. C   Newest to the front

RATIONALE: The medical record is a chronologic system for recording a patient's medical care. Its continuity ensures the best medical care. By filing the most current information to the front, it provides a quick current reference of the patient's care and management.

27. C   Another physician

RATIONALE: The person answering the telephone is expected to screen all incoming calls. Good judgment in deciding whether to put through a call comes with experience. Calls from other physicians should be put through at once if the physician is available to take the call.

28. D   In consecutive order without large gaps

RATIONALE: Appointment scheduling is the process that determines which patients will be seen by the provider, dates and times of the appointments, and how much time will be allotted to each patient based on the complaint and the availability of the provider. Most providers find that efficient scheduling and time management is one of the most important factors in the success of the practice.

29. E   Diagnosis

RATIONALE: At an initial visit, the patient's diagnosis may not be made. At the first visit, the patient may complete a patient information form that will include name, address, telephone number, insurance information, business information, and referral information.

30. A   8½ × 11; no. 10 envelope

RATIONALE: A standard-size letter (8½ in × 11 in) is used for general business and professional correspondence. Standard ways of folding and inserting letters are used so the letter fits properly and is easy to remove. A size no. 10 envelope is used for a standard-size letter.

31. C   In a separate ledger file

RATIONALE: A ledger card is prepared for each patient (or family) at the time of the first visit. It is the record of all charges and payments for each patient and is kept in a separate file for ease of access and billing purposes.

32. A   The checkbook

RATIONALE: A bank statement is periodically sent by the bank to the customer. It shows the status of the account on a given date. The bank statement balance and the checkbook balance should be the same or they will need to be reconciled (disclosure of any errors in the checkbook or bank statement).

33. D   Minutes

RATIONALE: The record of the proceedings of a meeting is called the minutes. The minutes contain a record of what was done at a meeting, not what was said by the members.

Minutes should be signed by the secretary and kept on file according to the procedure of the organization.

34. C Backing up
RATIONALE: Backing up is the process of using a tape, floppy disk, or compact disk for storage of files to prevent their loss in the event of hard drive failure.

35. C Grouping
RATIONALE: Grouping or clustering allows the provider to make good use of time by seeing patients with the same needs at the same time. An example of grouping may be that the provider only performs complete physical examinations on Wednesday mornings.

36. A Information about the scope of the practice
RATIONALE: Each office should have an attractive brochure that can be used to welcome new patients and to furnish general information about the practice. This brochure can include name and type of practice; name or names of physicians; address and location map; appointment procedures; office hours; comments on billing, charges, and insurance; and a statement concerning the confidentiality of medical records. Any more specific information should be discussed with the appropriate person.

37. B W-4 Form
RATIONALE: The W-4 Form is the Employee's Withholding Allowance Certificate. It is filled out by the employee and allows him or her to determine the number of withholding allowances.

38. D HGB
RATIONALE: The correct abbreviation for hemoglobin is Hgb.

39. C Invasion of privacy
RATIONALE: Invasion of privacy is the act of divulging patient information that has been acquired through privileged interaction (provider-patient communication) without the consent of the patient, which is an intentional tort. Information shared between the provider and the patient is confidential. A release of information form must be signed before this information can be shared.

40. A Omission of all punctuation
RATIONALE: The U.S. Postal Service attempts to read, code, sort, and cancel all mail electronically. The success of this system depends on the correct format that can be read by the automatic equipment. This format includes all addresses typed in block format in the correct area of the envelope, everything in the address capitalized, all punctuation eliminated, states abbreviated using the standard two-letter code, and ZIP code must be included in the last line.

41. B A subpoena
RATIONALE: A *subpoena duces tecum* is an order to provide records or documents to the court. Authority to release information from the medical record lies solely with the patient unless required by law.

42. B Daily log
RATIONALE: The double-entry system provides a comprehensive picture of the medical practice and its effect on the physician's net worth. It requires skill and time and is not frequently used in a small practice. The medical assistant generally maintains only the daily log.

43. B Enclosure
RATIONALE: The enclosure notation identifies any material that may be accompanying the correspondence. The notation is placed two lines below the signature line. If more than one enclosure is included, then specify the number (e.g., Enclosures 2).

44. A Insurance claim
RATIONALE: A superbill is a combination charge slip, statement, and insurance reporting form. It is completed and given to the patient at each visit.

45. E All of the above
RATIONALE: Complete and accurate records are essential to a well-managed medical practice. Health information management includes not only the assembling of the record, but also having an efficient system for saving, retrieving, protecting, transferring, storing, retaining, and destroying these records.

46. B *International Classification of Diseases,* ninth edition, Clinical Modification (ICD-9-CM)
RATIONALE: ICD-9-CM is the coding system used to code diagnosis or disease conditions. CPT, HCPCS, RVS, and RBRVS are systems used to code medical procedures.

47. C Initials come before complete names
RATIONALE: Indexing rules are standardized and are based on current business practices. The rule that applies to initials states, "that initials precede a name beginning with the same letter." For example, the chart for M. Johnson would be filed *before* the chart for Mary Johnson.

48. E V-codes
RATIONALE: V codes (V01 to V82) are the codes that refer to factors that influence the health status of the patient. A definite diagnosis cannot be stated, but a valid reason for seeing the provider exists (e.g., well-baby check-up, annual physical examination).

49. B Bit
RATIONALE: A bit is a binary digit. It is the smallest piece of information that can be processed by a computer.

50. D Directory
RATIONALE: The directory is the index of files on a disk. It shows the names of the documents that are saved on that disk. The operator can then choose a file and open it.

51. E B and C only
RATIONALE: The scheduling system chosen by the facility must be individualized for each specific practice. Important factors that determine the best system include patient need, physician preferences and habits, and the facilities available.

52. B Mixed punctuation
RATIONALE: Mixed (standard) punctuation is appropriate for use with block or modified block letter styles. It places

a colon after the salutation and a comma after the complimentary closing. It is the most commonly used punctuation pattern.

53. C Operating manuals

RATIONALE: An inventory of all capital items (equipment) should be prepared every year. For each item, the name, serial number, date of purchase, price, and any warranty information are included. Operating manuals should be kept separate and readily accessible.

54. B Operative notes

RATIONALE: Operative notes are considered to be part of the physician's records and can only be released by the physician. Nurse's notes, laboratory reports, radiology reports, and billing are hospital generated documents and belong to the institution.

55. C Preexisting condition

RATIONALE: A preexisting condition is a physical condition of a person that existed before the insurance policy was issued.

56. D Inactive files

RATIONALE: Inactive files generally are those of patients whom the provider has not seen for 6 months or longer. When the patient returns for care, his or her chart is moved to the active file.

57. A Patient confidentiality

RATIONALE: The patient is entitled to complete confidentiality with regards to his or her medical records and release of information. Computer technology allows for the gathering and storage of vast amounts of information. This information can then be accessible to a variety of individuals. The monitor displays information and should be positioned away from others that may be at the desk.

58. E All of the above

RATIONALE: All patients should be escorted to the examination or treatment room. All patients are generally more cooperative and less anxious if they understand what is expected of them.

59. B Name of the assisting physician

RATIONALE: Surgery is scheduled by type of procedure and availability of facilities. Important information includes the name of the procedure, expected length of the procedure in hours, type of anesthesia, and the patient's name, age, and telephone number.

60. B A copy of the letter is sent to Dr. Jones

RATIONALE: The copy notation (c:) indicates that a copy of the document was sent to a third party or parties. The notation is placed one to two lines below the enclosure notation.

61. A Results of laboratory tests

RATIONALE: The history and physical are valuable tools in diagnosis. They are a way for the physician to gather information about the physical and psychological condition of the patient. The history is the record of the information provided by the patient. The physical involves a thorough examination of the patient from head to toe. Laboratory tests may be ordered after the physical if needed for diagnosis.

62. B Accept predetermined fees

RATIONALE: Managed care is a type of prepaid health plan. It was developed to provide health care services at a low cost. Managed care includes Health Maintenance Organizations (HMOs) and Independent Practice Associations (IPAs). The traditional HMO builds a group of physicians who agree to be paid on a per-patient basis instead of a fee-for-service basis.

63. D Preferred provider organization

RATIONALE: The preferred provider organization uses a fee-for-service concept. Providers agree on a predetermined list of charges for all services. Care is not prepaid. The patient must pay deductibles.

64. A Cost of services

RATIONALE: E&M codes include basic diagnostic and treatment services such as office visits and examinations. The type of history, the type of examination, and the complexity of medical decision making must be determined to select the correct code properly.

65. E Deposit slip

RATIONALE: Deposit slips are itemized documents of cash, checks, and other funds that a depositor presents to the bank with the items to be credited to an account. All deposits must be accompanied by a deposit slip. A copy of the slip is kept on file.

66. D Patient's surname

RATIONALE: One system of color-coding files is the alphabetical color-coding system. This system uses different colored tabs to represent a different segment of the alphabet. The chart is coded by the patient's last name (surname).

67. B The patient

RATIONALE: The physician owns the medical record, but the patient owns the information contained in the record. Any information concerning the contents of the medical record requires consent from both the patient and the physician before it can be released.

68. C Times not available

RATIONALE: To develop the matrix in the appointment book, block out the times the physician or physicians will be unavailable. All else revolves around the physicians' availability.

69. D Group scheduling

RATIONALE: Grouping is scheduling similar appointments together during a day. For example, all complete physical examinations are scheduled for Friday morning. This type of scheduling is a method of time management.

70. A Extensive editing capability

RATIONALE: The computer, as a document production tool, permits efficient preparation and editing of written documents. Spell-check and column layout are simply added benefits. Storage capacity relates to the computer as a whole and is not specific to word processing.

71. A Insurance coverage is available

RATIONALE: Certified mail requires the receiver's signature as proof of delivery and receipt. Any mail in which first-class postage is paid can be accepted as certified mail.

72. D Personal letters and postcards

RATIONALE: First-class mail includes sealed or unsealed handwritten or typed material, such as letters, postcards, and business reply mail. A variety of mailing options is available for other mailable materials.

73. E The estate is billed

RATIONALE: Estate claims are made against the estate of a deceased patient. Once the office receives notification of the patient's death, the office must submit a claim for the unpaid balance to the administrator of the estate. Each state has different rules and regulations concerning the filing of estate claims.

74. A Immediately

RATIONALE: Endorsement is a signature or writing on the back of a check by which the endorser transfers all rights of the check to another party. All checks received as payments should be restrictively endorsed (for deposit only) immediately to safeguard against loss or theft.

75. E Andrew Stephen

RATIONALE: In alphabetic filing, a person's name is indexed with the surname as unit 1, the given name as unit 2, and the middle name as unit 3. Names are alphabetized according to the first unit letter by letter.

76. E David Roberts, M.D.

RATIONALE: The inside address includes the name, title, and address of the receiver. When addressing a letter to a physician, omit the courtesy title, and type the physician's name followed by his or her academic degree.

77. E A license must be obtained from the post office

RATIONALE: A postage meter is an efficient way of stamping large amounts of mail. Postage is prepaid and applied directly to the envelope or on adhesive strips. The other choices are all true about postage meters.

78. B NE

RATIONALE: The use of standard two-letter abbreviations aids in the reading, coding, sorting, and canceling of the mail. The U.S. Postal Service has issued a list of two-letter state abbreviations to be used with zip codes. None of the other choices represent a U.S. state abbreviation.

79. C Full block style

RATIONALE: The full block style places all lines flush at the left margin. The other choices vary indentation of the margin or margins.

80. C Complimentary close

RATIONALE: A memorandum is a written communication among persons within an office or organization. It uses guide words that indicate the date, sender, receiver or receivers, and subject.

81. C Name, page number, and date

RATIONALE: The second and continuous pages of a letter or report are placed on plain paper that matches the letterhead in weight, color, and fiber content. The heading of the subsequent pages must contain the name of the addressee, page number, and date.

82. A Two

RATIONALE: The complimentary close is placed on the second line below the last line of the body of the letter.

83. D Physician charges

RATIONALE: A fee profile is established by compiling and averaging the usual charges for services of the physician over a given period. This profile is then used to determine the amount of third-party liability.

84. B Date of birth

RATIONALE: Demographics relate to the statistical characteristics of a population. It includes the name, date of birth, marital status, children, occupation, education, and social information of the patient.

85. D Irritable bowel syndrome

RATIONALE: ICD-9-CM assigns numeric codes to diseases, illnesses, injuries, and health-related conditions. The coding system is used to establish medical necessity to facilitate payment for health care services and to translate written terminology or descriptions into numbers to provide a universal common language.

86. B 1:00 PM

RATIONALE: The United States is divided into four time zones: (1) Pacific time (WA, OR, NV, and CA), (2) Mountain time (MT, UT, ID, WY, CO, NM, AZ, and parts of ND, SD, NE, and KS), (3) Central time (MN, WI, IA, MO, AR, OK, TX, LA, MS, IL, AL, and parts of TN, KY, ND, SD, NE, and KS), and (4) Eastern time (all others). Central, Mountain, and Pacific time zones are 1 or more hours behind Eastern time. Pacific time is 3 hours behind Eastern time; when it is 1:00 Pacific time, it is 4:00 Eastern time.

87. B Third ring

RATIONALE: If possible, the telephone should be answered on the first ring and always by the third ring.

88. A Refers to external causes

RATIONALE: An E-code is a classification of ICD-9-CM coding. It is used to describe environmental events, circumstances, and conditions as the external cause of injury, poisoning, and other adverse effects.

89. D CMS-1500

RATIONALE: The CMS-1500 is a universal claim form developed by the HCFA that standardizes the data required by most insurance carriers to process insurance claims.

90. D At the end of the day

RATIONALE: Patients who are habitually late for appointments should be scheduled at the end of the day so as not to disrupt the workflow.

91. C Draw a single line through the error, write the word *error,* make the correction, and date and initial the entry

RATIONALE: Corrections are made in the medical record by drawing a single line through the error, writing the word *error* next to it, making the correction, and dating and initialing the correction (SLIDE rule).

92. D Problem-oriented progress notes

RATIONALE: SOAP is an organized way of charting progress notes. SOAP stands for *subjective, objective, assessment,* and *plan.*

93. A A referral to another physician

RATIONALE: The physician must notify the patient of his or her intention to terminate the relationship to protect the physician against abandonment. The physician is not required to refer to another physician.

94. E Should be squeezed in for a brief visit so the physician can decide what the next treatment step should be

RATIONALE: If the patient requires immediate attention, then he or she should be accommodated. If the patient does not need immediate care, then a brief visit with the physician and a scheduled appointment at a later date may be the best policy. The patient should be told that the office runs on an appointment basis.

95. B Immediately offer a new appointment time

RATIONALE: Attempt to reschedule the appointment while the patient is on the telephone. Patients with advance appointments may fill canceled appointments.

96. B Low-pitched and expressive voice

RATIONALE: The telephone voice should be warm, friendly, and natural. Pronunciation and enunciation should be clear and distinct. A normal tone of voice carries best. Variance in tone brings out the meaning of words and adds vitality to what is said. The other choices present opportunities for disconcertion, confusion, or miscommunication.

97. B To deal with the collection agency

RATIONALE: After an account has been released to a collection agency, the medical office makes no further attempts at collection. No more statements are sent. The patient's ledger is marked so that the office knows it is in the hands of an agency. Refer the patient to the agency if he or she contacts the office in regard to the account. Any payments should be reported to the agency.

98. D Word processing

RATIONALE: Word processing is the system used to process written communications. It is a document production tool. Telecommunications involve verbal communication; documentation, interfacing, and formatting are not types of computer systems.

99. B Enclosed packing slip

RATIONALE: All orders received should be compared with the original purchase order and the invoice included with the shipment. The order should be checked for correct items, sizes, styles, and amounts.

100. C The patient pays in advance

RATIONALE: A credit balance is the amount of advance payment or overpayment on an account. The amount of receipts exceeds the amount charged.

Pre-Test 3 Answer Key

1. C All patients

RATIONALE: *Standard precautions* apply to the handling of all potentially infectious body fluids and tissues. Health care workers should take nondiscriminatory precautions to protect themselves.

2. E B and C

RATIONALE: Gloves are considered to be a barrier precaution and should be used when contact with blood or other body fluids is anticipated.

3. C 98.6°F

RATIONALE: Normal adult oral temperature is between 97° and 99° F.

4. B 14 to 20 breaths per minute

RATIONALE: Normal adult rate can be from 14 to 20 breaths per minute.

5. E B and C

RATIONALE: Temperature, pulse, respiration, and blood pressure are considered to be the vital signs. They are the measurements that indicate the state of general health of the patient.

6. B Usually higher in children than in adults

RATIONALE: The normal pulse rate for a child is between 80 and 120 beats per minute. Normal values for an adult are between 60 and 80 beats per minute.

7. E All of the above

RATIONALE: The pulse rate is decreased by conditions such as depression, chronic pain, central nervous system disorders, and hypothyroidism.

8. D 103° to 105° F

RATIONALE: Fever is a temperature over 100° F. A high fever is over 103° F. Untreated high fever can result in brain damage or death.

9. A The difference between the systolic and the diastolic blood pressure

RATIONALE: The pulse pressure is the difference between the systolic and the diastolic blood pressures. It reflects the volume of circulating blood. Less than 30 mm Hg or more than 50 mm Hg is considered normal.

10. B 99

RATIONALE: To convert kilograms to pounds, multiply the number of kilograms by 2.2 (45 kg × 2.2 = 99 lb).

11. A 6 feet

RATIONALE: Height is measured in inches. Using the conversion factor of 12 inches equals 1 foot, divide 72 inches by 12 inches (72 ÷ 12 = 6).

12. A Chest and back

RATIONALE: Percussion is the use of tapping or striking the body to elicit sounds, usually done with the fingers or small hammer. Percussion aids in the determination of the size, position, and density of the underlying organ or cavity.

13. D Social history

RATIONALE: The social history gives information regarding the patient's lifestyle, hobbies, education, occupation, sleeping habits, methods of exercise, sex life, and coping skills.

14. D All of the above

RATIONALE: Subjective findings (symptoms) are perceptible only to the patient or known only to the patient.

15. E Clearness of vision

RATIONALE: Visual acuity using the Snellen eye chart is a common distance acuity screening test.

16. C Rectum

RATIONALE: Proctoscopy is the use of a scope to examine the rectum and the distal portion of the colon.

17. B Left side and chest, with right leg flexed

RATIONALE: The Sims' position is one in which the patient lies on the left side with the right knee and thigh drawn up toward the chest. It is sometimes called the lateral position and can be used for rectal examinations and some pelvic examinations.

18. D Prone position

RATIONALE: The prone position is one in which the patient is lying face down on the table.

19. A Ophthalmoscope

RATIONALE: The ophthalmoscope is an instrument used to inspect the inner structures of the eye. It has a handle containing batteries and an attached head equipped with a light and magnifying lenses.

20. B Sitting

RATIONALE: In the sitting position, the patient is sitting upright on the examination table. This position is useful in examining and treating the head, neck, and chest.

21. A Glucose and protein

RATIONALE: On all subsequent visits, a urine sample is obtained and tested for the presence of sugar (glucose) and albumin (protein). The presence of glucose might be a warning sign of a prediabetic state or diabetes. The presence of protein might be an early warning sign of toxemia. Both of these conditions would require careful medical supervision and treatment.

22. A 1 week after her period

RATIONALE: A monthly breast self-examination can detect early signs of breast cancer. The examination should be performed once a month and approximately 1 week after the menstrual period because the breasts are usually not tender or swollen at this time.

23. A Acute

RATIONALE: Disease is a pathologic process that in some way alters the normal function, structure, or metabolism of an organism. An acute disease process or acute infection begins abruptly with sharp intensity and then subsides after a short period.

24. C 21 to 28 days

RATIONALE: Double-wrapped sterile packs are considered sterile up to 28 days from the date of sterilization. They should be stored in a clean, dry, and dust-free place. When a pack expires, the contents must be reprocessed.

25. E Unwrap the pack, rewrap the pack, replace the indicator, and resterilize

RATIONALE: A sterilization indicator shows that the proper combination of steam, time, and temperature has been achieved. It does not prove that the contents are sterile. Failure of an indicator to change color might indicate that an error has occurred in the sterilization process. The pack should be reprocessed to correct any problem that may have caused the improper sterilization.

26. B Sanitization

RATIONALE: Instruments and other items used in the office must be carefully cleaned before proceeding with disinfection or sterilization. This cleaning process is sanitization. It is used to remove microorganisms, blood, and debris that might interfere with the sterilization process.

27. C Acquired active

RATIONALE: Immunity is the body's resistance to pathogenic microorganisms. It is classified as either natural or acquired. Natural immunity is a genetic feature specific to a person's race, sex, and ability to respond. Acquired immunity means that the body has developed an ability to defend itself. Acquired immunity can be active or passive. Active immunity results when a person has been exposed to or has had the disease. Passive immunity is gained from receiving immune substances, thus bypassing the body's immune system.

28. B Away from the body

RATIONALE: Unfolding the top flap away from the body avoids the necessity of reaching over the sterile field and causing contamination. It also helps avoid touching a person or uniform.

29. E 8–0

RATIONALE: The size or gauge of most sutures is labeled in terms of 0s; 0 is the thickest, and the numbers of 0s decrease up to 10–0, which is the thinnest. (The more 0s, the thinner the material.)

30. D Forceps

RATIONALE: Forceps are instruments of varied sizes and shapes used for grasping, compressing, or holding tissues and/or objects. They are two-pronged instruments with either a spring handle or a ring handle with a ratchet closure.

31. C Iodine

RATIONALE: Betadine is an antiseptic solution often used to disinfect the skin before a minor surgical procedure. It contains iodine, and a patient who is allergic to iodine will have a reaction to the solution.

32. E Purulent

RATIONALE: When a dressing is changed, it and the wound must be inspected for the amount and character of drainage. Drainage that is described as purulent consists of or contains pus.

33. A 10 to 15 degrees

RATIONALE: The objective of an intradermal injection is to inject a minute amount of solution between the layers of the skin. The needle is inserted at a 10 to 15 degree angle to deliver the solution to the correct area. When given correctly, the injection produces a wheal on the skin surface.

34. C Sublingual

RATIONALE: A sublingual route of administration places the drug under the patient's tongue. It is then left to dissolve and be absorbed.

35. B   1½ inch, 21 gauge

RATIONALE: The main objective when administering an intramuscular injection is to inject the medication into deep muscle tissue for gradual and optimal absorption. The longer length of the needle allows this level of administration to occur. The gauge allows for thick medications to be injected easily.

36. B   Diuretic

RATIONALE: Diuretic medications promote the formation and excretion of urine. They can be prescribed to reduce the volume of extracellular fluid in the treatment of many disorders, including hypertension, edema, and congestive heart failure.

37. A   0.5 mL

RATIONALE: Use the following formula:

$$\frac{\text{dose ordered}}{\text{available strength}} \times \text{dose form} = \text{dose given}$$

$$\frac{250\ \text{mg} \times 1\ \text{mL}}{500\ \text{mg}} = 0.5\ \text{mL}$$

38. B   Directly opposite from the specimen

RATIONALE: A centrifuge is a piece of laboratory equipment used to separate specimens by using centrifugal force. When a specimen tube is placed in the centrifuge, it must be counterbalanced with a tube of similar design and weight for balance. An unbalanced load can cause the centrifuge to vibrate and ruin the specimen.

39. A   Within ½ hour of collection

RATIONALE: The microscopic examination of urine consists of categorizing and counting cells, casts, crystals, and miscellaneous constituents of the sediment. Chemical and cellular components change rapidly in a urine sample if they are allowed to sit at room temperature. These changes can be avoided by refrigerating the specimen if the analysis cannot be performed within 30 minutes after collection.

40. A   Anuria

RATIONALE: Normal volume of urine produced every 24 hours is approximately 750 to 2000 mL, with an average of 1500 mL. Anuria is the complete suppression of urine formation by the kidney. It can be caused by renal obstruction or renal failure.

41. E   1.010 and 1.025

RATIONALE: Specific gravity is the weight of a substance compared with the weight of an equal volume of distilled water. In urinalysis, specific gravity is the rough measurement of the concentration of substances dissolved in urine. Most urine samples fall between 1.010 and 1.025. This reading indicates the ability of the kidney to concentrate the specimen, and a reading outside this range might indicate kidney disease.

42. D   All of the above

RATIONALE: A complete blood count (CBC) is one of the most common laboratory tests ordered on blood. It gives a complete look at the blood components, thus giving a wealth of information about a patient's condition. Tests performed in a CBC include red blood cell count, white blood cell count, hemoglobin and hematocrit, differential, platelet number estimation, and red blood cell morphology.

43. A   From a skin puncture

RATIONALE: Capillary or peripheral blood is obtained by performing a skin puncture on the fingertip, earlobe, or great toe or heel of an infant. This method allows for a minimal amount of blood to be collected but is sufficient for many laboratory tests.

44. C   Gallbladder

RATIONALE: A cholecystogram is an x-ray of the gallbladder. It is made after the ingestion or injection of a radiopaque substance. The test is useful in diagnosing cholecystitis (inflammation of the gallbladder), cholelithiasis (gallstones), and tumors.

45. A   Dilates blood vessels

RATIONALE: Thermotherapy (application of heat) produces local vasodilation and increases circulation. These results of heat application speed up the inflammatory process, promote local drainage, relax muscles, and relieve pain.

46. A   P

RATIONALE: Electrocardiography is the procedure that records the electrical activity of the heart. The electrocardiogram records a series of waves or deflections above or below a baseline. Each wave or deflection corresponds to a particular part of the cardiac cycle. The P wave reflects contraction of the atria.

47. B   Sinoatrial node

RATIONALE: The sinoatrial node is a specialized tissue found in the right atrial wall near the superior vena cava. It initiates each heartbeat and sets its pace (pacemaker).

48. D   12

RATIONALE: The standard electrocardiogram consists of 12 separate leads or recordings of the electrical activity of the heart from different angles. Each lead must be marked or coded for the physician to know which angle has been recorded. The 12 leads include leads I, II, and III (standard or bipolar leads); leads aVR, aVL, and aVF (augmented leads); and leads V_1, V_2, V_3, V_4, V_5, and V_6 (chest or precordial leads).

49. D   25 mm/sec

RATIONALE: The paper used in an electrocardiographic machine is a specialized graph paper with internationally accepted increments for measuring the cardiac cycle. As the paper advances, the heat-sensitive stylus moves along the vertical line and intersects with a vertical line. The paper advances at a speed of 25 mm/sec.

50. A   Silver nitrate

RATIONALE: Silver nitrate ($AgNO_3$) is a caustic solution that is used to promote the healing process after surgery. It is available in solution form or coated on an applicator stick.

51. A   Prothrombin time

RATIONALE: The drug Coumadin (warfarin sodium) is an anticoagulant and keeps the blood from clotting. The prothrombin time (pro time) is a test for detecting coagulation deficits. A prolonged pro time can indicate a deficiency in the normal blood clotting mechanism and can help monitor anticoagulation therapy.

52. C Catgut

RATIONALE: The purpose of sutures is to hold the edges of a wound together until healing can occur. Absorbable sutures, usually used on deeper tissues, do not have to be removed because they are absorbed or digested by body fluids and tissues during the healing process. An example of this type of suture material is surgical gut (catgut). Nonabsorbable sutures used on outer skin surfaces are removed after the wound is healed.

53. B 100

RATIONALE: The differential white blood cell count is a test that determines the percentage of each of the five different types of white blood cells in the blood. The procedure involves examining a specific area of a stained blood smear under the microscope. One hundred cells are counted and classified, and a tally is kept.

54. C 30%

RATIONALE: Hemoglobin and hematocrit values are related. Each 1% hematocrit contains 0.34 g of hemoglobin. The hematocrit should equal three times the hemoglobin within 3%.

55. D Erythrocyte sedimentation rate: 30 mm/hr

RATIONALE: The normal value for a sedimentation rate is 0 to 20 mm/hr. An increased erythrocyte sedimentation rate might indicate inflammation.

56. A Gram stain

RATIONALE: Because bacteria are small and possess little color, staining is necessary to observe them under the microscope. The Gram stain is used most often. The dyes in the stain are taken up differently in each type of bacterial cell, and they stain different colors. Bacteria are identified as gram negative (stain red) or gram positive (stain purple).

57. B Alkaline

RATIONALE: pH expresses the degree of acidity or alkalinity of a solution. Usually, freshly voided urine is acidic. After sitting, bacteria contaminate the sample and cause it to become alkaline.

58. D Red-stoppered (serum separator tube [SST], tiger)

RATIONALE: Blood collection tubes are color-coded, depending on the additive it contains or does not contain. Red-stoppered (SST, tiger) tubes contain no additives, therefore the blood collected in these tubes clot and serum can be removed.

59. E All of the above

RATIONALE: Surgical instruments have clearly identifiable parts and can easily be differentiated from one another. Instruments are classified according to their uses, and most belong to one of four main groups: (1) cutting and dissecting instruments, (2) grasping and clamping instruments, (3) retractors, and (4) probes and dilators.

60. A Assess the victim's airway

RATIONALE: Check the victim for responsiveness. If unconscious, assess the ABC: airway, breathing, and circulation.

61. E All of the above

RATIONALE: A complete urinalysis is composed of three parts: (1) the physical examination that includes assessment of color, clarity, odor, amount, and specific gravity; (2) the chemical examination that can include using a reagent strip to test for the presence of glucose, ketones, leukocytes, blood, nitrates, pH, urobilinogen, protein, and bilirubin; and (3) the microscopic examination for cells, bacteria, casts, and artifacts.

62. D Liver

RATIONALE: After a drug is absorbed into the body and transported to the cells or tissues for which it is intended, it is again picked up by the bloodstream and transported to the liver, the site of metabolism and/or biotransformation. In the liver, the drug is broken down and prepared for elimination from the body.

63. C Tests for color-blindness

RATIONALE: Color-blindness is tested using Ishihara plates. The Ishihara color test uses a series of plates on which are printed round dots in a variety of colors and patterns. Patients with normal color vision are able to discern specific patterns on the plates. Patients with a deficiency in color perception cannot do so.

64. E Polyuria

RATIONALE: Signs and symptoms of a myocardial infarction (heart attack) is an occlusion of a coronary artery that results in loss of blood flow and necrosis to the myocardium. The onset is characterized by crushing chest pain. The patient becomes ashen, clammy, short of breath, and nauseated.

65. A Forceps

RATIONALE: Hemostatic forceps are a type of clamping instrument used to stop bleeding, clamp severed vessels, and hold tissue.

66. C 1 to 4

RATIONALE: A fairly constant ratio of four pulse beats to one respiration exists. As a general rule, both pulse and respiration rates normally respond to exercise or emotional upsets. Normal pulse rate for an adult is between 60 and 80 beats per minute. Normal respiratory rate for an adult is between 14 and 20 breaths per minute.

67. E All of the above

RATIONALE: Insulin shock is caused by too much insulin intake, decrease in food intake, or excessive exercise. It is characterized by sweating, trembling, chills, nervousness, irritability, hunger, hallucinations, and pallor. If uncorrected, it can progress to convulsions, coma, and death. Treatment requires an immediate dose of glucose.

68. A Kidneys

RATIONALE: The kidneys are the most important route for the excretion (elimination) of drugs from the body. Most drugs are filtered out of the circulation, broken down into harmless substances, and then excreted in the urine.

69. C   Antidepressant

RATIONALE: Drugs can be classified according to their actions in the body. An antidepressant medication is used as a mood elevator and is used to treat depression. Prozac (fluoxetine) is an example of an antidepressant.

70. B   Friction and running water

RATIONALE: Hands must be washed, using the correct technique, before and after each patient is examined or treated. Proper hand washing depends on two factors: (1) running water and (2) friction. Friction is the firm rubbing of skin surfaces to loosen debris. Running water washes away the debris.

71. D   12 months

RATIONALE: The vaccination for mumps, measles, and rubella is recommended that the first dose be given between 12 and 15 months of age. The second dose is recommended between ages 6 and 12 years.

72. B   Migraine

RATIONALE: Migraine headaches are paroxysmal attacks of headaches that may be completely incapacitating. They are frequently characterized by nausea, vomiting, visual disturbances, throbbing pain in one side of the head, and an aura. An aura is some type of visual disturbance such as lines or spots across the visual field.

73. D   To carry oxygen and carbon dioxide

RATIONALE: Hemoglobin, which is made up of iron and protein, is a main constituent of red blood cells. It carries oxygen to the cells from the lungs and carbon dioxide away from the cells to the lungs for excretion. Normal hemoglobin values vary throughout life and are affected by age, gender, diet, altitude, and disease.

74. A   Ensures the accuracy of results

RATIONALE: Quality assurance is a major component of the Clinical Laboratory Improvement Acts of 1988 (CLIA '88) regulations relating to laboratory standards. It is a comprehensive set of policies and procedures developed to ensure the quality of laboratory testing and includes quality control, personnel orientation, laboratory documentation, knowledge of instrumentation, and enrollment in a proficiency-testing program.

75. B   48 to 72 hours after it is performed

RATIONALE: The Mantoux test is used for routine screening and diagnosis of tuberculosis. The test uses a purified protein derivative from a live tuberculin culture to test for antibodies. The results should be read 48 to 72 hours after the test is performed by intradermal injection. The extent of induration is measured and recorded.

76. C   AU

RATIONALE: The abbreviation for both ears is AU. It comes from the Latin *auris unitas*.

77. D   O

RATIONALE: Patients with type O blood are considered to be universal donors. Type O blood contains no antigens on the red blood cells, thus it will not agglutinate in the presence of anti-A and anti-B antibodies in the plasma.

78. E   Colon

RATIONALE: A lower gastrointestinal series (barium enema) is an x-ray examination of the colon. Contrast medium (barium) is instilled into the colon through an enema. The colon can then be visualized by x-ray examination.

79. B   Computed tomographic scan

RATIONALE: A computed tomographic scan is a radiographic technique that produces a film that represents a detailed cross-section of a tissue structure. The technique uses a narrow beam of x-ray that rotates in a continuous 360-degree motion around the patient. The pictures obtained from this method are highly detailed and simulate a three-dimensional appearance.

80. A   Cancer

RATIONALE: Massive or excessive exposure to radiation can cause tissue damage and various side effects, which can include damage to blood cells, skin cells, eyes, and reproductive cells. Overexposure can result in decreased red and white blood cell counts, burns, and an increased incidence of cancers.

81. B   Leads I, II, and III

RATIONALE: The first three leads recorded are the standard or bipolar leads (leads I, II, and III). They each use two limb electrodes to record electrical activity.

82. B   Chains

RATIONALE: Bacteria may be classified by morphology (size and shape). Streptococci are bacteria that are spherical in shape and arranged in chains.

83. D   Increasing age

RATIONALE: Normal pulse rates normally vary as a result of a person's gender, age, body size, posture, activity level, health status, nervous system function, emotional state, and the volume and composition of the blood. Pulse normally decreases with age.

84. D   RL

RATIONALE: The leads of an electrocardiogram measure the electrical activity from the frontal and horizontal planes of the body. The right leg acts as the grounding as electrical activity is recorded from the right arm, left arm, and left leg.

85. A   OSHA

RATIONALE: The Occupational Safety and Health Act was established by the federal government in 1970 to set standards and protocols for occupational health and safety. The regulations must be known and followed. They include hazard exposure plans, medical waste management, personal protective measures, general safety precautions, fire safety, staff development, and blood-borne pathogen regulations.

86. E   Cost

RATIONALE: A drug reference provides information about medications. Most references include the following information about the medication: action, indication, side effects, adverse effects, precautions, contraindications, doses, and administration. These references include the *Physician's Desk Reference*, package inserts, *U.S. Pharmacopeia/National Formulary*, and other published references.

87. E   All of the above

RATIONALE: An analgesic medication lessens the sensory function of the brain. They are used for pain relief. Analgesics can be classified as narcotic (morphine, codeine, Demerol) or nonnarcotic (aspirin, Tylenol, ibuprofen).

88. C   Keep a written record of all daily activities

RATIONALE: A Holter monitor is a portable monitoring system used to record the cardiac activity of the patient for a 24-hour period. Keeping a written diary of all activities during the day that causes stress is important for the patient. Examples of these activities include driving in traffic, stair climbing, and bowel movements. Symptoms associated with possible heart problems should also be included.

89. D   Peristalsis

RATIONALE: Peristalsis is the involuntary wavelike movement that moves food downward through the gastrointestinal tract. Peristalsis is activated when the food mass is swallowed and enters the esophagus.

90. A   2 months

RATIONALE: The schedule for childhood immunizations begins with the first doses of DTP (DtaP), IPV, *Haemophilus influenzae* type b (HiB) vaccine, and hepatitis B (HepB) vaccine being administered at age 2 months.

91. C   Histology

RATIONALE: Histology involves the preparation and study of specimens of tissue from any source in the body. Changes in the tissue form and/or structure are observed microscopically.

92. C   A nonsterile person entering the room

RATIONALE: Surgical asepsis, or sterile technique, is the practice used when an area and supplies in that area are to be made and kept sterile. The goal of surgical asepsis is to prevent the introduction of microorganisms into the body. Talking over the sterile field can introduce microorganisms onto it. Hair that is not pulled back or inside a cap might also introduce microorganisms. Moisture contaminates the sterile field. A 1-inch edge around the entire sterile field is considered not sterile.

93. C   Benadryl

RATIONALE: An antihistamine drug counteracts the effects of histamine by blocking the action in the tissues. Antihistamines are used for relief of allergies. An example of an antihistamine is diphenhydramine (Benadryl).

94. D   qod (every day)

RATIONALE: The abbreviation *qod* means every other day. The abbreviation *qd* means every day.

95. D   Needle biopsy

RATIONALE: Surgical asepsis is defined as the destruction of organisms before they enter the body. The technique is used for any procedure that punctures, pierces, or incises the skin or mucous membranes. Everything that comes in contact with the patient should be sterile, including instruments, drapes, and gloved hands. A needle biopsy is a procedure that breaks the skin and thus requires surgical asepsis.

96. A   Daily

RATIONALE: Quality control is the operational procedure used to implement the quality assurance program. The objective of quality control is to ensure accuracy of test results while detecting errors. It is mandated by law. Specially prepared quality control samples are tested daily. The results of these samples must be within a preestablished range before patient results can be reported.

97. B   Impetigo

RATIONALE: Impetigo is a highly infectious bacterial infection of the skin. It is caused by *Staphylococcus* or *Streptococcus* and is characterized by vesicles that rupture and form a honey-colored crust. Lesions form primarily on the face, especially around the mouth and nose. Impetigo is treated with antibiotic ointment. Proper hand washing can help prevent its spread.

98. C   Osteoporosis

RATIONALE: Osteoporosis is a disorder of the skeletal system characterized by porous, brittle bones. These bones then become susceptible to fractures. Osteoporosis occurs most frequently in postmenopausal women. It is treated with calcium supplements, hormone replacement therapy (estrogen), exercise, and medications.

99. D   Presbyopia

RATIONALE: Presbyopia is a disorder of accommodation. It is due to the loss of elasticity of the lens of the eye as a result of aging. It can be corrected with bifocals or trifocals.

100. A   Otitis media

RATIONALE: Otitis media is an inflammation (infection) of the middle ear. Fluid collects behind the tympanic membrane. Otitis media is often associated with an upper respiratory infection. The patient will experience pain and fever. The infected canal and eardrum appear red and swollen, and a purulent discharge may be present. It is treated with antibiotics and analgesics.

Post-Test Answer Key

General

1. B Uniform Anatomical Gift Act

RATIONALE: The Act states that any person of sound mind and of the age of 18 or older may give all or part of his or her body after death for research, transplantation, or placement in a tissue bank.

2. B Thyroid

RATIONALE: Calcitonin is secreted by cells found between the follicles in the thyroid gland. Calcitonin regulates the plasma levels of calcium.

3. B The patient is human immunodeficiency virus (HIV) positive

RATIONALE: Even though the physician is charged with safeguarding patient confidentiality, state laws require certain disclosures. All states require sexually transmitted diseases to be reported, including confirmed cases of acquired immunodeficiency syndrome. Most states, but not all, require that patients who are HIV positive be reported.

4. C Registered nurse

RATIONALE: The registered nurse (RN) is licensed in the state in which he or she practices. This license must be renewed on a regular basis, or the nurse cannot practice as an RN.

5. B Ask the patient to calm down

RATIONALE: The medical assistant can help calm an angry patient by speaking calmly and refusing to return the emotion. Calmly ask the person to take a deep breath and stop talking for a few moments. Gradually lowering the volume of the voice will cause the angry person to lower his or her own voice so he or she can hear what the medical assistant is saying.

6. B The formation of new blood cells

RATIONALE: *Hemat/o* is the combining form for blood. The suffix-*poiesis* means formation or to make.

7. A Notify the patient that her medical care is being terminated

RATIONALE: The patient-physician relationship is an implied contract. Both parties must uphold their part of the contract.

Not following physician's orders would be grounds to terminate the contract. The physician must notify the patient by sending a certified letter.

8. C Explain the delay and offer another appointment if the patient requests one

RATIONALE: Explaining the situation briefly and offering another appointment can reduce the frustration and stress that the patient may be feeling.

9. D State government

RATIONALE: The MD, DO, or DC degree is conferred on graduation from the medical or chiropractic school. The license to practice medicine is granted by a state board, also known as the state board of medical examiners.

10. D Durable power of attorney

RATIONALE: A durable power of attorney is a legal document that allows the patient to appoint someone who is trusted to make medical decisions for the patient in the event that the patient cannot make those decisions.

11. C Closed-ended

RATIONALE: The closed-ended question asks for specific information. It limits the answer to one or two words. A *yes* or *no* answer may be enough.

12. A Health Insurance Portability and Accountability Act

RATIONALE: This federal Act consists of several components, one of which contains provisions to protect a patient's privacy.

13. B Adolescence

RATIONALE: Adolescence (age 11 to 19 years) begins with the onset of menses in young women and sperm production in young men. The psychosocial characteristics of this age group include the need for privacy, acceptance by a group, and peer pressure, as well as egocentric, self-absorbed, and rebellious behaviors.

14. B Scoliosis

RATIONALE: Scoliosis is the abnormal lateral curvature of the spine. Mild scoliosis generally causes no problems. Severe curvature can cause back pain and heart and lung problems resulting from decreased space in the thoracic cavity.

15. A Fax

RATIONALE: A fax machine is a time and labor saver in conveying patient information from physician to physician or physician to hospital. However, precautions must be taken to ensure security of the information arriving by fax. This goal can be accomplished by telephoning ahead to alert the receiver that sensitive information will be arriving.

16. D Encourage questions

RATIONALE: Being elderly is not an impairment. Many older patients are mentally sharp and do not expect special treatment. Asking questions helps clarify understanding.

17. C Lack of blood flow to tissue

RATIONALE: Ischemia is reduced or lack of blood flow to tissue that results in impairment of cell function.

18. C Serous

RATIONALE: Serous drainage is the thin, watery, serum-like drainage that is present in a wound during the healing process.

19. A "Please tell me more about those feelings."

RATIONALE: Using an open-ended statement encourages the patient to open up and expand on his or her thoughts.

20. E Performing medical research without the consent of the patient

RATIONALE: Performing research on a patient without the patient's consent is a breach of patient confidentiality and invasion of privacy, which is considered to be unprofessional conduct and can result in the revocation of the physician's license.

21. E Transient ischemic attack

RATIONALE: Transient ischemic attacks are temporary episodes of impaired neurologic functioning caused by inadequate flow of blood to a portion of the brain. Signs and symptoms may include sudden weakness, numbness and tingling on one side of the body, dizziness, confusion, and vision disturbances.

22. B Denial

RATIONALE: Denial is a defense mechanism in which confrontation with a personal problem or with reality is avoided by denying the existence of the problem or reality. The person, for whatever reason, is unable to cope with the situation and completely pushes it or any person or thing representing it away.

23. C Quotation marks

RATIONALE: The chief complaint is a concise account of the patient's symptoms explained in the patient's own words. This information is set apart from the other charting information by placing the words in quotes.

24. A -penia

RATIONALE: The suffix -penia means deficiency, lack of, or too few.

25. D Lines body cavities that open to the outside of the body

RATIONALE: Mucous membranes line all body cavities that open to the exterior of the body. They secrete mucus, a substance that keeps the membrane moist and lubricated.

26. A There was no recurrence of the tumor

RATIONALE: The sentence is grammatically correct.

27. B Encourage nonverbal communication

RATIONALE: With non–English-speaking patients, the medical assistant may need to use gestures and more body language to convey messages. Having a bilingual staff member is always helpful.

28. B Ringworm

RATIONALE: *Tinea corporis* (ringworm) is a chronic superficial fungal infection of the skin characterized by lesions that are round, ringed, and scaled with vesicles.

29. C Dorsal

RATIONALE: The dorsal surface of the body is located toward the back. It is another word for posterior.

30. A Femur

RATIONALE: The femur is the thighbone. It is the longest and strongest bone in the body.

31. B Seminiferous tubules

RATIONALE: The seminiferous tubules are tightly coiled structures located in each testis. Sperm are formed in the epithelium of these tubules.

32. A Impetigo

RATIONALE: Impetigo is a common, contagious, superficial skin infection. Early lesions can be blister-like or pustular that rupture and form thick yellow crusts. It is caused by either group A *Streptococcus* or *Staphylococcus aureus*.

33. D Occipital

RATIONALE: The occipital bone is located at the base of the skull. It contains a large opening (foramen magnum) where the spinal cord exits the cranium.

34. B Liver

RATIONALE: Bile is a green-yellow secretion produced by the liver and stored in the gallbladder. Bile plays an important role in the digestion of fats.

35. A Survival

RATIONALE: Psychologist Abraham Maslow created what he called the *hierarchy of needs*. This hierarchy categorizes these needs into five levels. The most basic of these needs are the physiologic needs: oxygen, food, water, excretion, shelter, and sexual expression.

36. D Alveoli

RATIONALE: The alveoli are tiny air sacs that form at the ends of the respiratory passages. A pulmonary capillary surrounds each alveolus. Oxygen and carbon dioxide are exchanged between the alveolar-capillary membranes.

37. A Aplastic

RATIONALE: Aplastic anemia results from the failure of the hematopoietic cells (stem cells) in the bone marrow. This condition can be caused by exposure to toxins, alkylating agents, certain drugs, and radiation.

38. C Hiatal hernia

RATIONALE: A hiatal hernia is a defect in the diaphragm that permits a segment of the stomach to slide into the thoracic cavity.

39. D "Can you tell me more about that?"

RATIONALE: An open-ended question requires more than a *yes* or *no* answer. It forces the patient to provide additional detail and expand on his or her thoughts.

40. B Abnormal condition

RATIONALE: The suffix *-iasis* means an abnormal condition or disease.

41. A A physician accidentally amputates the wrong finger from a patient

RATIONALE: *Res ipsa loquitur* means *the thing speaks for itself*. It describes a situation in which the nature of the injury can implicate negligence.

42. B Fee splitting

RATIONALE: If a physician accepts payment from another physician solely for the referral of a patient, then both are guilty of the unethical practice of fee splitting.

43. E All of the above

RATIONALE: Heartbeat, breathing, peristalsis, and pupil dilation are all controlled by the autonomic nervous system. A person has no conscious control over these actions.

44. A Gloss/o

RATIONALE: The combining form for tongue is *gloss/o* and *lingu/o*.

45. B Invasion of privacy

RATIONALE: Giving out patient information without the patient's consent is an invasion of the patient's privacy, which is an intentional tort.

46. D Controlled Substance Act

RATIONALE: The Controlled Substance Act of 1970 is regulated by the Drug Enforcement Administration. This agency addresses and regulates the issues of drug use and abuse in the United States. Under the Controlled Substance Act, drugs are categorized into schedules that define their potential for abuse and addiction.

47. B Glucagon

RATIONALE: Glucagon, which is produced in the alpha cells in the pancreas, stimulates the conversion of glycogen to glucose in the liver. Its primary function is to increase blood glucose levels.

48. C Cholecystectomy

RATIONALE: *Cholecyst-* is the root word meaning gallbladder. The suffix *-ectomy* means surgical removal.

49. B Villi

RATIONALE: The wall of the small intestine forms circular folds with finger-like projections called villi (*sing.* villus). The villi increases the amount of digested food that can be absorbed.

50. B Antibodies

RATIONALE: Foreign substances to which the body (lymphocytes) respond are called antigens. Antigens are found on pathogens, such as bacteria and viruses. Lymphocytes make antibodies to counteract the antigens, putting the antigen-antibody reaction in motion. Antibodies destroy antigens, which helps protect the body against disease.

51. E May refuse to accept a patient if he or she chooses

RATIONALE: A physician has the right to limit the size of his or her practice or the number of patients that he or she treats.

52. D Is a detailed outline of a trip

RATIONALE: Necessary information includes the date and time of departure; flight numbers; mode of transportation to the hotel; name, address, and telephone number of the hotel; and the date and time of return.

53. B Staying calm when dealing with angry patients

RATIONALE: Professionalism is defined as exhibiting a courteous, conscientious, and business-like manner in the workplace. It is characterized by the technical and ethical standards of a certain profession.

54. B Empathy

RATIONALE: Empathy is sensitivity to the individual needs and reactions of patients or others.

55. B Hyster/o

RATIONALE: The combining forms for uterus include *hyster/o, metr/i, metr/o, metri/o, uter/i,* and *uter/o*.

56. A Denial

RATIONALE: Denial is a defense mechanism in which confrontation with a personal problem or with reality is avoided by denying the existence of the problem or reality. The person, for whatever reason, is unable to cope with the situation and completely pushes it or any person or thing representing it away.

57. E All of the above

RATIONALE: Personality is defined as the composite of the behavioral traits and characteristics by which one is recognized as an individual. A person's age, life experience, heredity, and environment all contribute to the composite.

58. B Impatience

RATIONALE: Many characteristics make up the professional qualities desirable in a medical assistant. These characteristics include loyalty, dependability, courtesy, initiative, flexibility, credibility, confidentiality, and attitude.

59. B Cecum

RATIONALE: The cecum is the first division of the large intestine. It is connected to the ileum of the small intestine. The appendix (vermiform) is attached to the cecum.

60. C   The patient must sign a release form

RATIONALE: The medical office must be extremely careful when releasing any type of medical information. The patient must sign a release for any information to be given to any third party.

61. B   Pulmonary artery

RATIONALE: Blood that is low in oxygen exits the right ventricle through the pulmonary artery where it enters the lungs and picks up oxygen.

62. A   Vital signs

RATIONALE: Objective data include anything that is measurable or observed.

63. A   Another physician

RATIONALE: A call from another physician or professional colleague should always be transferred to the physician immediately.

64. B   Small intestines

RATIONALE: *Enter/o* is the combining form for small intestines.

65. D   Delay treatment and inform or consult with the physician

RATIONALE: A physician must have consent from the patient to treat the patient, even though the consent is usually implied. A patient has the right to refuse treatment at any time.

66. E   All of the above

RATIONALE: A contract is an agreement that creates an obligation. To be valid or enforceable, the contract must have four basic elements: (1) an offer or acceptance, (2) consideration, (3) capacity, and (4) legality.

67. A.   -ectomy

RATIONALE: The suffix *-ectomy* means cutting into, surgical removal, or excision.

68. E   All of the above

RATIONALE: Informed consent must be obtained from the patient before a procedure can be performed. Informed consent implies an understanding of what is to be done, why it should be done, the risks involved, the expected outcomes, and alternative treatments, including consequences of failure to treat.

69. C   Peristalsis

RATIONALE: Food material is moved through the digestive tube by means of a wavelike, rhythmic contraction of the smooth muscle in the tube. This movement is called peristalsis.

70. B   Ureter

RATIONALE: Urine drains out of the collecting tubules of each kidney into the renal pelvis and down through the ureter into the urinary bladder.

71. C   Health Insurance Portability and Accountability Act (HIPAA)

RATIONALE: HIPAA was developed in 1996 to help ensure the confidentiality of medical records and patient information.

72. B   Humerus

RATIONALE: The humerus is the largest bone of the upper arm.

73. A   Deltoid

RATIONALE: The deltoid is a large, thick, triangular-shaped muscle that covers the shoulder.

74. A   Atherosclerosis

RATIONALE: Atherosclerosis, a thickening and hardening of the arteries, occurs when plaques of cholesterol and lipids form on the walls of the arteries.

75. B   -tripsy

RATIONALE: The suffix *-tripsy* means to crush.

76. E   All of the above

RATIONALE: The liver is the largest gland in the body. Its main functions include production of bile, detoxification, metabolism of proteins and carbohydrates, storage of vitamins and glycogen, production of heparin, and the recycling of worn-out red blood cells.

77. B   A referring physician when it pertains directly to the course of treatment

RATIONALE: The medical record and the information it contains must be protected. The original should be retained in the facility where it originated. A summary or photocopy of the information may be sent to another physician.

78. C   Epithelial

RATIONALE: Epithelial tissue (epithelium) forms large, continuous sheets. It helps form the skin, lines most of the inner cavities of the body, and makes up glands.

79. B   Bacteria

RATIONALE: In medical language, if the term ends in *um,* the plural is formed by changing the *um* to *a.*

80. D   Allow the child to answer the questions in his or her own words

RATIONALE: The federal Child Abuse Protection and Treatment Act states that all threats to a child's physical and/or mental welfare must be reported. When communicating with a child, always use language the child understands. Speak in quiet tones and at the child's physical level.

81. A   The employee

RATIONALE: The mission of this Act, since its creation in 1970, is to ensure workplace safety and a healthy environment within the workplace.

82. C Decreases blood sugar levels

RATIONALE: Insulin is a hormone manufactured by the beta cells in the pancreas. Its main function is to metabolize glucose and thereby reduce blood sugar levels.

83. D Leukopenia

RATIONALE: Leukopenia is an abnormal decrease in the number of white blood cells to fewer than 5000 cells/mm^3 of blood. *Leuko-* means white or white blood cell; *-penia* means decrease, deficiency, lack of, or too few.

84. B Stat

RATIONALE: *Stat* is the abbreviation for *statim,* which means immediately.

85. E All of the above

RATIONALE: The physician has a legal duty to report information that may have an effect on the health, safety, or welfare of the public. This information includes births, deaths, communicable diseases, abuse, criminal acts, and professional misconduct.

86. A Slow

RATIONALE: The prefix *brady-* means slow.

87. C Deep

RATIONALE: Superficial pertains to the skin or another surface. *Deep* refers to away from the surface.

88. B An advanced directive

RATIONALE: An advanced directive is a legal document that gives a person the right to determine what medical procedures they want provided if they become unable to make those decisions for themselves.

89. B Denial

RATIONALE: Unconscious defense mechanisms protect the mind from guilt or anxiety. Denial is the unconscious avoidance of the reality of an unpleasant or disturbing feeling, thought, or event.

90. D Glycogen

RATIONALE: Glycogen is a polysaccharide similar to plant starch. It is the form in which humans store glucose, primarily in the liver and skeletal muscles.

91. C Etiology

RATIONALE: Etiology is the study of all factors that may be involved in the development of a disease process.

92. E All of the above

RATIONALE: Nonverbal communications are messages conveyed without the use of words, primarily through body language.

93. B An eating disorder

RATIONALE: Bulimia is an insatiable craving for food characterized by binge eating followed by self-induced vomiting.

94. D Stroke

RATIONALE: A cerebrovascular accident or brain attack is an abnormal condition of the blood vessels of the brain. It is characterized by an occlusion that results in ischemia of the brain tissue.

95. C Measles

RATIONALE: Measles (rubeola) is an acute, highly contagious viral infection transmitted by droplets.

96. C Trichomoniasis

RATIONALE: Trichomoniasis is a vaginal infection caused by the protozoan *Trichomonas vaginalis*. It is transmitted through sexual intercourse.

97. D Potassium

RATIONALE: Potassium is necessary to the life of all animals. It is the major cellular cation and helps regulate neuromuscular excitability and muscle contraction.

98. B Emphysema

RATIONALE: Emphysema is an abnormal condition of the respiratory system. It is characterized by overinflation and destructive changes of the alveoli, which results in a loss of lung elasticity and a decrease in gas exchange.

99. D Otorhinolaryngologist

RATIONALE: This physician (ear, nose, and throat [ENT]) treats diseases and conditions that affect the ear, nose, throat, and structures related to the head and neck. Problems that affect the voice and hearing are also referred to this physician.

100. A Taking the patient's arm to guide him or her without speaking

RATIONALE: When caring for a visually impaired patient, the medical assistant should always ask how best to assist the patient.

Administrative

101. C Overbooking

RATIONALE: Overbooking may result in a prolonged waiting time for the patient to see the provider, and it may cause dissatisfaction with the practice.

102. D Itinerary

RATIONALE: An itinerary contains the details of a trip. Necessary information includes the date and time of departure; flight numbers; mode of transportation to the hotel; name, address, and telephone number of the hotel; and the date and time of return.

103. D A scanner

RATIONALE: A scanner is a device that reads text or illustrations on a printed page and translates the information on the page into a form that the computer can understand.

104. C Extended warranty agreement

RATIONALE: A warranty is agreement with a company to repair or replace a product if it does not function correctly within a specified amount of time (limited warranty). An extended warranty allows the owner to purchase additional time for the coverage to be in effect.

105. A $5,630

RATIONALE: Using the income statement, net income equals revenue minus expenses. An asset is anything of value that is owned, not just revenue.

106. A Full block

RATIONALE: In the full block (block) style format, all lines begin flush with the left margin.

107. C Holmes-Mathis, Jennie

RATIONALE: Hyphenated elements of a name, whether first name, middle name, or surname, are considered to be one unit.

108. C Price list

RATIONALE: A fee schedule is a list of services and procedures that a physician usually performs with the amount charged for each.

109. D Postage meter

RATIONALE: The postage meter is the most efficient way of stamping the mail in a large business office. The machine can be purchases or leased; the postage is purchased from the U.S. Postal Service. The date must be changed daily.

110. B Buffer time

RATIONALE: Leaving times open in the morning and afternoon allows the physician and staff a short rest time and catch-up time.

111. C Below the return address

RATIONALE: Any notation on the envelope directed toward the addressee, such as *Personal* or *Confidential,* should be typed and underlined on the third line below the return address and aligned with the return address.

112. A The claim will be denied

RATIONALE: Incomplete or inaccurate codes may result in insurance denial because of lack of medical necessity.

113. B An OUTguide

RATIONALE: An OUTguide is a heavy guide that is used to replace a folder that has temporarily been removed or moved from a filing space. It should be of a distinctive color for easy identification.

114. B Current Procedural Terminology (CPT)

RATIONALE: Morbidity is the relative incidence of disease, which plays a role in the complexity of the decision-making process used when treating a patient. This factor must also be considered when choosing an Evaluation and Management (E&M) level to assign to a patient on a given encounter.

115. A When the patient calls for an appointment

RATIONALE: As a business, a medical office must charge competitive and fair prices for services and must receive payment for the services in a timely fashion. Patients should be fully informed about a practice's fees and payment policies before they receive treatment.

116. D Future events arranged in chronologic order

RATIONALE: A tickler file is a chronologic file used as a reminder that something must be done on a certain date.

117. A Diarrhea

RATIONALE: CPT is a listing of descriptive terms and identifying codes used for reporting medical services and procedures performed by the provider.

118. D Treatment plan

RATIONALE: The problem-oriented medical record (POMR) method is a system that provides a logical, organized, and systematic approach to patient care management. It has four essential sections: (1) database, (2) problem list, (3) treatment plan, and (4) progress notes. The treatment plan includes management, additional work-ups, and therapy.

119. C Endocrine

RATIONALE: The thyroid gland is a major gland in the endocrine system.

120. C Cost of items

RATIONALE: The cost of the item has to be determined before all other additional costs can be calculated.

121. B Employee's marital status

RATIONALE: The amount of money withheld from each paycheck is based on the information the employee provides on Form W-4. The Employer's Tax Guide has tables showing how much tax must be withheld based on the pay period and the employee's marital status.

122. E All of the above

RATIONALE: E&M descriptors are part of the CPT coding system. They include basic diagnostic and treatment services such as office visits and physical examinations.

123. C Numeric

RATIONALE: In the numeric filing system, each file is assigned a number, starting with the lowest number and moving up. Files are organized in numeric order. A cross-reference with the patient's name is kept elsewhere.

124. D To make documents available to all staff members

RATIONALE: Files in the medical office need to be organized systematically so that everyone can locate and replace files accurately and efficiently.

125. D The mission statement

RATIONALE: A policy manual describes the office philosophy and goals. The office mission statement reflects the reasons for the existence of the practice.

126. C Newest to the front

RATIONALE: The medical record is a chronologic system for recording a patient's medical care. By filing the most current information to the front, a current reference is quickly provided.

127. C Another physician

RATIONALE: The person answering the telephone is expected to screen incoming calls. Calls from other physicians should be put through immediately if the provider is available to take the call.

128. A Syringe

RATIONALE: An expendable item is one that is consumable, disposable, or able to be thrown away after use.

129. B Properties owned by the business

RATIONALE: Anything not owed is an asset. Anything owed is a liability.

130. A 8½ × 11; no. 10 envelope

RATIONALE: A standard-size letter (8½ in × 11 in) is used for general business and professional correspondence. Standard ways of folding and inserting letters are used so the letter fits properly and is easy to remove. A size no. 10 envelope is used for a standard-size letter.

131. D W-4

RATIONALE: The Form W-4 is the Employee's Withholding Allowance Certificate. It is filled out by the employee and allows him or her to determine the number of withholding allowances.

132. B Express mail

RATIONALE: Express mail is the fastest delivery in the U.S. Postal Service system. Overnight, second-day, and Saturday delivery options are available. Rates vary with weight, distance, and delivery options.

133. D Minutes

RATIONALE: A record of the proceedings of a meeting is called the minutes. They contain a record of what was done at the meeting. Minutes should be signed and kept on file according to the policy of the organization.

134. D Five

RATIONALE: Each chapter in the tabular list classifies diseases and injuries according to cause and organ system, dividing them into groups: category codes (three-digit code), subcategory code (fourth digit), and subclassification code (fifth digit).

135. C Grouping

RATIONALE: Grouping or clustering allows the provider to use time efficiently by seeing patients with the same needs at the same time.

136. C Medications the patient has taken

RATIONALE: Subjective information is perceived only by the patient. This information would include past medical information or information about which the provider may not know.

137. C Photocopier

RATIONALE: Capital equipment is equipment used to generate revenue.

138. D HGB

RATIONALE: The correct abbreviation for hemoglobin is Hgb.

139. D 99

RATIONALE: CPT lists and codes procedures and services performed by the provider. The CPT book is divided into six sections. The E&M section codes are 99200 to 99499.

140. A Liability

RATIONALE: Liability insurance includes benefits for medical expenses payable to individuals who are injured on the insured person's property or vehicle without regard to the insured person's actual legal liability for the accident.

141. A A subpoena

RATIONALE: The physician and medical assistant may never release confidential information without the consent of the patient except when it is legally required. A *subpoena duces tecum* is a legally binding request to provide records or documents to appear in court.

142. C 090432

RATIONALE: In the terminal digit system, patients are assigned consecutive numbers. The digits are separated into groups of twos or threes and are read from right to left instead of from left to right.

143. B Enclosure

RATIONALE: The enclosure notation identifies any material that may be accompanying the correspondence. The notation is placed two lines below the signature line.

144. D Substance Abuse and Mental Health Services Administration

RATIONALE: The Substance Abuse and Mental Health Administration is an agency of the U.S. Department of Health and Human Services with local offices and hotlines nationwide.

145. E All of the above

RATIONALE: Complete and accurate records are essential to a well-managed medical practice. Health information management includes not only the assembling of the record, but also the saving, retrieving, protecting, transferring, storing, retaining, and destroying of these records.

146. B ICD-9-CM

RATIONALE: ICD-9-CM is the coding system used to code diagnosis or disease conditions.

147. C Initials come after complete names

RATIONALE: Indexing rules are standardized and are based on current business practices. The rule that applies to initials states, "that initials precede a name beginning with the same letter." (M. Johnson would be filed before Mary Johnson.)

148. D V-codes

RATIONALE: V-codes are the codes that refer to factors that influence the health status of the patient.

149. A Chief complaint

RATIONALE: The patient's history relates to the patient's clinical picture and depends on the patient for answers to specific questions. The history is composed of the chief complaint or the reason why the patient is being seen. This information is usually in the patient's own words.

150. D Subject

RATIONALE: Subject filing is used for correspondence, invoices, and research. Within each file, documents are arranged either alphabetically or in chronologic order.

151. E Unemployment tax

RATIONALE: Federal unemployment taxes, based on the Federal Unemployment Tax Act (FUTA) are paid entirely by the employer. The FUTA tax provides unemployment payments to workers who lose their job.

152. E In reverse chronologic order

RATIONALE: The source-oriented medical record (SOMR) method consists of chronologic listings in the medical record. The encounters are filed in the record in reverse chronologic order—today's encounter in the front.

153. D Accounting

RATIONALE: A spreadsheet is a software program for inputting and manipulating numeric data to facilitate a wide variety of financial activities.

154. B Contact a travel agent

RATIONALE: A travel agent can help search for a particular flight, specific departure or arrival times, or the best fares. They can also assist for ground transportation, hotel accommodations, sightseeing tours, and other recreational bookings.

155. C Preexisting condition

RATIONALE: A preexisting condition is a condition or disease that was present before an insurance policy was issued.

156. D Identifying and reporting diagnoses

RATIONALE: The ICD-9-CM is used for coding diagnoses on insurance claim forms.

157. C $1,137.50

RATIONALE: A medical assistant who is paid biweekly at the rate of $13.00/hr would gross $1,040 per paycheck ($13.00 × 80 hours = $1,040). The time-and-a-half rate would be $19.50 per hour ($13.00 × 1.5 = $19.50). Overtime pay for that pay period would be $97.50 ($19.50 × 5 hours = $97.50). The gross pay would be $1,137.50 ($1,040 + $97.50 = $1,137.50).

158. C Extremities

RATIONALE: The radial pulses are located in the wrists (extremities).

159. C Write-protect

RATIONALE: Write-protect is a process or code that prevents overwriting of data or programs on a disk.

160. C The central processing unit

RATIONALE: The central processing unit is the main chip that runs the computer and directs the processing of the data. It is also responsible for interpreting and carrying out instructions in the software.

161. B Holmes, Jen

RATIONALE: Indexing rules are standardized based on current business practices. Last names are considered first in filing, first name is second, and middle name or initial is third.

162. C Draw a single line through the misspelled word

RATIONALE: Correct errors in charting by using the SLIDE rule: draw a single line through the entry, write *error* above the entry, correct the entry, and date and initial the entry.

163. E Quarterly

RATIONALE: Every 3 months, the employer must file an Employer's Quarterly Federal Tax Return (Form 941) with the IRS. This form lists the amounts withheld from employee paychecks.

164. B Numeric

RATIONALE: In the numeric filing system, the file is given a number and filed in numeric order. A master list with the corresponding names is kept elsewhere.

165. B A retirement complex with individual apartments

RATIONALE: Autonomy is the quality of having the ability or tendency to function independently. A community where a senior can interact with persons of the same age and participate in activities but keep his or her own apartment would allow independence.

166. E Special delivery

RATIONALE: Mail of any class can be marked *special delivery*. The designation does not speed up the normal travel time between two cities, but it does ensure immediate delivery of the item when it arrives at the designated post office.

167. E A postage meter

RATIONALE: The postage meter machine can be leased or purchased. The postage is purchased through the U.S. Postal Service.

168. B Two

RATIONALE: Level one CPT codes are developed by the American Medical Association and contained in the current CPT manual. They are five-digit codes and two-digit modifiers.

169. A A subject line

RATIONALE: A memorandum is an effective way to communicate information with employees. It should contain the following information: *To, From, Date,* and *Subject*.

170. B The delete key

RATIONALE: The keyboard is the most common means of inputting data. The *delete* function removes characters on the right side of the cursor.

171. C Spreadsheet

RATIONALE: A spreadsheet is a software program for inputting and manipulating data to facilitate a wide variety of activities.

172. C Doing a patient flow analysis

RATIONALE: The main goal in scheduling is to achieve a steady flow of patients that will make efficient use of the provider's time. A time study or patient flow analysis may help determine the office's needs. This study may assess the patient's waiting time and downtime of office members resulting from cancellations or no-shows.

173. D It is a direct filing system

RATIONALE: Alphabetical filing by name is the oldest, simplest, and most commonly used system. It is a direct filing system because the person filing only needs to know the name to find the desired file.

174. A Aging accounts

RATIONALE: An aging account report is a list of overdue accounts showing the length of time each one is overdue based on the date of the transaction.

175. B Browser

RATIONALE: The browser allows the user to locate a web address, call up the site, and view it on the screen.

176. D 260

RATIONALE: Taking into consideration that 52 weeks are in 1 calendar year, 10 reams would be used 26 times during that year (26 weeks × 10 reams = 260 reams).

177. D Subtracted from the bank statement balance

RATIONALE: A bank statement must be reconciled (making the balances on the bank statement and in the checkbook agree). It must account for deposits made and checks written after the ending date of the statement. The total of all outstanding checks not listed on the bank statement should be subtracted from the checkbook balance.

178. D Salary

RATIONALE: Salaried employees are paid a specific amount of money per pay period, regardless of the number of hours they work.

179. C June 15, 2006

RATONALE: The date line consists of the name of the month written in full, followed by the day and year. This arrangement is the most appropriate form for business correspondence.

180. A Accounts payable

RATIONALE: Accounts payable are debts incurred and not yet paid.

181. D Give the patient written instructions on the procedure

RATIONALE: When possible, all patient instruction should include a handout or some type of printed material. This form will reinforce the information and can be used by the patient as a resource.

182. B Medicaid

RATIONALE: The federal government provides for the medically indigent through a program known as Medicaid. Assistance is provided through the state and may have different names in different states.

183. C ICD-9-CM

RATIONALE: The ICD-9-CM is used for coding diagnoses.

184. D Modified wave

RATIONALE: The wave schedule can be modified in several ways. One application would have patients scheduled to arrive at given intervals.

185. E Participating

RATIONALE: A provider who enters into a contract with a specific insurance company or program, and by doing so, agrees to abide by certain rules and regulations set forth by that third-party payor.

186. B 10040-69979

RATIONALE: CPT lists and codes procedures and services performed by the provider. The CPT book is divided into six sections. The surgery section codes are 10000 to 69999.

187. A Stop sending statements to the patient

RATIONALE: Bankruptcy laws are federal and are applicable in all states. The laws were passed to secure equal distribution of the assets of the individual among the individual's creditors. When notified that a patient has declared bankruptcy, do not send any statements or attempt to collect on the account.

188. D Open hours

RATIONALE: With open office hours, the facility is open at given hours of the day or evening, and patients arrive during these times. Patients are usually seen in the order they arrive.

189. A Truth in Lending Act

RATIONALE: The Truth in Lending Act, which is enforced by the Federal Trade Commission, requires that when an agreement exists between the patient and physician to accept payments, the physician is required to provide disclosure of information regarding finance charges.

190. D Suggest alternative methods of payment

RATIONALE: Aggressively attempting to collect the balances that patients owe the physician may be necessary. Persuasive collection procedures include telephone calls, collection reminders and letters, and personal calls or interviews. Convey the impression that the patient intended to pay and doing so may only be a matter of working out some suitable arrangement.

191. C   Medicare Part A

RATIONALE: Retired people 65 years and older and people who receive monthly Social Security or railroad retirement checks are automatically enrolled for hospital insurance benefits (Part A) and pay no premiums for this coverage.

192. D   Patient information form

RATIONALE: The medical record begins with routine personal information, which the patient usually supplies on the first visit. This personal information (demographics) is obtained either by patient interview or by the completion of a personal information form by the patient.

193. E   Professional liability insurance policies

RATIONALE: The physician carries professional liability insurance to cover his or her practice of medicine in the event of a lawsuit. Old policies should never be discarded in case a lawsuit is filed years after the event, and the old policies must be available to prove coverage.

194. D   The daytime telephone number of the patient

RATIONALE: Canceling or rearranging the schedule in a hurry may become necessary, and precious time can be saved if the telephone number is available.

195. D   The number of exemptions the employee has claimed

RATIONALE: The amount of money withheld from each paycheck is based on the information the employee provides on Form W-4. This form includes the number of withholding allowances.

196. D   ICD-9-CM

RATIONALE: A V-code refers to factors that influence health status, such as annual physicals or well-baby checks.

197. A   "How many wet diapers do you change in a day?"

RATIONALE: If the baby is urinating on a regular basis, it is receiving enough fluid.

198. D   Sit with back curved and with the keyboard on the lap

RATIONALE: Correct ergonomics and position are essential in preventing fatigue and injury while inputting data. This technique includes keeping the feet flat on the floor, keeping eyes on the source copy, and curving the fingers over the home row of keys.

199. C   Physician, patient, and insurance company

RATIONALE: A third-party payor is someone other than the patient, spouse, or parent who is responsible for paying all or part of the patient's medical costs.

200. E   All of the above

RATIONALE: If a claim form is not sufficiently detailed, complete, and accurate, it may be rejected by the insurance company. Reasons for rejection may include missing or incomplete diagnosis; charges not itemized; patient's group, member, or policy number missing; patient signature missing; patient date of birth missing; or physician signature missing.

CLINICAL

201. B   Antineoplastic

RATIONALE: An antineoplastic agent (cancer drug) inhibits the growth of malignant cells.

202. B   1½ in, 22 G

RATIONALE: The goal of an intramuscular injection is to deliver the medication into muscle tissue. The length of the needle can be up to 2 inches, depending on the size of the patient and the consistency of the medication. The gauge of the needle can be from 22 G to 25 G, depending on the consistency of the medication.

203. B   Diuretic

RATIONALE: A diuretic promotes or increases urination.

204. C   2 mL

RATIONALE: Use the following formula:

$$\frac{\text{Dose ordered}}{\text{Available strength}} \times \text{dose form} = \text{dose given}$$

$$\frac{1000 \text{ mg}}{500 \text{ mg}} \times 1 \text{ mL} = 2 \text{ mL}$$

205. A   Rinse contaminants from the lip of the bottle

RATIONALE: Pouring a small amount of the solution into a waste receptacle rinses any contaminants off the bottle lip. If the bottle has a double cap, then this step can be skipped.

206. C   Read the label on the bottle, and check the expiration date

RATIONALE: Three label checks *("The Three Befores")* should be performed before administering any solution or medication.

207. D   Eating

RATIONALE: The postprandial blood sugar (2-hr PPBS) is a screening test for diabetes mellitus. A fasting blood sugar level is obtained. If the results are within an acceptable range, then the patient eats a meal and is retested after 2 hours.

208. B   1.010 and 1.025

RATIONALE: The specific gravity measures the amount of particles that are dissolved in the urine sample and indicates the ability of the kidneys to concentrate the urine. The normal range for specific gravity usually falls between 1.010 and 1.025.

209. C   Nonsterile gloves, laboratory coat, and goggles

RATIONALE: Sigmoidoscopy is used to diagnose polyps, hemorrhoids, and diverticular disorders. The sigmoidoscope is a flexible fiberoptic instrument that allows the physician to complete the examination without much discomfort to the patient. Nonsterile gloves, laboratory coat, and goggles are adequate personal protection equipment for assisting with the procedure.

210. C   Aspiration of a breast cyst

RATIONALE: Aspiration involves inserting a sterile needle into a cyst or mass and withdrawing fluid or other material. This procedure would be performed under sterile conditions because the skin is broken.

211. C   Gallbladder

RATIONALE: *Cholecyt/o* is the combining form for gallbladder, and *-gram* is the suffix meaning record.

212. A   Audiometer

RATIONALE: Audiometry measures the lowest intensity of sound that a person can hear. The machine used for this testing is an audiometer. The results can be printed on a graph called an audiogram.

213. A   1 mL

RATIONALE: The cubic centimeter (cc) and the milliliter (mL) are interchangeable units of measure in the metric system.

214. B   Prilosec (omeprazole)

RATIONALE: Prilosec (omeprazole) is classified as an anti-ulcer agent. It is used to manage ulcers, gastroesophageal reflux disease (GERD), heartburn, indigestion, and gastric hyperacidity. It helps prevent the accumulation of acid in the stomach.

215. A   Alanine aminotransferase

RATIONALE: Alanine aminotransferase is an enzyme found in highly metabolic tissues such as the heart muscle, liver, and skeletal muscle. Levels increase after a myocardial infarction.

216. B   Gastrointestinal

RATIONALE: Hematemesis is vomiting of bright red blood, indicating upper gastrointestinal bleeding. This bleeding might be associated with esophageal varices or peptic ulcer.

217. A   Silver nitrate

RATIONALE: Topical silver nitrate ($AgNO_3$) solution or an applicator coated with $AgNO_3$ can be used to stop localized bleeding. The applicators must be kept in lightproof brown containers. The applicators are convenient for use in the mouth and nose.

218. A   Prothrombin time

RATIONALE: The Clinical Laboratory Improvement Amendments of 1988 testing method for monitoring a patient's coagulation time is called the prothrombin time (pro time) test. This test is useful to monitor patients receiving anticoagulation therapy, such as Coumadin.

219. C   Staphylococci

RATIONALE: Pathogenic bacteria are classified by their shape and arrangement. *Staphyl/o* means clusters or bunch (as in bunch of grapes).

220. C   Vastus lateralis

RATIONALE: The vastus lateralis muscle is part of the quadriceps group of the thigh. It is well developed at birth and considered to be the safest intramuscular injection site for infants.

221. C   30%

RATIONALE: Hemoglobin and hematocrit values are related. Each 1% hematocrit contains 0.34 g of hemoglobin. The hematocrit should equal three times the hemoglobin within 3%.

222. C   Palliative

RATIONALE: A palliative drug does not cure but provides relief from pain or symptoms related to the disorder.

223. B   1.0 mL

RATIONALE: Use the following formula:

$$\frac{\text{Dose ordered}}{\text{Available strength}} \times \text{dose form} = \text{dose given}$$

$$\frac{50 \text{ mg}}{50 \text{ mg}} \times 1 \text{ mL} = 1.0 \text{ mL}$$

224. C   Blood urea nitrogen (BUN)

RATIONALE: Urea is the main nonprotein nitrogen in the blood. It is formed in the liver and excreted by the kidneys. By observing the increases in BUN, the physician can see when the kidney has become impaired.

225. C   Reduces the number of contaminants to a safe level

RATIONALE: Sanitization is the cleansing process that decreases the number of microorganisms to a safe level as dictated by public health guidelines. This process removes debris so that later sterilization can penetrate all surfaces of the item.

226. B   The jewelry can harbor microorganisms

RATIONALE: Jewelry can harbor and conceal microorganisms and is not permitted in surgical asepsis.

227. A   Facing away from the examiner

RATIONALE: Audiometry measures the lowest intensity of sound that a person can hear. The patient places headphones over both ears. A single frequency is delivered to each ear. The patient is asked to signal when he or she hears the sound. To reduce human error, the patient should be seated facing away from the examiner so the patient cannot see the examiner push the button to deliver the sound.

228. A   Permeable to steam but protective against airborne contaminants

RATIONALE: Maintenance of sterility depends completely on the method of wrapping and the wrapper itself. The wrapping material must be permeable to steam but impervious to contaminants such as dust and insects.

229. C   Ecchymosis

RATIONALE: Ecchymosis is a hemorrhagic skin discoloration commonly called a bruise. The skin is not broken, thus the wound is closed.

230. C   Hyaline

RATIONALE: The hyaline cast, the most frequently seen cast, is made up of protein. Conditions such as strenuous exercise, dehydration, heat exposure, and emotional stress can cause hyaline casts to be present in the urine.

231. D Bronchodilator

RATIONALE: A bronchodilator is used to manage reversible airway obstruction caused by asthma and chronic obstructive pulmonary disease (COPD). It helps relax the smooth muscle of the respiratory tract, resulting in bronchodilation.

232. D Axillary

RATIONALE: When recording the temperature reading in the patient's medical record, the site (rectal [R], tympanic [T], axillary [A]) must be noted to clarify the temperature site because values are not the same at each site.

233. A Schedule I

RATIONALE: Schedule I drugs have no accepted medical use and a high potential for abuse. Possession of these drugs is illegal. Examples of schedule I drugs include heroin, d-lysergic acid diethylamide (LSD), mescaline, and amphetamine variations.

234. D Lithotomy

RATIONALE: In the lithotomy position, the female patient is placed on her back with the knees sharply flexed, the buttocks to the edge of the table, and the feet supported in table stirrups.

235. C Do not eat red meat for 48 hours before collection

RATIONALE: Eating red meat and taking iron supplements and certain medications (e.g., aspirin, vitamin C, steroids, anticoagulants) can cause a false-positive result.

236. B 1:10

RATIONALE: Disinfection is the process of killing pathogenic organisms or rendering them inactive. For equipment and countertops, the cheapest and most reliable method is the use of a 1:10 bleach solution.

237. A Anisocytosis

RATIONALE: In a diseased state, red blood cells may become altered in appearance. They can vary in size (anisocytosis), shape (poikilocytosis), and/or color (polychromia, hypochromia, hyperchromia).

238. C Bread

RATIONALE: Carbohydrates are organic compounds that are primarily plant products in origin. They are divided into groups based on the complexity of their molecules. Their main function is to supply fuel for energy. Breads, pasta rice, corn, and barley are classified as complex carbohydrates.

239. D Urobilinogen

RATIONALE: Urobilinogen results from the breakdown of bilirubin in the intestines. It travels to the liver where it is sent back to the intestines and excreted in feces. Urine levels may be increased in conditions of the liver.

240. C Claritin (loratadine)

RATIONALE: Claritin (loratadine) is classified as an antihistamine agent. Antihistamines are used to relieve symptoms associated with allergies (rhinorrhea and itchy eyes, nose, and throat). They help block the effects of histamine at histamine receptor sites.

241. B Pink or red

RATIONALE: The Gram stain is the method of staining microorganisms, which serves as a primary means of classifying and identifying bacteria. Using this method, bacteria will be either gram-positive (retaining the purple color of the stain) or gram-negative (retaining the color of the counterstain).

242. B Up and back

RATIONALE: Gently pulling the pinna up and back straightens the ear canal and allows the medication to reach its designated area.

243. C AU

RATIONALE: The abbreviation *AU (aures unitas)* means both ears.

244. A Intradermal

RATIONALE: An intradermal injection places the medication within the skin layers. The site is used primarily for allergy testing and tuberculin screening (Mantoux test).

245. B Disinfection

RATIONALE: Disinfection is the process of killing pathogenic organisms or rendering them inactive. The process is used on surfaces and equipment by chemical means (bleach solution, Cidex, alcohol, Betadine) and by boiling (212° F).

246. A Brachial

RATIONALE: Blood pressure is a reflection of the pressure of the blood against the walls of the arteries. The brachial artery in the arm is easily accessible.

247. D Tilt the patient's head forward

RATIONALE: Nosebleed (epistaxis) is a hemorrhage from the nose usually caused by the rupture of small blood vessels within the nose. Mild to moderate bleeding can be controlled by having the patient sit upright, lean forward, and applying direct pressure to the nose.

248. B Leads I, II, and III

RATIONALE: An electrocardiogram consists of 12 leads. The standard (bipolar) limb leads are recorded first. These leads each use two limb electrodes to record the heart's electrical activity.

249. B 1:10 bleach solution

RATIONALE: Disinfection is the process of killing pathogenic organisms or rendering them inactive. For equipment and countertops, the cheapest and most reliable method is the use of a 1:10 bleach solution.

250. B   10

RATIONALE: Standardization has been determined by international agreement so that an electrocardiogram can be interpreted in the same way anywhere in the world. This standardization requires calibration according to universal standards. When the machine is in standard, 1 mV of electricity causes the stylus to move vertically 10 mm (10 small squares).

251. A   Two drops in both ears every 4 hours as needed

RATIONALE: The abbreviation for drops is *gtt, AU* is the abbreviation for both ears, *q4h* is the abbreviation for every 4 hours, and *prn* is the abbreviation for as needed.

252. B   Intramuscular

RATIONALE: Intramuscular injections are given into the muscle when the volume of medication to be injected is large, when the drugs may irritate the subcutaneous tissue, or when a rapid absorption is desired. This route is the preferred route for antibiotics.

253. A   Ethylenediaminetetraacetic acid (EDTA)

RATIONALE: The anticoagulant EDTA is used for hematology studies. It prevents the aggregation of platelets and allows preparation of blood smears with minimal distortion of white blood cells.

254. C   Myelogram

RATIONALE: *Myel/o* is the combining form for spinal cord and bone marrow, and *-gram* is the suffix meaning to record or recording.

255. D   Leukocytes: ++

RATIONALE: The normal range for leukocytes in a sample should be negative. The presence of white bloods cells usually indicates a urinary tract infection.

256. D   Occupational Safety and Health Administration (OSHA)

RATIONALE: OSHA mandated the *blood-borne pathogens standard,* which covers all employees who might "reasonably anticipate as the result of performing their job duties to face contact with blood and other potentially infectious materials."

257. D   Measure blood pressure

RATIONALE: The instrument used to measure blood pressure is called a sphygmomanometer. It consists of an inflatable cuff, an inflation bulb with a control valve, and a pressure gauge. (*Sphygm/o* means pulse; *manometer* refers to an instrument used to measure the pressure of a liquid or a gas.)

258. A   Carbohydrates

RATIONALE: Carbohydrates are organic compounds that are primarily plant products in origin. They are divided into groups based on the complexity of their molecules. Their main function is to supply fuel for energy.

259. B   Auscultation

RATIONALE: In auscultation, the examiner uses a stethoscope to listen to the sounds made by the body.

260. C   Injection

RATIONALE: A parenteral medication is administered with a sterile needle and syringe.

261. A   Forced vital capacity

RATIONALE: The forced vital capacity (FVC) is the amount of air that can be forcefully exhaled from a maximal inhalation. FVC is measured through spirometry (pulmonary function test).

262. A   bid (twice a day)

RATIONALE: The abbreviations are bid (twice a day), tid (three times a day), OD (right eye), and ac (before meals).

263. D   20

RATIONALE: Distance visual acuity is frequently part of a complete physical examination. It is widely used in schools and industry and is the best single test available for visual screening. The procedure uses the Snellen eye chart. The patient is positioned 20 feet from the chart (standard testing distance), either standing or sitting.

264. B   5 minutes

RATIONALE: A microscopic examination of urine consists of examining, counting, and categorizing the solid material. It consists of centrifuging a standard amount of urine (5 minutes at 1500 rpm), pouring off the liquid, and placing the sediment on a slide for examination.

265. D V_4

RATIONALE: The chest (precordial) leads are unipolar and designated V_1, V_2, V_3, V_4, V_5, and V_6. These leads measure the electrical activity between six specific points on the chest wall and a point within the heart. Lead V_4 is placed in the fifth intercostal space at the left midclavicular line.

266. B   Perform the Heimlich maneuver

RATIONALE: Choking is usually caused by a foreign object lodged in the upper airway. If the victim is unable to speak, is coughing weakly, and/or is wheezing, then the airway is obstructed, resulting in poor air exchange. The obstruction must be removed before respiratory arrest occurs. This task may be accomplished by performing the abdominal thrust procedure (Heimlich maneuver) to dislodge the obstruction.

267. D   Red

RATIONALE: A red-stoppered tube contains no additive (anticoagulant). Blood will coagulate in this tube and produce serum when spun and separated.

268. C   Osteoporosis

RATIONALE: Osteoporosis is a common but serious bone disease. The disease is characterized by excessive loss of calcified bone matrix. The bone becomes porous, which can cause it to be easily broken.

269. D   Sterilization

RATIONALE: Sterilization is the complete destruction of all forms of microbial life. Surgical asepsis is the complete destruction of organisms before they enter the body.

270. C 36

RATIONALE: Examination of the child during routine well-child visits includes measurement of the circumference of the infant's head to determine normal growth and development. Routine head measurement is recommended in children until age 36 months when 75% of brain growth should be completed.

271. C Right arm and left arm

RATIONALE: An electrocardiogram consists of 12 leads. The standard (bipolar) limb leads are recorded first. These leads each use two limb electrodes to record the heart's electrical activity. Lead I records the electrical activity between the right arm and the left arm.

272. A Intradermal

RATIONALE: An intradermal injection places the medication within the skin layers. The site is used primarily for allergy testing and tuberculin screening and is routinely used in the medical office. The other types of injections (intralesional delivers medication directly into a lesion, intrathecal into the spinal canal, and intravenous into the vein) are not routine and require special training to perform.

273. B Pain

RATIONALE: Pain is a general sense, with receptors located throughout the body. Pain serves as a protective function and is described in universal terms, including, but not limited to, acute, stabbing, burning, intractable, and excruciating.

274. A Manipulation

RATIONALE: Manipulation is the forceful, passive movement of a joint to determine the range of extension or flexion.

275. C Hepatitis B

RATIONALE: Hepatitis B vaccine #1 can be administered from birth to 1 month of age. The schedule is updated periodically and serves only as a guideline.

276. B Guaiac test

RATIONALE: Routine screening of stool specimens for occult blood is frequently performed in the medical office. The guaiac slide test is most often used and is available commercially by the name of Hemoccult and ColoScreen. Guaiac is a wood resin that reacts with blood.

277. A Chief complaint

RATIONALE: The chief complaint is the reason for the patient's seeking medical care. It is recorded in the patient's own words and is set off from the rest of the chart notes by quotation marks.

278. B Prevent the entry of microorganisms into the patient's body

RATIONALE: The skin cannot be sterilized; therefore it must be cleansed and disinfected in some manner to keep resident and transient microorganisms from entering the body when the skin is broken.

279. D Patient's name, date of collection, and source of specimen

RATIONALE: Collection containers must be labeled properly at the time of collection. Labels should include the patient's full name, date, and type or source of specimen.

280. B Multipara

RATIONALE: The root word -para indicates full-term infants delivered. The prefix multi- indicates more than one (multiple).

281. C Antipyretic

RATIONALE: Acetaminophen is classified as an analgesic and antipyretic agent that contains no aspirin. It is often prescribed for mild to moderate pain and fever.

282. A Hyperglycemia

RATIONALE: Hyperglycemia is an abnormally high level of glucose in the blood. People with diabetes need insulin to decrease the amount of glucose in the blood.

283. E All of the above

RATIONALE: Microorganisms can be transmitted through person-to-person contact, by a vector (insect, rodent), by contaminated objects, or by contaminated food and water. The simplest way of preventing the transmission of pathogens is proper hand washing.

284. C Verify the number of refills

RATIONALE: The medical assistant should always ask when any question about an order exists. Given that two different numbers are written for the number of refills, the medical assistant should clarify which number is correct.

285. B Corn oil

RATIONALE: Fat is the storage form of fuel in the body. It is more concentrated than carbohydrates. Vegetable fats (corn, olive, avocado, nuts, beans, and their oils) are unsaturated types of fats and are less dense than the animal fats and less likely to raise serum lipid levels.

286. C Dilution of the blood sample with tissue fluid

RATIONALE: Squeezing tissue at the puncture site opens up the tissue and allows tissue fluid to flow into the sample, which might dilute the sample and cause inaccurate results. Gently milking the finger and applying gentle pressure is recommended.

287. B Place the patient in a supine position with legs elevated

RATIONALE: Shock is a state of collapse resulting from failure of the circulatory system to deliver enough oxygenated blood to the body's vital organs. Place the patient supine with the legs elevated to return the blood from the legs to the vital organs.

288. C Hands of employees

RATIONALE: The most effective way to break the chain of infection is proper hand washing.

289. C 4

RATIONALE: The American Academy of Pediatrics recommends four doses of inactivated poliovirus (IPV, poliomyelitis) vaccine to be given at ages 2 months, 4 months, between 6 and 18 months, and at 4 to 6 years.

290. A Sigmoidoscopy

RATIONALE: Proctology is the branch of internal medicine concerned with the diseases and disorders of the colon, rectum, and anus. The anal area is examined using an anoscope or a proctoscope. The rectum and sigmoid colon are examined with a flexible sigmoidoscope. The descending, transverse, and descending colon are examined with a colonoscope.

291. A Color vision

RATIONALE: Defects in color vision are either congenital or acquired. The Ishihara color vision test is a simple, convenient, and accurate procedure that detects total colorblindness, as well as red-green blindness. It consists of a test booklet with polychromatic plates that the patients view.

292. C Scalpel

RATIONALE: A scalpel is classified as a cutting instrument that is used to cut, scrape, or dissect. It consists of a handle and an attached blade.

293. B Instructions to the patient

RATIONALE: *Sig (signatura)* is the Latin term for write or label. It indicates the information that is to be included on the medication label.

294. A Hematocrit

RATIONALE: Hemoglobin and hematocrit values are related. Each 1% hematocrit contains 0.34 g of hemoglobin. The hematocrit should equal three times the hemoglobin within 3%.

295. D Oral

RATIONALE: A patient with dyspnea has difficulty breathing. Placing a thermometer in the patient's mouth might further obstruct the airway. A better method for this patient would be axillary or aural.

296. B Perineum

RATIONALE: The perineum is the pelvic floor. It extends from the anus to the vulva in women and from the anus to the scrotum in men.

297. C High-density lipoprotein (HDL)

RATIONALE: HDL is the *good* or *healthy* cholesterol. It has the lowest fat content and protects against the accumulation of fatty deposits on the blood vessels. It is also capable of removing excess cholesterol from the blood and transporting it back to the liver for excretion.

298. D Cytologic fixative

RATIONALE: Vaginitis is an inflammation of the vagina usually caused by a microorganism. It is characterized by an abnormal discharge. A specimen is collected and evaluated for the invading organism, usually with a wet preparation. This slide would not be fixed, therefore fixative is not needed.

299. A Sweat

RATIONALE: Standard precautions must be followed at all times when handling body fluids. Sweat has not been shown to transmit blood-borne pathogens.

300. A Fever

RATIONALE: An antipyretic agent reduces fever. Widely used agents include acetaminophen and aspirin.